HANDBOOK OF
NEURORADIOLOGY

HANDBOOKS IN RADIOLOGY SERIES

Series Editors

ANNE G. OSBORN, M.D.

Professor, Department of Radiology,
University of Utah School of Medicine,
Salt Lake City, Utah;
Sterling Visiting Professor in Diagnostic Imaging,
Armed Forces Institute of Pathology,
Washington, D.C.

DAVID G. BRAGG, M.D.

Professor and Chairman, Department of Radiology,
University of Utah School of Medicine,
Salt Lake City, Utah

Other Volumes in This Series

Head and Neck Imaging
H. Ric Harnsberger, M.D.

Skeletal Radiology
B.J. Manaster, M.D., Ph.D.

Chest Radiology
Howard Mann, M.D., David G. Bragg, M.D.

Nuclear Medicine
Frederick L. Datz, M.D.

Interventional Radiology and Angiography
Myron M. Wojtowyez, M.D.

HANDBOOK OF NEURORADIOLOGY

ANNE G. OSBORN, M.D.

Professor, Department of Radiology,
University of Utah School of Medicine,
Salt Lake City, Utah;
Sterling Visiting Professor in Diagnostic Imaging,
Armed Forces Institute of Pathology,
Washington, D.C.

*With **38** Illustrations*

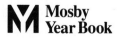

Mosby
Year Book

St. Louis Baltimore Boston Chicago London Philadelphia Sydney Toronto

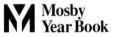
Mosby
Year Book
Dedicated to Publishing Excellence

Editor: Anne S. Patterson
Assistant Editor: Maura K. Leib
Project Manager: Patricia Tannian
Book and Cover Design: Gail Morey Hudson

Mosby–Year Book, Inc.
11830 Westline Industrial Drive, St. Louis, Missouri 63146

Library of Congress Cataloging in Publication Data

Osborn, Anne G., 1943-
    Handbook of neuroradiology / Anne G. Osborn.
        p.   cm. —(Handbooks in radiology series)
    Includes bibliographical references and index.
    ISBN 0-8151-6578-1
    1. Central nervous system—Imaging—Handbooks, manuals, etc.
    2. Central nervous system—Radiography—Handbooks, manuals, etc.
    I. Title. II. Series.
        [DNLM: 1. Central Nervous System—radiography—handbooks.
    WL 39
    081h]
    RC349.D5208   1991   91-8801
    616.8′04757—dc20   CIP
    DNLM/DLC
    for Library of Congress

CL/MA   9   8   7   6   5   4   3

Contributors

CAROL M. ANDREWS, M.D.

Resident,
Department of Radiology,
University of Utah,
Salt Lake City, Utah

RICHARD S. BOYER, M.D.

Clinical Assistant Professor of Radiology,
Department of Radiology,
University of Utah,
Salt Lake City, Utah

H. RIC HARNSBERGER, M.D.

Director of Neuroradiology and
Associate Professor of Radiology,
Department of Radiology,
University of Utah and
Primary Children's Medical Center,
Salt Lake City, Utah

M. JUDITH DONOVAN POST, M.D.

Professor of Radiology,
University of Miami School of Medicine,
Miami, Florida

WENDY R.K. SMOKER, M.D.

Professor of Radiology and
Director of ENT/Neuroradiology,
Medical College of Virginia,
Richmond, Virginia

TO RON

My brain may belong to neuroradiology,
but my heart definitely belongs to you

Preface

This book is designed as a handy reference guide to neuroradiology. Intended for radiology and neuroscience residents, fellows, clinicians, and practicing radiologists who perform neuroimaging procedures, it summarizes the basic normal and pathologic anatomy of the central nervous system. It is organized into major sections that include the brain vasculature and its diseases; normal and pathologic anatomy of the skull and cranial nerves; normal and abnormal development of the brain; ventricles, cisterns, and subarachnoid spaces; brain pathology by disease process; disease processes by location; and spine and cord. Each section is divided into chapters covering specific topics and disease entities.

For quick review and ready reference, each chapter begins with a key concepts box that briefly summarizes some important features of the subject discussed.

Although not meant to be all inclusive, this handbook is comprehensive. For more in-depth study of given topics, the reader should consult the suggested readings at the end of each chapter. These have been updated to within 3 months of publication.

I hope readers will find this volume both interesting and useful.

Anne G. Osborn, M.D.

Contents

SECTION I

BRAIN VASCULATURE: NORMAL AND ABNORMAL

CHAPTER 1

Aortic arch and great vessels

KEY CONCEPTS

1. Major branches arising directly from the arch (in order) are the innominate artery (brachiocephalic trunk), left common carotid artery, and left subclavian artery (Fig. 1-1).
2. Common anomalies are an arch origin of the left vertebral artery (5%) and an aberrant right subclavian artery (0.5% to 1%).
3. Common carotid (CCA) bifurcation into the internal (ICA) and external (ECA) carotid arteries usually occurs at the C4 or C5 level but may be as high as C2 or as low as C6. The ICA is usually posterolateral to the ECA; 10% are medial to the ECA.
4. The CCA bifurcation and proximal ICA are the most common sites of significant atherosclerosis involving the aortic arch and great vessels.

I. Normal anatomy, anatomic variants.
   A. Aortic arch (Fig. 1-1).
      1. Normal origins of great vessels (in order).
         a. Innominate artery (brachiocephalic trunk).
         b. Left common carotid artery.
         c. Left subclavian artery.
      2. Common anomalies.
         a. Left vertebral artery arises directly from arch (5%).
         b. Aberrant right subclavian artery (0.5% to 1%).
   B. Right common carotid artery.
      1. Normal origin: innominate bifurcation.
      2. Anomalous origins.
         a. From right subclavian artery (SCA).

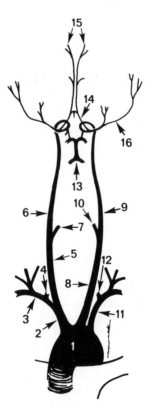

Fig. 1-1 Anatomic drawing of aortic arch and great vessels with their major branches.

1. Aortic arch
2. Innominate artery (brachiocephalic trunk)
3. Right subclavian artery
4. Right vertebral artery
5. Right common carotid artery
6. Right internal carotid artery
7. Right external carotid artery
8. Left common carotid artery
9. Left internal carotid artery
10. Left external carotid artery
11. Left subclavian artery
12. Left vertebral artery
13. Vertebral arteries uniting to form basilar artery
14. Circle of Willis
15. Anterior cerebral arteries
16. Middle cerebral arteries

   b. If right SCA is aberrant, right CCA has separate origin as first vessel arising from aortic arch.

 C. Left common carotid artery.

  1. Normal origin: directly from aortic arch.

  2. Variants.

   a. Common origin with innominate artery (25%).

   b. Directly from proximal innominate artery.

 D. CCA bifurcation.

  1. Normal.

   a. Bifurcation into ECA and ICA about C4 or C5 level.

   b. ICA initially posterolateral to ECA; courses medial to ECA as it ascends.

   c. No normal ICA branches in neck.

  2. Variants.

   a. Bifurcation may be as high as C2, as low as C6.

   b. ICA arises medial to ECA in 10%.

   c. Some ECA branches (ascending pharyngeal and superior thyroidal arteries) can arise from distal CCA or CCA bifurcation.

  3. Anomalies.

   a. Very rarely, ICA and ECA arise directly and separately from aortic arch.

   b. If aberrant ICA is present, ECA branches may arise directly from ICA and no CCA bifurcation is seen. (Anomaly is also called "nonbifurcating" carotid artery.)

 E. Techniques for visualizing CCA bifurcation.

  1. Catheter angiography (cut film, digital subtraction).

  2. Color-flow Doppler.

  3. Magnetic resonance angiography.

II. Pathology.

 A. General.

  1. Irregularity of vessel lumen most commonly caused by atherosclerosis.

  2. Narrowing of aortic arch or its branches caused by atherosclerotic disease, dissecting aneurysm, arteritis (Takayasu's; rarely, giant cell arteritis).

  3. Occlusion of one or more arch vessels at their origin is uncommon. Occlusion of subclavian artery proximal to vertebral origin "steals" flow from contralateral vertebral artery via posterior fossa to supply subclavian circulation distal to stenosis or occlusion (subclavian steal syndrome). So-called bald aorta is rare and occurs when all three major arch vessels are occluded. In this situation collateral flow to head and neck is via intercostal and muscular branches.

B. Atherosclerosis (see Chapter 11).
   1. Great vessel origins and CCA bifurcation are common locations.
   2. Proximal ICA and ECA stenosis and occlusion are also common.
   3. If both ICA and ECA are occluded, retrograde thrombosis of CCA to origin may occur.
C. Trauma (see Chapter 17) may cause:
   1. Dissection.
   2. False aneurysm.
   3. Thrombosis.
D. Arteritis, miscellaneous nonatheromatous stenoses (see Chapter 12).
   1. Takayasu's arteritis.
      a. Usually affects aortic arch and great vessels.
      b. May involve ECA and cervical ICA.
   2. Fibromuscular dysplasia: usually spares CCA and bifurcation and proximal ICA.
E. Neoplasms.
   1. Can displace or encase CCA and its branches.
   2. Occlusion uncommon.
   3. Carotid body tumor (paraganglioma).
      a. Densely vascular.
      b. Well delineated.
      c. Splays CCA bifurcation apart.

SUGGESTED READINGS

Carroll BA: Carotid sonography, *Radiology* 178:303-313, 1991.

Edelman RR, Mattle HP, Atkinson DJ, Hoogewoud HM: MR angiography, *AJR* 154:937-946, 1990.

El Gammal T, Brooks BS: Conventional MR neuroangiography, *AJR* 156:1075-1080, 1991.

Erickson SJ, Mewissen MW, Foley WD, et al: Stenoses of the internal carotid artery: assessment using color Doppler imaging compared with angiography, *Am J Roentgenol* 152:1299-1305, 1989.

Foley WD, Erickson SJ: Color Doppler flow imaging, *AJR* 156:3-13, 1991.

Litt AW, Eidelman EM, Pinto RS, et al: Diagnosis of carotid artery stenosis: comparison of 2DFT time-of-flight MR angiography with contrast angiography in 50 patients, *AJNR* 12:149-154, 1991.

Morimoto T, Nitta K, Kazekawa K, Hashizume K: The anomaly of a non-bifurcating cervical carotid artery, *J Neurosurg* 72:130-132, 1990.

Osborn AG: *Introduction to cerebral angiography,* New York, 1980, Harper & Row, Chapters 2 to 4.

Steinke W, Kloetzsch C, Hennerici M: Carotid artery disease assessed by color Doppler flow imaging: correlation with standard Doppler sonography and angiography, *ANJR* 11:259-266, 1990.

Zamir M, Sinclair P: Origin of the brachiocephalic trunk, left carotid, and left subclavian arteries from the arch of the human aorta, *Invest Radiol* 26:128-133, 1991.

CHAPTER 2
External carotid artery

KEY CONCEPTS

1. Initials of the major external carotid artery (ECA) branches spell "SALFOPS+M":
   - **S** Superior thyroidal
   - **A** Ascending pharyngeal
   - **L** Lingual ⎫ frequently share common trunk
   - **F** Facial ⎭
   - **O** Occipital
   - **P** Posterior auricular
   - **S** Superficial temporal
   - **M** Maxillary (internal)
2. Several cranial nerves (CNs V, VII, IX, X, XI, and XII) are supplied principally by ECA branches, especially the maxillary (via meningeal branches), posterior auricular, and ascending pharyngeal arteries. CNs III, IV, and VI may derive some supply from ECA meningeal branches.
3. The three most common vascular tumors supplied by the ECA are paragangliomas, angiofibromas, and meningiomas. The *center* of most meningiomas is supplied by the ECA; intracranial internal carotid artery (ICA) branches typically supply the periphery.

I. Normal anatomy: As smaller of two terminal common carotid branches, ECA usually arises from bifurcation at about C4 or C5. It is medial and anterior to ICA but then courses posterolaterally.
   A. Major ECA branches and their classic areas of supply (Figs. 2-1 and 2-2).
      1. Superior thyroid artery: larynx, thyroid.

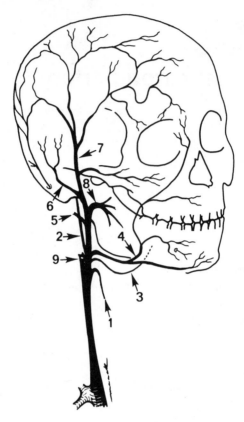

Fig. 2-1 Anatomic drawing of right common carotid bifurcation with the external carotid artery and its major branches. Oblique view.

1. Superior thyroidal artery
2. Ascending pharyngeal artery
3. Lingual artery
4. Facial artery
5. Occipital artery
6. Posterior auricular artery
7. Superficial temporal artery
8. Maxillary artery
9. Internal carotid artery

2. Ascending pharyngeal artery: nasopharynx and oropharynx, tympanic cavity, hypoglossal and jugular branches (CNs IX, X, XI), some meningeal supply, muscular branches (branches anastomose with vertebral artery at C3 level).
3. Lingual artery: tongue, floor of mouth, submandibular gland.

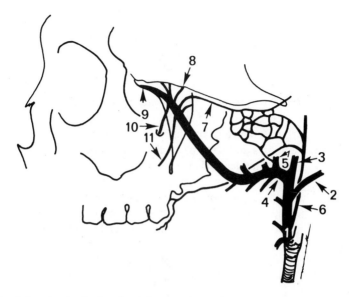

Fig. 2-2 Anatomic drawing of external carotid artery, its distal branches, and major branches of maxillary artery. Lateral view.

1. External carotid artery
2. Occipital artery
3. Superficial temporal artery
4. Maxillary artery
5. Middle meningeal artery
6. Ascending pharyngeal artery
7. Vidian artery
8. Artery of the foramen rotundum
9. Infraorbital artery
10. Descending palatine artery
11. Buccal artery

4. Facial artery: face, palate, pharynx, cheek, lip, anastomotic arteries to internal maxillary system.
5. Occipital artery: scalp, upper cervical musculature, posterior fossa meninges; anastomoses with vertebral artery at C1-2 level.
6. Posterior auricular artery: scalp, pinna, tympanic cavity.
7. Superficial temporal artery: scalp, ear, may supply part of face and buccal (cheek) area (transverse facial branch).
8. Internal maxillary artery: middle and accessory meningeal arteries, muscles of mastication, palate, teeth, part of nose and orbit. Several small branches of distal maxillary artery also anastomose with ophthalmic artery and ICA branches in cavernous sinus.

B. Hemodynamic balance of ECA branches: Vascular distribution of ECA is highly variable, with its component branches existing in hemodynamic balance. For example, blood supply to face can be derived primarily from either facial or internal maxillary artery. Ascending pharyngeal system can anastomose with cavernous ICA or vertebral artery. Occipital artery can anastomose with vertebral artery and superficial temporal artery system. Before therapeutic embolization of vascular lesions, each vascular territory must be carefully and precisely mapped with anastomoses and patterns of collateral circulation determined.
C. Extracranial to intracranial anastomoses: Number of anastomoses between ECA and intracranial circulation (via both ICA and vertebral artery) are possible (see box below). These are important sources of collateral flow in persons with vascular occlusive disease. They also represent potential hazards when therapeutic embolization procedures are performed on face and neck vessels.
D. Cranial and peripheral nerve supply.
  1. ECA supplies nerves:
    a. Directly via ECA branches.
    b. Indirectly by dural and transosseous collaterals to ICA branches.

MAJOR EXTRACRANIAL TO INTRACRANIAL VASCULAR ANASTOMOSES

1. Maxillary artery to internal carotid artery (ICA) via:
   a. Middle meningeal artery to ethmoidal branches of ophthalmic artery
   b. Artery of the foramen rotundum to inferolateral trunk of ICA
   c. Accessory meningeal artery to inferolateral trunk
   d. Vidian artery to intratemporal ICA
   e. Anterior and middeep temporal arteries to ophthalmic artery via lacrimal, palpebral, or muscular branches
2. Occipital artery to vertebral artery (via muscular and radicular branches) arteries of the first and second cervical spaces
3. Ascending pharyngeal artery to vertebral artery (via musculospinal branches) at C3 level
4. Ascending pharyngeal artery to internal carotid artery (via petrous and cavernous branches)
5. Facial artery to internal carotid artery (via angular branch of facial to orbital branches of ophthalmic artery)
6. Posterior auricular artery to internal carotid artery (via stylomastoid artery)
7. Extracranial-intracranial surgical bypass (typically superficial temporal or occipital artery to middle cerebral); rarely performed

2. CNs III, IV, V, and VI.
   a. ICA cavernous branches.
   b. Middle and accessory meningeal (pterygomeningeal) arteries of ECA.
   c. Ascending pharyngeal artery (CN VI, gasserian ganglion).
   d. Artery of foramen rotundum, a branch of maxillary artery (CN V_2).
3. CN VII.
   a. Anteroinferior cerebellar artery (acoustic branch); this vessel also supplies CN VIII.
   b. Middle meningeal artery (petrosal branch).
   c. Occipital or posterior auricular arteries (stylomastoid branch).
   d. Peripheral CN VII based on territory.
4. CNs IX, X, XI.
   a. Ascending pharyngeal artery.
   b. Occipital artery.
   c. Anterior cervical arteries (vertebral artery branches).
5. CN XII.
   a. Ascending pharyngeal artery.
   b. Vertebral artery branches.

II. Pathology.
 A. Vascular lesions.
   1. Pial (brain parenchyma) arteriovenous malformation (AVM) (see Chapter 14).
      a. Virtually any pial AVM has potential to parasitize dural vasculature if it becomes large enough.
      b. Most pial AVMs with ECA supply are in posterior fossa or adjacent to skull base.
      c. Supply: meningeal, dural branches (from middle meningeal, superficial temporal occipital arteries, etc.).
      d. Congenital.
   2. Dural AVMs.
      a. Involve predominantly meningeal branches of ECA, vertebral artery, or cavernous ICA.
      b. Supply depends on location of AVM:
         (1) Cavernous sinus: dural branches of ICA, meningeal branch of internal maxillary (middle and accessory meningeal arteries; artery of foramen rotundum) ascending pharyngeal artery.
         (2) Petrous/jugular foramen: dural branch of cavernous sinus, posterior meningeal branch of vertebral artery, middle meningeal artery.
         (3) Anterior location: ethmoidal, anterior falx artery, etc.

  c. Acquired; probably caused by thrombosis of dural sinus with subsequent fistulization.

 3. Capillary telangiectasias.

  a. Osler-Weber-Rendu disease.

  b. Small nests of abnormal vessels in mucosa and scalp.

  c. Usually multiple.

  d. May cause intractable epistaxis.

 4. Cavernous angiomas (port-wine stain).

  a. Spontaneous occurrence or with Sturge-Weber syndrome.

  b. Grapelike puddling of contrast media in late venous phase following long, slow injections of contrast media in moderately large amounts.

 5. Carotid-cavernous fistulas (see Chapter 17).

  a. Usually supplied by ICA.

  b. Sometimes dural supply from ECA branches (rami of maxillary, middle and accessory meningeal, and ascending pharyngeal arteries; artery of foramen rotundum).

 6. Aneurysm of ECA and its branches.

  a. Rare.

  b. Common causes: trauma (pseudoaneurysm), atherosclerosis.

 7. Atherosclerosis.

  a. ECA less commonly affected than ICA.

  b. Rich collateral supply from vertebral artery, ICA, and contralateral ECA usually present; consequently, occlusion is typically asymptomatic.

  c. ECA stenosis can produce carotid bruit, occasionally is cause of pulsatile tinnitus.

B. Tumors of head and neck: involve ECA by displacing vessels or deriving vascular supply from them.

 1. Squamous cell carcinoma.

  a. Angiographic findings.

   (1) Avascular mass.

   (2) Vessel encasement or displacement.

   (3) "Beading" of affected vessels, pseudoaneurysm, and neovascularity less common.

   (4) Rare: frank arterial occlusion.

  b. Angiography usually not performed unless therapeutic embolization for cataclysmic hemorrhage is contemplated.

 2. Paraganglioma ("glomus" tumor, chemodectoma).

  a. Angiographic findings.

   (1) Well-delineated dense vascular stain that persists into late arterial or capillary phase.

   (2) Arteriovenous shunting can occur.

(3) Arterial supply: If tumor is monocompartmental, one artery (usually ascending pharyngeal) supplies all of tumor; if tumor is polycompartmental, more than one artery supplies it.
  b. Carotid body tumor nestles in common carotid artery (CCA) bifurcation and splays ECA and ICA around it.
  c. Glomus vagale and jugulare tumors can have both intracranial and extracranial components.
  d. Glomus tympanicum and jugulotympanicum tumors.
   (1) Middle ear.
   (2) Ascending pharyngeal artery supply most common.
3. Angiofibroma (juvenile nasopharyngeal angiofibroma [JNA]).
  a. Adolescent males.
  b. Originates in sphenopalatine foramen, pterygopalatine fossa; spreads via natural foramina and fissures.
  c. Angiography.
   (1) Maxillary artery typically main supply, although numerous other vessels can contribute.
   (2) Dense, well-demarcated vascular stain.
   (3) "Spoke-wheel" appearance on arterial phase.
   (4) Vascular stain persists into capillary phase.
   (5) Look for extension into cavernous sinus, orbit, and cranial cavity.
  d. Preoperative embolization can dramatically reduce intraoperative blood loss.
  e. Megavoltage radiation therapy has been advocated for advanced or recurrent JNA by some investigators.
4. Meningioma.
  a. ECA and other dural vessels supply nidus of these dura-derived tumors.
  b. Angiographic findings.
   (1) Enlarged, nontapering meningeal arteries.
   (2) "Sunburst" of dense, reticular accumulation of contrast media.
   (3) Early draining veins not uncommon.
   (4) ICA may supply tumor via its dural branches (to nidus), or pial vessels may be parasitized (anterior, middle, and posterior cerebral arteries then supply periphery of lesion).
  c. Preoperative embolization via superselective catheterization can dramatically reduce operative time and blood loss.
5. Nerve and nerve sheath tumors.
  a. Can mimic glomus tumors but often are less vascular.
  b. Usually found in carotid space or at skull base.

SUGGESTED READINGS

Ahn HS, Kerber CW, Deeb ZL: Extra- to intracranial arterial anastomoses in therapeutic embolization: recognition and role, *Am J Radiol* 1:71-75, 1980.

Berenstein A, Lasjavnias P, Kricheff II: Functional anatomy of the facial vasculature in pathologic conditions and its therapeutic application, *Am J Radiol* 4:149-153, 1983.

Bonna M, Lasjaunias P: The arteries of the lingual thyroid: angiographic findings and anatomic variations, *AJNR* 11:730-732, 1990.

Fields JN, Halverson KJ, Devineni VR, et al: Juvenile nasopharyngeal angiofibroma: efficacy of radiation therapy, *Radiology* 176:263-265, 1990.

Lasjaunias PL, Berenstein A: *Surgical neuroangiography,* vol 1, Baltimore, 1987, Williams & Wilkins, pp 1-153.

Osborn AG: *Introduction to cerebral angiography,* New York, 1980, Harper & Row, Chapter 3.

Remley KB, Coit WE, Harnsberger HR, et al: Pulsatile tinnitus and the vascular tympanic membrane: CT, MR, and angiographic findings, *Radiology* 174:383-389, 1990.

Russell EJ: Functional angiography of the head and neck, *Am J Radiol* 7:927-936, 1986.

Vitek JJ: Accessory meningeal artery, *AJNR* 10:569-573, 1989.

Wilner HI, Lazo A, Metes JJ, et al: Embolization in cataclysmal hemorrhage caused by squamous cell carcinomas of the head and neck, *Radiology* 163:759-762, 1987.

CHAPTER 3

Internal carotid artery: cervical and petrous segments

KEY CONCEPTS

1. The internal carotid artery (ICA) has no named branches in the neck. Aberrant ICA course through the middle ear is an important anomaly.
2. Persistent (embryonic) carotid-vertebrobasilar anastomoses are, in descending order of frequency, trigeminal artery, hypoglossal artery, proatlantal intersegmental artery, and persistent otic (acoustic) artery.
3. Atherosclerosis is the most common cause of ICA narrowing.
4. The most common nonatheromatous causes of narrowed ICA are fibromuscular dysplasia (FMD), spontaneous dissection, trauma, spasm, and cerebral hypoperfusion or arrest ("brain death"). Arteritis, tumor encasement, and more distal high-grade stenosis (e.g., siphon disease) are less common causes of ICA narrowing.

I. Normal anatomy: ICA has four radiographically identifiable segments: cervical, petrous, cavernous (juxtasellar), and intracranial (supraclinoid). Latter two segments are discussed in Chapter 4.
   A. Normal course (Fig. 3-1).
      1. Originates from common carotid artery at bifurcation.
      2. Is initially posterolateral to external carotid artery (ECA), then courses medially as it runs cephalad (90% of persons).
      3. Enters carotid canal of petrous temporal bone.
         a. Initially anterior to jugular fossa and bulb.
         b. Turns anteromedially in front of middle ear cavity.
      4. Emerges from carotid canal near apex of petrous temporal bone.
      5. Lies above foramen lacerum.
      6. Passes into cavernous sinus.

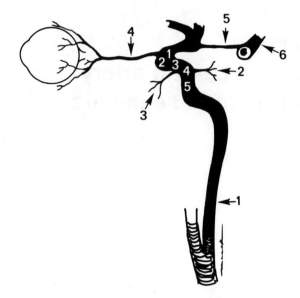

Fig. 3-1 Internal carotid artery and its branches. Lateral view. White letters denote cavernous carotid segments. Black letters:

1. Cervical ICA
2. Meningohypophyseal trunk
3. Lateral mainstem artery
4. Ophthalmic artery
5. Posterior communicating artery
6. Posterior cerebral artery

B. Branches.
   1. Cervical portion usually has no named branches (see below for anomalies and persistent carotid-vertebral anastomoses).
   2. Petrous segment.
      a. Anterior and posterior tympanic branches.
      b. Vidian artery (artery of pterygoid canal).
         (1) Seen in 25% of angiograms.
         (2) Distinct anterior horizontal course through foramen lacerum.
         (3) Joins petrous ICA with maxillary artery (ECA branch).
      c. Caroticotympanic artery.
C. Variants and anomalies.
   1. ICA agenesis.
      a. Very rare (fewer than 100 cases in English literature).
      b. Absent or hypoplastic carotid canal.
      c. Intercarotid anastomotic vessels at skull base frequently seen in these rare cases.
      d. High incidence of associated intracranial aneurysms.

2. Anomalous branches: A number can occur, most often:
   a. Occipital, ascending pharyngeal arteries from cervical ICA. Rarely, all branches normally supplied by ECA can originate from a nonbifurcating carotid artery.
   b. Persistent mandibular artery from cervical ICA.
   c. Persistent stapedial artery from petrous ICA (can supply middle meningeal territory; in this case foramen spinosum is absent).
3. Aberrant course.
   a. Retropharyngeal course of cervical ICA (can be present as pulsatile oropharyngeal submucosal mass).
   b. Aberrant course of ICA through middle ear.
      (1) ICA more posterior and lateral than normal.
      (2) Traverses hypotympanicum (can be seen on computed tomography [CT], magnetic resonance [MR]).
      (3) One cause of pulsatile tinnitus and vascular or "blue" tympanic membrane.
      (4) Clinical importance: If aberrant course is unrecognized, biopsy or puncture can result in fatal hemorrhage or catastrophic stroke.
4. Carotid-vertebral anastomoses: represent persistent embryonic circulatory patterns that link carotid and vertrobasilar systems (Fig. 3-2). With exception of extracranial proatlantal intersegmental arteries, these are named according to cranial nerves they parallel. From cephalad to caudad they are:
   a. Persistent trigeminal artery.
      (1) Most common carotid-vertebral anastomosis (85% of all persistent carotid-vertebrobasilar vessels).
      (2) Angiographic incidence of 0.6% in some series.
      (3) Connects precavernous or intracavernous ICA with basilar artery (between superior and anterior inferior cerebellar arteries).
      (4) Associated aneurysms not uncommon.
      (5) Clinical significance: surgical hazard in sellar and parasellar operations.
      (6) Can be seen on MR, sometimes CT.
   b. Persistent otic artery.
      (1) Extremely rare (handful of documented cases).
      (2) Connects petrous ICA with proximal basilar artery.
      (3) Clinical significance: projects medially through internal auditory canal.
   c. Hypoglossal artery.
      (1) Second most common carotid-vertebral anastomosis.
      (2) Connects cervical ICA with basilar artery.
      (3) Courses through hypoglossal canal.

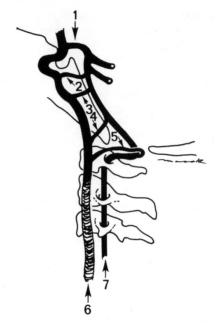

Fig. 3-2   Potential embryonic carotid-vertebrobasilar anastomoses. Lateral
view.

1. Posterior communicating artery
2. Persistent trigeminal artery
3. Acoustic (otic) artery
4. Hypoglossal artery
5. Proatlantal intersegmental artery
6. Internal carotid artery
7. Vertebral artery

    d. Proatlantal intersegmental artery.
       (1) Connects cervical ICA or ECA with vertebral artery.
       (2) Courses between arch of C1 and occiput.

NOTE: Presence of any one of these embryonic connections is a relative con-
traindication to WADA testing (intracarotid injection of sodium amylbarbital to
determine cerebral dominance before temporal lobectomy for intractable seizures), since it may disturb brainstem function.

II. Pathology.
   A. Atherosclerotic vascular disease (ASVD) usually involves common ca-
      rotid bifurcation and proximal ICA, as well as carotid siphon. Cervical
      and petrous segments are less often affected. In addition to traditional
      catheter angiography, color Doppler flow imaging and MR angiography
      are useful (and noninvasive) methods for evaluating ASVD.

B. Nonatheromatous causes of cervical or petrous ICA stenosis or occlusion are less common than ASVD but include:
1. Congenital hypoplasia (rare).
2. Fibromuscular dysplasia.
3. Cerebral circulatory arrest or hypoperfusion, high-grade upstream stenosis.
4. Arteritides such as Takayasu's disease.
5. Spontaneous dissection.
6. Trauma (blunt, torsion, penetrating injury).
7. Spasm (secondary to subarachnoid hemorrhage or catheter manipulation).
8. Encasement by neoplasm (may narrow ICA but rarely occludes it).
C. Miscellaneous.
1. Aneurysms of the cervical ICA are uncommon and usually related to penetrating injury or atherosclerosis. ICA pseudoaneurysms may also be associated with spontaneous dissection, FMD, and rarely tumor. Aneurysms of petrous segment are also uncommon. When present they are usually congenital or traumatic. Intracranial aneurysms with subarachnoid hemorrhage appear to have increased incidence of cervical vascular anomalies such as fibromuscular dysplasia and vascular loops.
2. Arteriovenous fistulas can also result from penetrating wounds or deceleration injury and are seen as direct communications from ICA to internal jugular vein.
3. Dural arteriovenous malformation at skull base may derive supply from enlarged intrapetrous and cavernous ICA branches.
4. Neoplasms of skull base (petroclival, temporal, cavernous sinus, parapharyngeal) may encase or, less commonly, actually invade ICA. Narrowing, beading, and pseudoaneurysm can be seen.

SUGGESTED READINGS

Bradac GB: Angiography in cerebral ischemia, *Riv Neuroradiol* 3(suppl 2):57-66, 1990.
Brant-Zawadzki M: Routine MR imaging of the internal carotid artery siphon: angiographic correlation with cervical carotid lesions, *AJNR* 11:467-471, 1990.
George B, Mourier KL, Belbert F, et al: Vascular abnormalities in the neck associated with intracranial aneurysms, *Neurosurgery* 24:499-508, 1989.
Kido DK, Barsotti JB, Rice LZ, et al: Evaluation of the carotid artery bifurcation: comparison of magnetic resonance angiography and digital subtraction arch aortography, *Neuroradiology* 33:48-51, 1991.
Kraemer JL, Schneider FL, Raupp SF, Ferreira NP: Anatomical correlation of the intersection of the carotid siphon with the dura mater, *Neuroradiology* 31:408-412, 1989.
Littooy FN, Baker WH, Field TC, et al: Anomalous branches of the cervical internal carotid artery: two cases of clinical importance, *J Vasc Surg* 8:634-637, 1988.
Morimoto T, Nitta K, Kozekawa K, Hoshizume K: The anomaly of a non-bifurcating cervical carotid artery, *J Neurosurg* 72:130-132, 1990.
Osborn AG: Introduction to cerebral angiography, New York, 1980, Harper & Row, Chapter 4.

Quint DJ, Boulos RS, Spera TD: Congenital absence of the cervical and petrous internal carotid artery with intercavernous anastomosis, *AJNR* 10:435-439, 1989.

Richardson DN, Elster AD, Ball MR: Intrasellar trigeminal artery, *AJNR* 10:205, 1989.

Schlenska GK: Absence of both internal carotid arteries, *J Neurol* 233:263-266, 1986.

Schuierer G, Laub G, Huk WJ: MR angiography of the primitive trigeminal artery: report on two cases, *AJNR* 11:1131-1132, 1990.

Steinke W, Kloetzsch C, Hennerici M: Carotid artery disease assessed by color Doppler flow imaging: correlation with standard Doppler sonography and angiography, *AJNR* 11:259-266, 1990.

Wismer GL: Circle of Willis variant analogous to fetal type primitive trigeminal artery, *Neuroradiology* 31:366-368, 1989.

CHAPTER 4

Internal carotid artery: cavernous and supraclinoid segments

KEY CONCEPTS

1. Cavernous and intradural internal carotid artery (ICA) branches are:
   a. Meningohypophyseal trunk
   b. Inferolateral trunk (lateral mainstem artery)
   c. Capsular arteries
   d. Ophthalmic artery (OA)
   e. Posterior communicating artery
   f. Anterior choroidal artery
   g. Anterior and middle cerebral arteries (terminal ICA bifurcation)
2. Important variants or anomalies are:
   a. "Fetal" origin of posterior cerebral artery (PCA)
   b. Persistent trigeminal artery
   c. Middle meningeal artery origin from ophthalmic artery
3. The most common cause of distal ICA narrowing is atherosclerosis. Some other nonatheromatous causes of siphon stenosis are:
   a. Spasm
   b. Sphenoid sinusitis, basilar meningitis
   c. Neurofibromatosis
   d. Dissection
   e. Radiation therapy
   f. Neoplasm (e.g., pituitary adenoma, craniopharyngioma, hypothalamic glioma)

I. Normal anatomy (see Fig. 3-1).
   A. Cavernous and supraclinoid segments of ICA form S-shaped loop, are collectively termed "carotid siphon." Segments and nomenclature are:
      1. Ascending cavernous or C5 portion: segment from exit at petrous apex to posterior genu.

2. Genu or C4 portion: segment between ascending and horizontal ICA.
3. Horizontal cavernous or C3 portion: segment between posterior and anterior genua.
4. Anterior genu or C2 portion: segment between horizontal segment and remainder of intradural ICA. (Recently statistical tables have been published on precise anatomoradiologic correlation between carotid siphon and its intersection with dura.)
5. C1 segment: remainder of intradural cavernous ICA.
6. Bifurcation into anterior (ACA) and middle (MCA) cerebral arteries.

B. Branches of cavernous ICA.
1. Meningohypophyseal (posterior) trunk.
   a. Present in 100% of anatomic dissections.
   b. Arises from C5 portion near junction with C4 segment.
   c. Supplies:
      (1) Posterior pituitary (inferior hypophyseal branch).
      (2) Tentorium via marginal tentorial branch (artery of Bernasconi and Cassinari).
      (3) Part of cavernous sinus dura (via dorsal meningeal branch).
      (4) Sometimes cranial nerves III, IV, V, and VI.
   d. Can be seen on high-quality distal or film magnification-subtraction studies.
2. Inferolateral trunk (also called lateral mainstem artery or artery of inferior cavernous sinus).
   a. Found in about two thirds of anatomic specimens.
   b. Arises from lateral aspect of C3 or C4 segment.
   c. Supplies:
      (1) Cavernous sinus dura.
      (2) Cranial nerves III to VII.
   d. Numerous important anastomoses with ECA branches through foramina ovale, rotundum, and spinosum and superior orbital fissure.
   e. Usually seen on lateral subtraction angiograms.
3. Capsular branches.
   a. Arise from C3 segment.
   b. Supply:
      (1) Sella.
      (2) Pituitary gland.
   c. Not usually seen with angiography.
4. Ophthalmic artery (see below): intradural in 90%; arises from cavernous ICA in 8% to 16% of cases.

C. Branches of supraclinoid ICA.
1. Ophthalmic artery.
   a. Arises from anterosuperior ICA just below anterior clinoid process.
   b. Course:
      (1) Exits skull through optic canal with optic nerve.
      (2) Initially below nerve, then crosses over.
   c. Supplies:
      (1) Globe (central retinal artery, ciliary arteries).
      (2) Orbit and contents (in balance with ECA supply).
      (3) Extraorbital soft tissues (reciprocal with ECA).
      (4) Dura (anterior falx artery, recurrent meningeal artery).
   d. Numerous anastomoses with ECA (facial, maxillary, and middle meningeal arteries).
   e. Circulatory variations common (reciprocity with ECA).
2. Posterior communicating artery (PCoA) (see Chapter 5).
   a. Arises from posterior aspect of intradural ICA.
   b. Course: posterior to PCA, superolateral to third cranial nerve.
   c. Joins ICA with P1 segment of PCA.
   d. Perforating branches from PCoA supply parts of thalamus, hypothalamus, and other structures at base of brain such as optic chiasm and mammillary bodies.
   e. If "fetal" type of circulation persists, PCA arises directly from ICA and is said to have "fetal origin."
3. Anterior choroidal artery (AChA).
   a. Arises from posterior ICA just above PCoA.
   b. Two radiographically distinct segments.
      (1) Cisternal (proximal) segment from ICA around medial temporal lobe in ambient cistern to choroidal fissure of temporal horn (abrupt kink or "plexal" point seen on lateral angiograms).
      (2) Plexal (intraventricular) segment courses in choroid plexus of temporal horn, curves posterolaterally around thalamus.
   c. Supply variable (reciprocal with posterior choroidal arteries) but usually:
      (1) Posterior limb and retrolenticular fibers of internal capsule.
      (2) Choroid plexus, part of temporal lobe.
      (3) Optic tract.
      (4) Parts of globus pallidus, thalamus, hypothalamus, caudate nucleus.
      (5) Cerebral peduncle, substantia nigra, red nucleus.
   d. Numerous anastomoses with posterior choroidal, PCoA, PCA, and MCA branches.

D. Terminal ICA branches.
   1. Anterior cerebral artery (see Chapter 6).
   2. Middle cerebral artery (see Chapter 7).
E. Variants and anomalies.
   1. "Fetal" origin of PCA from ICA occurs in 20% of cases.
   2. Persistent trigeminal artery (see Chapter 3); 0.1% to 0.6% of cases.
   3. Carotid origin of various posterior fossa vessels (e.g., superior, anterior inferior, and posterior inferior cerebellar arteries).
   4. Middle meningeal artery origin from OA; 0.5% of cases.
II. Pathology.
   A. Aneurysms (see Chapter 13).
      1. Locations.
         a. PCoA origin for 30% of all intracranial aneurysms.
         b. Paraclinoid or infraclinoid (cavernous ICA) for 1% to 5%.
         c. AChA origin rare.
   B. Atherosclerosis (see Chapter 11).
   C. Nonatheromatous causes of ICA narrowing or stenoses (see Chapter 12).
      1. Meningitis, sphenoid sinusitis.
      2. Spasm (secondary to subarachnoid hemorrhage).
      3. Severe increased intracranial pressure (reduced runoff).
      4. Arteritis (uncommon).
      5. Neurofibromatosis.
      6. Trauma (dissection at level of anterior clinoid process or circle of Willis).
      7. Sickle cell disease (although usually affects smaller vessels).
      8. Radiation therapy.
      9. Neoplasms (encase ICA; most common in pituitary adenoma).
      10. "Moya-moya" or idiopathic progressive arteriopathy of childhood.
      11. Menkes' kinky hair syndrome.
      12. Fibromuscular dysplasia (intracranial FMD is rare).
   D. Magnetic resonance (MR) imaging.
      1. Normal-appearing lumen, normal signal void seen in most patients (does not exclude significant *cervical* stenosis, cervical fibromuscular dysplasia, etc.).
      2. Isointense signal: severe compromise of flow but not necessarily occlusion (carotid angiography can distinguish very slow flow from complete occlusion, but whether MR angiography can do this is still in question).
      3. Narrowed irregular siphon.
         a. Atheromatous involvement.
         b. Dissection (high signal of blood degradation products in vessel wall, particularly in lower sections).

SUGGESTED READINGS

Brant-Zawadzki M: Routine MR imaging of the internal carotid artery siphon: angiographic correlation with cervical carotid lesions, *AJNR* 11:467-471, 1990.

Grossman, RI, Davis KR, Taveras JM: Circulatory variations of the ophthalmic artery, *AJNR* 3:327-329, 1982.

Halbach VV, Higashida RT, Hieshima GB, Hardin CW: Embolization of branches arising from the cavernous portion of the internal carotid artery, *AJNR* 10:143-150, 1989.

Hamada J-I, Kitamura I, Kurino M, et al: Abnormal origin of bilateral ophthalmic arteries, *J Neurosurg* 74:287-289, 1991.

Helgason CM: A new view of anterior choroidal artery territory infarction, *J Neurol* 235:387-391, 1988.

Knosp E, Muller G, Perneczky A: The paraclinoid carotid artery: anatomical aspects of a microsurgical approach, *Neurosurgery* 22:896-901, 1988.

Kraemer JL, Schneider FL, Raupp SF, Ferreira NP: Anatomoradiological correlation of the intersection of the carotid siphon with the dura mater, *Neuroradiology* 31:408-412, 1989.

Osborn AG: *Introduction to cerebral angiography,* New York, 1980, Harper & Row, Chapter 5.

Rhoton AL Jr, Hardy DG, Chambers SM: Microsurgical anatomy and dissection of the sphenoid bone, cavernous sinus and sellar region, *Surg Neurol* 12:63-104, 1979.

Sterbini GLP, Agatiello LM, Stocchi A, Solivetti FJ: CT of ischemic infarctions in the territory of the anterior choroidal artery, *AJNR* 8:229-232, 1987.

Takahashi S, Suga T, Kawata Y, Sakamoto K: Anterior choroidal artery: angiographic analysis of variations and anomalies, *AJNR* 11:719-729, 1990.

Timurkaynak E, Rhoton AL Jr, Barry M: Microsurgical anatomy and operative approaches to the lateral ventricles, *Neurosurgery* 19:685-723, 1986.

Tran-Dinh H: Cavernous branches of the internal carotid artery: anatomy and nomenclature, *Neurosurgery* 20:205-209, 1987.

CHAPTER 5

Circle of Willis

KEY CONCEPTS

1. Less than 20% of persons have a classic circle of Willis in which no segment is hypoplastic or absent.
2. Common normal variants are:
   a. Absent or hypoplastic A1 segment
   b. Hypoplasia of one or both posterior communicating arteries (PCoAs)
   c. "Fetal" origin of the posterior cerebral artery (PCA) from the internal carotid artery (ICA) instead of the vertebrobasilar system

---

I. Normal anatomy and variants.
  A. Components (Fig. 5-1).
    1. ICA.
    2. Horizontal, or A1, segments of right and left anterior cerebral arteries (ACAs).
    3. Anterior communicating artery (ACoA).
    4. Right and left PCoAs.
    5. Horizontal, or P1, segments of both PCAs.
    6. Basilar artery (BA) tip.
  B. Branches.
    1. Medial lenticulostriate arteries.
      a. Arise from A1 segment of ACA.
      b. Supply:
        (1) Basal ganglia.
        (2) Internal capsule.
        (3) Hypothalamus.

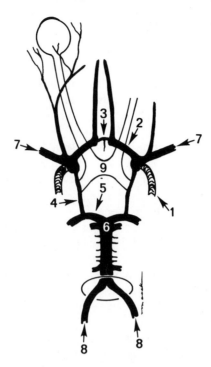

Fig. 5-1   Circle of Willis as seen from above.
1. Internal carotid artery
2. Horizontal (A1) segment of anterior cerebral artery
3. Anterior communicating artery
4. Posterior communicating artery
5. P1 segment of posterior cerebral artery
6. Basilar artery bifurcation
7. Middle cerebral artery (not part of circle of Willis)
8. Vertebral arteries (not part of circle of Willis)
9. Optic chiasm, tracts, and nerves

    (4) Optic chiasm, infundibulum, and other vital structures at base of brain.
2. Thalamoperforating arteries.
  a. Arise from PCoA, basilar tip, P1 segment of PCA.
  b. Supply:
    (1) Thalamus and hypothalamus (limbic system).
    (2) Posterior limb of internal capsule (efferent motor pathways, especially arm).
    (3) Midbrain (efferent motor pathways in cerebral peduncles, ocular movements via cranial nerve III nucleus, arousal via reticular formation).

      3. Thalamogeniculate arteries.
        a. Arise from proximal PCA.
        b. Supply lateral thalamus (sensory function).
      4. Persistent carotid-vertebrobasilar anastomosis (see Chapter 3).
  C. Variants: Circle of Willis variants are almost the rule.
      1. Only 25% of persons have complete circle (no segments hypoplastic or absent).
      2. Anomalies of posterior half of circle in 46%.
        a. "Fetal" origin of PCA in 22% (PCA arises from ICA in embryo; fails to regress and form PCoA); P1 segment of PCA usually hypoplastic.
        b. PCoA hypoplastic in 34%.
      3. A1 hypoplastic in 10%; absent in 1% to 2%; rarely duplicated.
      4. ACoA hypoplastic in 15%; double or triple ACoAs in 40%.
  D. Infundibula are funnel-shaped junctional dilatations at origin of ICA branches. They are most commonly seen at PCoA origin (7% to 10% of cases), although infundibula of ophthalmic and anterior choroidal arteries have been reported. Differences between infundibula and true aneurysms are:
      1. Infundibulum is less than 3 mm in diameter.
      2. Infundibulum is symmetric, funnel-shaped enlargement of PCoA at its origin from ICA.
      3. Infundibulum has smooth dome with PCoA arising from its apex, whereas aneurysm has asymmetric PCoA origin.
      4. Infundibulum is not lobulated and does not have "tit."
  E. Blood flow through circle of Willis can be demonstrated with catheter angiography, magnetic resonance angiography, or color Doppler imaging (especially in newborns).
II. Pathology.
  A. Aneurysms (see Chapter 13): Most intracranial aneurysms are congenital saccular ("berry") aneurysms that arise from circle of Willis, usually at bifurcation between two vessels.
      1. Most common sites on circle of Willis are:
        a. ACoA (30%).
        b. PCoA origin from ICA (20% to 30%).
        c. Basilar tip (5% to 15%).
        d. Middle cerebral artery (20%; this artery is not part of circle of Willis).
      2. Between 15% and 20% of patients have multiple aneurysms.
      3. Congenital anomalies of circle of Willis are associated with increased incidence of aneurysms (e.g., azygous ACA [see Chapter 6], hypoplastic ACA).

B. Atherosclerotic disease, vascular ectasias (see Chapter 11): Although atherosclerotic disease distal to circle of Willis is common, isolated fusiform ectasias are not.

C. Tumors at base of brain (e.g., pituitary adenoma, craniopharyngioma, hypothalamic glioma) may sometimes be large but produce little or no distortion of circle. However, such lesions nearly always displace lenticulostriate and thalamoperforating branches. If tumor is highly vascular, these vessels may also be significantly enlarged.

SUGGESTED READINGS

Barkhof F, Valk J: "Tip of the basilar" syndrome: a comparison of clinical and MR findings, *Neuroradiology* 30:293-298, 1988.

Dervin J, Kendall BE: Ectasia of arteries beyond the circle of Willis, *Neuroradiology* 31:483-485, 1990.

Mitchell DG, Merton DA, Mirsky PJ, Needleman L: Circle of Willis in newborns, *Radiology* 172:201-205, 1989.

Pedroza A, Dujovny M, Artero J, et al: Microanatomy of the posterior communicating artery, *Neurosurgery* 20:228-234, 1987.

Perlmutter D, Rhoton AL Jr: Microsurgical anatomy of the anterior-cerebral-anterior communicating-recurrent artery complex, *J Neurosurg* 45:259-272, 1976.

Pernicone JR, Siebert JE, Potchen EJ, et al: Three-dimensional phase-contrast MR angiography in the head and neck: preliminary report, *AJNR* 11:457-466, 1990.

Ruggieri PM, Laub GA, Masaryk TJ, Modic MT: Intracranial circulation: pulse-sequence consideration in three dimensional volume MR angiography, *Radiology* 171:785-791, 1989.

Saeki N, Rhoton AL Jr: Microsurgical anatomy of the upper basilar artery and the posterior circle of Willis, *J Neurosurg* 46:563-578, 1977.

CHAPTER 6

Anterior cerebral artery

KEY CONCEPTS

1. Since the A1 segment of one anterior cerebral artery (ACA) may be hypoplastic or absent, both ACAs may be supplied by the other internal carotid artery (ICA).
2. The ACA supplies the anterior two thirds of the medial hemisphere plus about I cm of the superolateral surface of the brain convexity.
3. The anterior communicating artery (ACoA) is a common site of saccular aneurysm (30% of all aneurysms).

I. Normal anatomy (Fig. 6-1).
   A. A1 or horizontal segment (from ICA bifurcation to ACoA).
      1. Medial lenticulostriate arteries.
         a. Arise from A1.
         b. Supply:
            (1) Basal ganglia.
            (2) Anterior limb of internal capsule.
      2. ACoA.
         a. Joins right and left A1 segments.
         b. Supplies:
            (1) Small branches to corpus callosum genu.
            (2) Head of caudate nucleus.
            (3) Basal ganglia.
      3. Recurrent artery of Heubner.
         a. Arises from A1 (25%) or A2 near ACoA (75%).
         b. Loops back and courses parallel to A1.
         c. Supplies head of caudate nucleus, rostral putamen, and anterior limb of internal capsule.

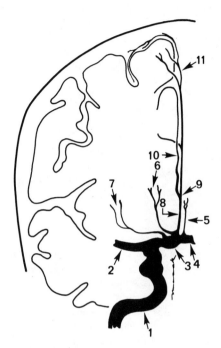

Fig. 6-1 Anteroposterior anatomic drawing of anterior cerebral artery (ACA) and its branches.

      1. Internal carotid artery
      2. Middle cerebral artery
      3. Horizontal (A1) segment of ACA
      4. Anterior communicating artery (ACoA)
      5. Small ACoA branch to basal ganglia, corpus callosum
      6. Medial lenticulostriate arteries
      7. Recurrent artery of Heubner
      8. A2 segment of ACA
      9. ACA bifurcation
    10. Pericallosal artery
    11. Callosomarginal artery

  B. A2 segment (from ACoA to bifurcation into pericallosal and callosomarginal arteries) runs around corpus callosum genu.
    1. Branches (Fig. 6-2).
      a. Orbitofrontal, frontopolar arteries.
      b. Callosomarginal artery.
      c. Pericallosal artery.
    2. Vascular distribution: anterior two thirds of medial hemisphere surface plus 1 cm of superomedial surface over convexity (Fig. 6-3).

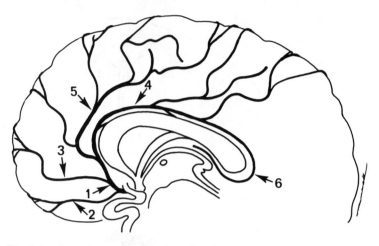

Fig. 6-2 Lateral anatomic drawing of medial surface of cerebral hemisphere showing anterior cerebral artery (ACA) and its major branches.

1. A2 segment of ACA
2. Orbitofrontal artery
3. Frontopolar artery
4. Pericallosal artery
5. Callosomarginal artery
6. Splenial artery

C. Anatomic variants (see Chapter 5).
  1. Al segment hypoplastic or absent.
  2. Absent ACoA; "accessory" or third A2 segment (4% to 10% of cases).
  3. Single ("azygous") ACA supplies both hemispheres. Accidental clipping of this vessel during aneurysm surgery results in bifrontal infarction.
  4. Infraoptic origin of ACA with low bifurcation of ICA (high incidence of associated aneurysm).
II. Pathology.
  A. Vascular displacements (subfalcine ACA herniations): Instead of its normal straight or gently undulating midline course, ACA is displaced in characteristic fashion by masses in particular locations (Fig. 6-4).
    1. Round shift: caused by anterior (frontal) mass.
    2. Square shift: characteristic of large temporal lobe lesions.
    3. Proximal shift: caused by low anterior frontal temporal masses that displace inferior part of A2 while distal ACA gradually courses back to midline more posteriorly.
    4. Distal shift: Proximal A2 is at or near midline. The more posterior the segment is, the more displaced across the midline it becomes.

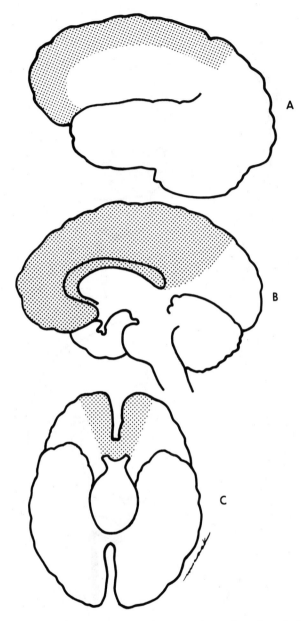

Fig. 6-3 Anterior cerebral artery vascular territory *(dotted area)*. **A,** Lateral view. **B,** Medial view. **C,** Base view.

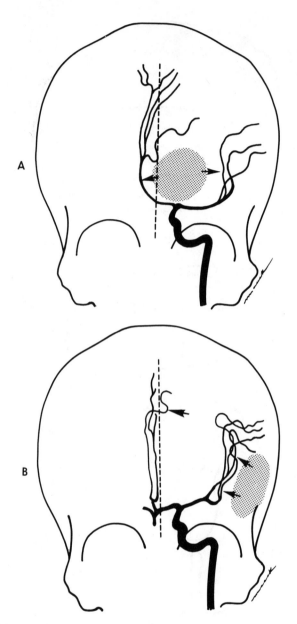

Fig. 6-4 **A,** Round shift of anterior cerebral artery (ACA) across midline caused by deep anterior (frontal) mass *(dotted area)*. **B,** Square shift of ACA across midline caused by holotemporal mass *(dotted area)*. Note where posterior part of ACA returns to midline under falx *(large arrow)*.

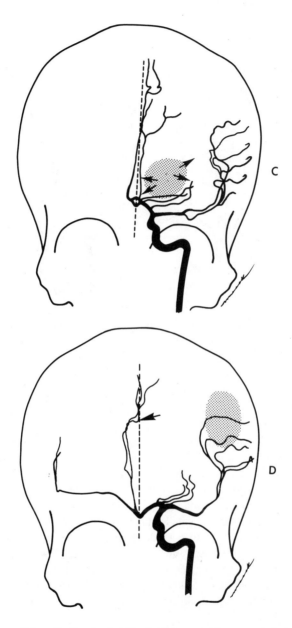

Fig. 6-4, cont'd. **C,** Proximal shift of ACA caused by anteroinferior mass. **D,** Distal ACA shift caused by posterior mass. Note sharply angulated point ("falx cut") where posterior part of ACA returns to midline under falx *(arrow)*. *Continued.*

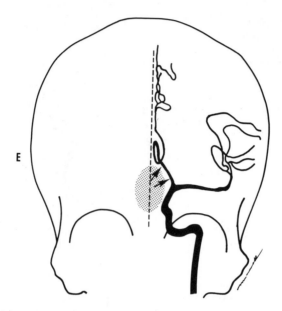

Fig. 6-4, cont'd.   **E,** A1 segment of ACA is elevated by extraaxial deep midline mass such as pituitary adenoma or craniopharyngioma. Thrombosed aneurysm could also have this appearance.

Finally, as inferior margin of falx cerebri approximates corpus callosum, distally displaced ACA must return to midline in sharply angulated step or "falx cut."

   5. A1 elevation: occurs with subfrontal or suprasellar masses. Elevation of orbitofrontal ACA branch is helpful in distinguishing extraaxial mass (such as meningioma) from intraaxial lesion.

B. Atherosclerotic disease: ACA is less frequently involved with significant atherosclerosis than are proximal middle or posterior cerebral arteries. Because ACA is smaller than middle cerebral artery, carotid emboli are also less likely to occlude it. Failure to visualize ACA on carotid injection usually means contralateral ICA supplies territory of both.

C. Aneurysms (see Chapter 13): Congenital or berry ACA aneurysms are nearly all on ACoA, although rarely such lesions occur at distal ACA bifurcation. More peripherally located aneurysms are usually traumatic or mycotic.

SUGGESTED READINGS

Berman SA, Hayman LA, Hinck VC: Correlation of CT cerebral vascular territories with function. I. Anterior cerebral artery, *Am J Neuroradiol* 1:259-263, 1980.

Caplan LR, Schmahmann JD, Kase CS, et al: Caudate infarcts, *Ann Neurol* 47:133-143, 1990.

Gibbons K, Hopkins LN, Heros RC: Occlusion of an "accessory" distal anterior cerebral artery during treatment of anterior communicating artery aneurysms, *J Neurosurg* 74:133-135, 1991.

Odake G: Carotid-anterior cerebral artery anastomosis with aneurysm: case report and review of the literature, *Neurosurgery* 23:654-658, 1988.

Osborn AG: *Introduction to cerebral angiography,* New York, 1980, Harper & Row, pp 189-237.

Savoiardo M: The vascular territories of the carotid and vertebrobasilar systems: diagrams based on CT studies of infarcts, *Ital J Neurol Sci* 7:405-409, 1986.

Taylor W, Miller JD, Todd NV: Long-term outcome following anterior cerebral artery ligation for ruptured anterior communicating artery aneurysms, *J Neurosurg* 74:91-94, 1991

CHAPTER 7

Middle cerebral artery

KEY CONCEPTS

1. The "sylvian triangle" is formed by middle cerebral artery (MCA) branches as they loop over the insula deep within the sylvian fissure.
2. The MCA bifurcation or trifurcation is the third most common site of saccular aneurysms overall (20% to 25% of all cases) and the most common location outside the circle of Willis.
3. The MCA and its branches are the most common sites for intracranial embolic occlusion (stroke).
4. Characteristic displacements of the sylvian triangle and point occur with intracranial masses and are valuable angiographic clues to their location.

I. Normal anatomy.
   A. MCA is the larger of the two terminal internal carotid artery (ICA) branches. MCA is divided into four major segments (Fig. 7-l).
      1. Horizontal (M1) segment: courses from origin at ICA bifurcation laterally toward insula, paralleling sphenoid wing. Lateral lenticulostriate branches arise from M1 to supply basal ganglia and anterior limb of internal capsule.
      2. Insular (M2) segment: At genu, MCA bifurcates (78% of cases) or trifurcates (12%). Branches loop over insula within sylvian fissure, forming "sylvian triangle" (Fig. 7-2).
      3. Opercular (M3) segment: MCA branches emerge from fissure (M3) and ramify over cortical surface (Fig. 7-2).
      4. Two groups of suprasylvian or terminal cortical (M4) branches:

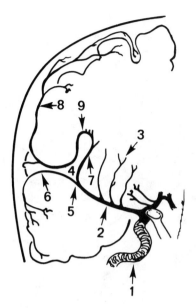

Fig. 7-1 Anteroposterior anatomic drawing of middle cerebral artery (MCA) and its branches.

        1. Internal carotid artery
        2. Horizontal (M1) segment of MCA
        3. Lateral lentriculostriate arteries
        4. Sylvian fissure
        5. MCA bifurcation
        6. Anterior temporal artery
        7. M2 (sylvian) segments of MCA branches
        8. M3 (opercular) branches
        9. Sylvian point

    a. Superior group (includes orbitofrontal, prefrontal, precentral, postcentral, anterior and posterior parietal, angular arteries) supplies frontal and parietal lobes.
    b. Inferior branches supply temporal lobe.
B. Vascular distribution: MCA and its branches supply most of lateral surface of hemisphere, insula, and anterior and lateral aspects of temporal lobe (Fig. 7-3).
C. Anatomic variations: MCA anomalies occur less frequently than variations in other major intracranial arteries.
    1. Most common variations:
        a. Quadrification (rather than bifurcation or trifurcation) of MCA trunk in 4% of anatomic specimens.

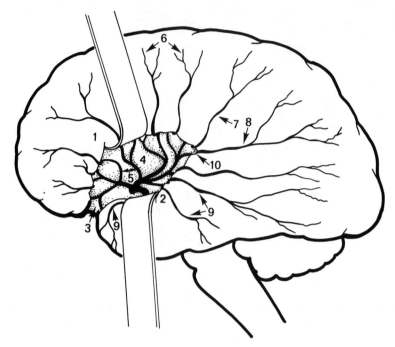

Fig. 7-2   Lateral anatomic drawing of brain showing middle cerebral artery (MCA) and its branches. Retractors have been applied and sylvian fissure widened by pulling apart frontal *(1)* and temporal *(2)* opercula. Insula is exposed within depths of sylvian fissure. MCA branches loop over surface of insula, then pass laterally through sylvian fissure to course over surface of brain.

1. Operculum of frontal lobe
2. Operculum of temporal lobe
3. Sylvian fissure (pulled apart)
4. Insula
5. Insular (M2) MCA branches
6. Precentral and postcentral sulcal MCA branches
7. Posterior parietal artery
8. Angular artery
9. Temporal branches
10. Sylvian point

    b. Single-trunk MCA (no division of main trunk) in 4%.
    c. Fenestration or partial duplication in 1%.
    d. Accessory MCA (origin from A1 segment of ACA) in 1% to 3%.
    e. Duplication (ICA gives origin to MCA branch) in 1% to 3%.
2. Clinical implications of variants: may complicate aneurysm surgery.

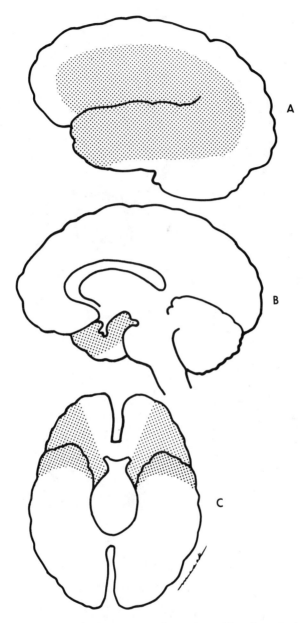

Fig. 7-3 Middle cerebral artery vascular territory *(dotted area)*. **A,** Lateral view. **B,** Medial view. **C,** Base view.

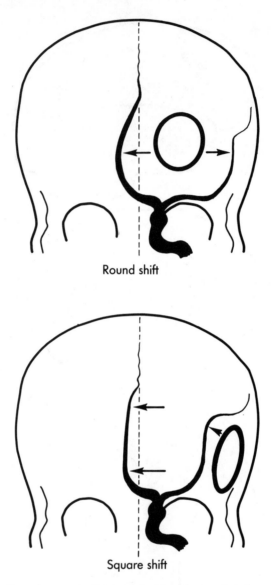

Fig. 7-4   Frontal anatomic diagrams showing characteristic in-out, up-down displacements of middle (MCA) and anterior (ACA) cerebral arteries caused by intracranial masses. Type of ACA shift is named.

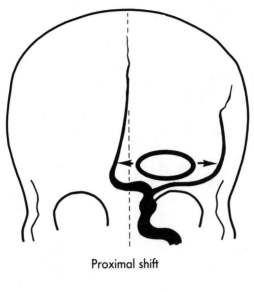

Proximal shift

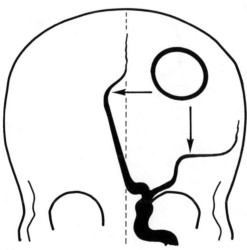

Distal shift

Fig. 7-4, cont'd.   For legend see opposite page.

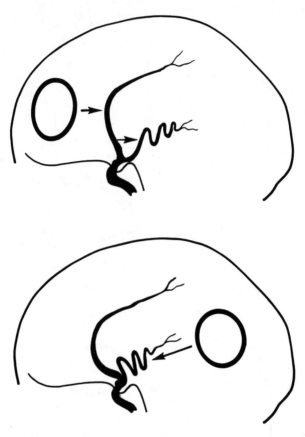

Fig. 7-5   Lateral anatomic diagrams showing some intracranial masses with front-back ACA and MCA displacements.

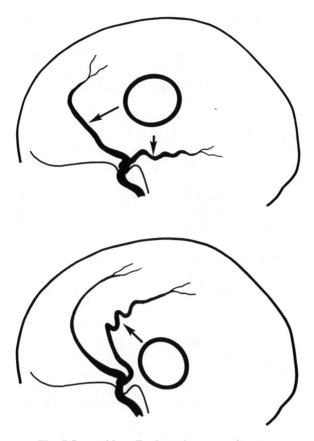

Fig. 7-5, cont'd. For legend see opposite page.

D. Normal angiographic measurements.
1. "Sylvian point" represents most medial extent of last insular loop and is 30 to 38 mm from inner table of skull on routine nonmagnified anteroposterior (AP) studies. It should also be about halfway between inner table of skull and orbital roof or petrous ridge (whichever is lower).
2. On lateral view, top of sylvian triangle should be about halfway between inner table and external auditory meatus. MCA axis posteriorly should also lie along line between anterior clinoid process and point about 9 cm (nonmagnified) above internal occipital protuberance.
II. Pathology.
A. Mass lesions: Distortions and displacements of MCA (sylvian triangle) occur along three axes (Figs. 7-4 and 7-5): up-down, in-out, front-back.
1. Basal ganglia, lateral ventricular masses: MCA bowed laterally on AP view.
2. Temporal lobe mass: on lateral view, MCA displaced medially and superiorly; on AP view, bowed up.
3. Frontal lobe mass: MCA displaced backward on lateral view.
4. Occipital lobe mass: MCA displaced forward on lateral view.
5. Posterior frontal–anterior parietal lobe mass: MCA displaced down on both AP and lateral views.
B. Aneurysms: 20% to 25% of intracranial aneurysms arise from MCA bifurcation or trifurcation (e.g., at MCA genu).
C. Occlusions: MCA and its branches are most common sites for intracranial occlusive vascular disease (usually embolic). Angiographic signs of stroke are:
1. Abrupt termination or tapering of a vessel.
2. "Bare" area (region of absent perfusion).
3. Slow antegrade flow.
4. Retrograde filling from collateral vessels.
5. Vascular blush ("luxury perfusion").
6. Early draining vein(s).
D. Stenosis: Causes include:
1. Atherosclerotic disease.
2. Arteritis or angiitis (e.g., giant cell arteritis, drug abuse angiitis).
3. Angiopathy (e.g., neurofibromatosis, radiation vasculitis, sickle cell disease).
4. Narrowing or spasm secondary to subarachnoid hemorrhage, tumor encasement, exudative meningitis.

SUGGESTED READINGS

Bradac GB: Angiography in cerebral ischemia, *Riv Neuroradiol* 3(suppl 2):57-66, 1990.
Gito H, Carver CC, Rhoton AL Jr, et al: Microsurgical anatomy of the middle cerebral artery, *J Neurosurg* 54:151-169, 1981.

Grand W: Microsurgical anatomy of the proximal middle cerebral artery and the internal carotid artery bifurcation, *Neurosurgery* 7:215-218, 1980.

Osborn AG: *Introduction to cerebral angiography,* New York, 1980, Harper & Row, pp 239-293.

Takahashi S, Hoshino F, Uemura K, et al: Accessory middle cerebral artery, *AJNR* 10:563-568, 1989.

Umansky F, Dujouny M, Ausman JI, et al: Anomalies and variations of the middle cerebral artery: a microanatomical study, *Neurosurgery* 22:1023-1027, 1988.

CHAPTER 8

Posterior cerebral artery

KEY CONCEPTS

1. Posterior cerebral artery (PCA) branches supply the diencephalon, midbrain, posterior one third of the medial hemisphere surface, and occipital pole.
2. The PCAs are usually visualized angiographically by injecting the vertebrobasilar system. PCAs not visualized most commonly arise from the ipsilateral internal carotid artery (ICA) ("fetal origin").

I. Normal anatomy (Figs. 8-1 and 8-2): PCA originates from basilar artery bifurcation. Its segments and major branches are:
   A. Pl (precommunicating or peduncular) segment: short segment from PCA origin to posterior communicating artery (PCoA) above oculomotor nerve (cranial nerve III).
      1. Branches.
         a. Thalamoperforating arteries (TPAs) arise from PCoA and Pl segment to supply diencephalon and midbrain.
   B. P2 (ambient) segment: runs in ambient cistern from PCoA to posterior aspect of midbrain.
      1. Branches.
         a. Medial posterior choroidal arteries (MPChAs).
            (1) Origin: proximal P2 segment.
            (2) Course: run medially around midbrain and forward along roof of third ventricle.
            (3) Supply colliculi, posterior thalamus, pineal gland, and part of midbrain.
            (4) Angiography: 3 configuration on lateral view.

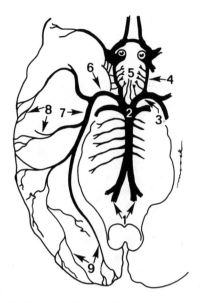

Fig. 8-1 Anatomic drawing of base of brain showing basilar artery, posterior cerebral artery (PCA), and circle of Willis.
1. Vertebral arteries
2. Basilar artery
3. P1 segment of PCA
4. Posterior communicating artery
5. Small branches from circle of Willis and basilar tip that supply base of brain
6. P2 segment of PCA
7. P3 segment of PCA
8. Temporal branches of PCA
9. Occipital branches with calcarine artery *(medial arrow)*

      b. Lateral posterior choroidal arteries (LPChAs).
         (1) Origin: from either PCA or its cortical branches.
         (2) Course: pass into choroid plexus of lateral ventricle, run over pulvinar of thalamus.
         (3) Supply: MPChAs and LPChAs anastomose with each other and anterior choroidal arteries (with which they have reciprocal relationship); variable areas of supply.
         (4) Angiography: on lateral view, LPChAs behind and above MPChA.
C. P3 (quadrigeminal) segment runs within quadrigeminal cistern behind brainstem. Branches (Fig. 8-2):
    1. Inferior temporal arteries supply undersurface of temporal lobe.

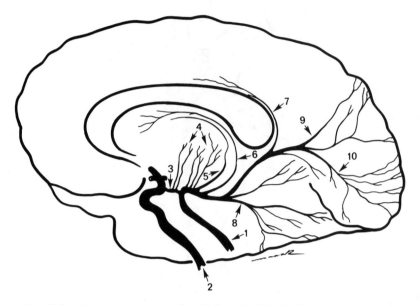

Fig. 8-2   Anatomic drawing of medial cerebral hemisphere showing posterior cerebral artery and its branches to occipital and temporal lobes and basal ganglia.

1. Basilar artery
2. Internal carotid artery
3. Posterior communicating artery
4. Thalamoperforating arteries
5. Medial posterior choroidal artery
6. Lateral posterior choroidal artery
7. Splenial artery
8. Posterior temporal artery
9. Posterior parietal artery
10. Occipital artery

    2. Parietooccipital artery runs in parietooccipital fissure to supply most of posterior one third of brain's medial surface, as well as small portion of lateral surface.
    3. Calcarine artery courses in calcarine fissure to supply visual cortex and occipital pole.
    4. Splenial arteries (posterior pericallosal arteries) supply posterior corpus callosum and anastomose with ACA branches.
  D. PCA vascular distribution (Fig. 8-3).
  E. Anatomic variants, anomalies.
    1. Fetal origins of PCA (see Chapter 5).
      a. P1 segment is hypoplastic or absent.

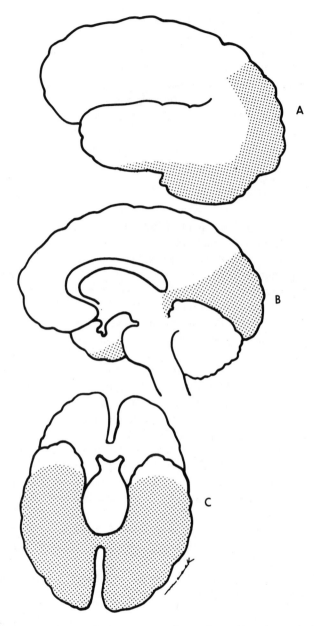

Fig. 8-3 Posterior cerebral artery vascular territory *(dotted areas).* **A,** Lateral view. **B,** Medial view. **C,** Base view.

b. PCA arises directly from ICA (15% to 22% of persons).
c. Fetal origin, *not* occlusive vascular disease, is most common reason a PCA is not visualized on vertebrobasilar studies. Injection of ipsilateral carotid artery demonstrates vessel.
2. Carotid-basilar anastomoses may result in carotid supply of PCAs via persistent trigeminal artery or other anomalous vessel.
3. Meningeal branch to tentorium (artery of Davidoff and Schechter) may arise from P2 segment. It is not normally seen on angiograms but may enlarge in presence of arteriovenous malformation (AVM), meningioma, or other highly vascular lesions with increased dural vascular supply.
II. Pathology.
  A. Vascular abnormalities.
    1. Atherosclerosis frequently affects distal basilar artery and proximal PCA segments (usually P2).
    2. Fibromuscular dysplasia is rare but occasionally affects intracranial vasculature.
    3. Aneurysms of PCAs themselves are uncommon and usually result from trauma or infection.
    4. AVMs affecting PCA are similar to those elsewhere. Special case is vein of Galen "aneurysm," in which enlarged choroidal arteries either feed directly into massively enlarged vein of Galen or supply thalamic AVM with secondary venous engorgement. Congestive heart failure and obstructive hydrocephalus are common signs.
  B. Angiographic mass effects and typical vascular displacements.
    1. Brainstem masses: if large enough, displace PCAs laterally.
    2. Posterior temporal masses: displace P2 medially.
    3. Descending transtentorial herniation: displaces P2 inferiorly and medially. Distal PCA downward kinking and occlusion against rim of tentorial incisura can occur, resulting in occipital lobe infarction.
    4. Tentorial meningioma: splays PCA and superior cerebellar arteries apart.
    5. Thalamic mass: stretches and bows LPChA posterosuperiorly.
    6. Suprasellar mass: thalamoperforating branches are stretched and bowed posteriorly and superiorly.
    7. Posterior fossa mass with upward transtentorial herniation: spreads PCAs apart and bows P2 segments superiorly.

SUGGESTED READINGS
Bojanowski WM, Rigamonti D, Spetzler RF, Flom R: Angiographic demonstration of the meningeal branch of the posterior cerebral artery, *AJNR* 9:808, 1988.
Marinkovic SV, Milisavljevic MM, Kovacevik MS: Anastomosis among the thalamoperforating branches of the posterior cerebral artery, *Arch Neurol* 43:811-814, 1986.

Milisavljevic MM, Marinkovic SV, Gibo H, Puskas LF: The thalamogeniculate perforators of the posterior cerebral artery: the microsurgical anatomy, *Neurosurgery* 28:523-530, 1991.

Ono M, Rhoton AL Jr, Barry M: Microsurgical anatomy of the region of the tentorial incisura, *J Neurosurg* 60:365-399, 1984.

Osborn AG: *Introduction to cerebral angiography,* New York, 1980, Harper & Row, pp 295-325.

Pedroza A, Dujovny M, Artero JC, et al: Microanatomy of the posterior communicating artery, *Neurosurgery* 20:228-234, 1987.

Seidenwurm D, Berenstein A, Hyman A, Kowalski H: Vein of Galen malformation, *AJNR* 12:347-354, 1991.

Zeal AA, Rhoton AL Jr: Microsurgical anatomy of the posterior cerebral artery, *J Neurosurg* 48:534-559, 1978.

CHAPTER 9

Cerebral venous system

KEY CONCEPTS

1. The cerebral venous system is highly variable, and anomalies are common.
2. The subependymal veins outline the lateral ventricular margins.
3. Dural sinus or cortical vein thrombosis can result from dehydration, mastoiditis, childbirth, and hypercoagulable states. Computed tomography is highly suggestive; magnetic resonance (MR) imaging and angiography are usually diagnostic.

I. Normal anatomy: Cerebral venous system is composed of dural sinuses plus superficial cortical and deep veins (Figs. 9-1 and 9-2). Posterior fossa venous anatomy is discussed in Chapter 10. Cerebral veins and dural sinuses can be delineated with either MR cerebral venography or catheter angiography (indirectly on late phases of arteriograms, directly by dural sinus catheterization).

A. Dural sinuses.

    1. Superior sagittal sinus (SSS).

        a. Midline structure formed by cranial vault and leaves of falx cerebri.

        b. SSS extends from its origin near crista galli to torcular Herophili.

        c. SSS may also end by becoming right transverse sinus.

        d. Occasionally rostral SSS is atretic and substitute parasagittal venous channels (usually prominent superficial cortical veins) are present.

    2. Inferior sagittal sinus (ISS).

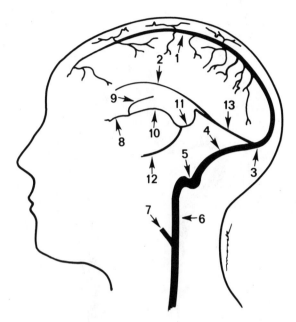

Fig. 9-1   Anatomic drawing of cerebral venous system. Lateral view.

1. Superior sagittal sinus
2. Inferior sagittal sinus
3. Torcular Herophili
4. Transverse sinus
5. Sigmoid sinus, jugular bulb
6. Internal jugular vein
7. External jugular vein
8. Septal vein
9. Thalamostriate vein
10. Internal cerebral vein
11. Vein of Galen
12. Basal vein of Rosenthal
13. Straight sinus

    a. Runs posteriorly in inferior (free) margin of falx to its junction with vein of Galen.

    b. Inconstantly seen at angiography.

3. Straight sinus (SS).

    a. Formed by vein of Galen and ISS.

    b. Runs posteroinferiorly in confluence of falx cerebri and tentorial leaves.

    c. Ends at internal occipital protuberance by joining with SSS to form torcular.

    d. Occasionally ends by becoming left transverse sinus.

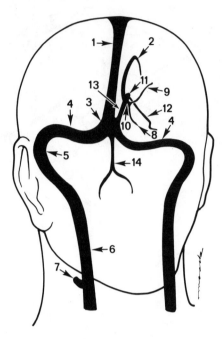

Fig. 9-2   Anatomic drawing of cerebral venous system. Frontal (anteroposterior) view. Superior sagittal sinus is shown running slightly off midline to demonstrate other paramedian structures, which are also depicted at slightly oblique angle.

1. Superior sagittal sinus
2. Inferior sagittal sinus
3. Torcular Herophili
4. Transverse sinus
5. Sigmoid sinus, jugular bulb
6. Internal jugular bulb
7. External jugular bulb
8. Septal vein
9. Thalamostriate vein
10. Internal cerebral vein
11. Vein of Galen
12. Basal vein of Rosenthal
13. Straight sinus
14. Occipital sinus

4. Torcular Herophili.
   a. Confluence of SSS and SS.
   b. Bifurcates into the two transverse sinuses (TSs).
5. Transverse sinuses.
   a. Paired structures.
   b. Extend from torcular along lateral tentorial attachments to sigmoid sinuses.
   c. Often (80%) asymmetric; usually right TS is larger than left TS with preferential drainage toward right jugular vein.
   d. Agenesis of part or all of a TS sometimes occurs.
   e. Determination of dominant venous drainage patterns and potential for collateralization is important in preoperative planning of extensive neurosurgical procedures.
6. Sigmoid sinuses: S-shaped anteroinferior continuation of TSs to jugular bulb.
7. Occipital sinus: small channel that courses posterosuperiorly from foramen magnum to torcular.
8. Cavernous sinuses.
   a. Complex multiseptated dural venous channels adjacent to sella and formed by numerous small groups of veins that have numerous interconnections.
   b. Important contents: internal carotid artery plus cranial nerves III, IV, V_1, V_2, and VI.
   c. Receives superior and inferior ophthalmic veins.
   d. Communicates medially via intercavernous sinuses, posteriorly with transverse sinuses via superior petrosal sinuses, and inferiorly via inferior petrosal sinuses to jugular bulbs.
B. Superficial veins: highly variable; most unnamed except for:
   1. Superficial middle cerebral (sylvian) vein.
      a. Course: along sylvian fissure.
      b. Numerous anastomoses with deep cerebral veins (such as basal vein of Rosenthal) and cavernous sinuses, facial veins via pterygoid plexus, etc.
   2. Veins of Trolard and Labbé: large anastomotic cortical veins that course from superficial middle cerebral vein to SSS or TS, respectively.
C. Deep veins: Most important are subependymal veins that receive medullary venous drainage from white matter via medullary veins that originate 1 to 2 cm below cortex and run through white matter toward ventricles. Subependymal veins outline margins of lateral ventricle on late venous phase angiograms.
   1. Thalamostriate vein (TSV).
      a. Course: over caudate nucleus.

b. With septal vein forms internal cerebral vein (ICV).

c. Angiography: Characteristic double curve on anteroposterior (AP) views resembles antler.

2. Septal vein.

a. Course: posteriorly from frontal horn along septum pellucidum.

b. With TSV forms ICV.

3. Internal cerebral veins.

a. Paired paramedian structures.

b. Course: posteriorly from foramen of Monro above third ventricle.

c. Together with basal veins they unite to form vein of Galen.

d. Angiography: shaped like shallow S on its side on lateral views.

4. Basal vein of Rosenthal (BVR).

a. Course: posterosuperiorly from deep sylvian fissure around midbrain to vein of Galen.

b. Angiography: characteristic "frogleg" appearance on AP view with "ankle" of frogleg representing medial aspect of uncus, "knee" where BVR turns laterally around cerebral peduncle.

5. Vein of Galen (great cerebral vein).

a. Short U-shaped vein.

b. Formed by union of ICVs.

c. Course: beneath corpus callosum splenium.

d. Ends at tentorial apex by uniting with ISS to form SS.

II. Pathology.

A. Congenital anomalies.

1. Chiari II malformation: small posterior fossa with low inion and low-lying torcular and TSs.

2. Dandy-Walker malformation: lambdoidal-torcular inversion (torcular is displaced above lambda). TSs angle steeply down to sigmoid sinuses.

3. Sturge-Weber syndrome (encephalotrigeminal angiomatosis): lack of superficial cortical veins with dilated medullary and subependymal veins.

4. High-riding jugular bulb: Congenital or surgical dehiscence of temporal bone causes dome of jugular bulb to appear as bluish mass in hypotympanum. This should not be mistaken for glomus tympanicum tumor.

B. Malformations, vascular anomalies.

1. Venous angioma (see Chapter 14): Sunburst or caput medusae of prominent medullary veins draining into dilated transcortical vein is pathognomonic. Some recent publications take the position that these are not true angiomas but should be regarded as extreme but normal variants of venous drainage, i.e., developmental venous anomalies.

2. Arteriovenous malformation (AVM): dilated, tortuous veins. These may enlarge sufficiently to produce mass effect. Ventricular obstruction can occur with aneurysmal dilation of vein of Galen, torcular, or both.

3. Sinus pericranii: large abnormal communication between intracranial and extracranial venous circulations (through frontal bone most common, followed by parietal and occipital locations).

C. Occlusions.

1. Tumor (e.g., meningioma): can invade and obstruct dural sinuses.

2. Thrombosis of cortical veins or dural sinuses.

   a. Occurs with dehydration, mastoiditis, hypercoagulable states (e.g., dehydration, post partum, polycythemia).

   b. Angiography: delayed emptying of cortical veins and occluded or absent dural sinuses with collateral drainage.

   c. Computed tomography: Clot in torcular or SSS can be seen as "empty triangle sign" on contrast-enhanced scans.

   d. Magnetic resonance: variable, depending on technique employed. In general, increased signal intensity on standard spin-echo images is seen with decreased or absent signal on partial flip angle scans.

D. Displacements.

1. Masses can displace both superficial and deep veins. Dural sinus displacement is uncommon but can occur with extradural masses (epidural tumor or hematoma). "Alpha sign" occurs when marked subfalcine herniation pushes TSV across midline. Anterior segment of ICV is also displaced, but ICV also returns to midline posteriorly.

2. Hydrocephalus is seen angiographically as stretching and spreading of subependymal veins (e.g., widening of TSVs on AP view).

E. "Early" draining veins: represent arteriovenous shunting. Many causes, some of which are:

1. Arteriovenous lesions: AVMs, fistulas, some angiomas.

2. Infarct (with loss of autoregulation, so-called luxury perfusion).

3. Primary brain tumors: Both malignant and benign lesions (e.g., meningioma) can have arteriovenous shunting.

4. Metastases.

5. Seizure focus.

6. Trauma (contusion).

7. Cerebritis (encephalitis).

SUGGESTED READINGS

Andrews BT, Dujovny M, Mirchandani HG, Ausman JI: Microsurgical anatomy of the venous drainage into the superior sagittal sinus, *Neurosurgery* 24:514-520, 1989.

Bonneville JF, Cattin F, Racle A, et al: Dynamic CT of the laterosellar extradural venous spaces, *AJNR* 10:535-542, 1989.

Goulao A, Alvarez H, Monaco RG, et al: Venous anomalies and abnormalities of the posterior fossa, *Neuroradiology* 31:476-482, 1990.

Lanzieri CF, Sacher M, Duchesneau PM, et al: The preoperative venogram in planning extended craniectomies, *Neuroradiology* 29:360-365, 1987.

Mattle HP, Wentz KU, Edelman RR, et al: Cerebral venography with MR, *Radiology* 178:453-458, 1991.

Miller DL, Doppman JL: Petrosal sinus sampling: technique and rationale, *Radiology* 178:37-47, 1991.

Osborn AG: *Introduction to cerebral angiography*, New York, Harper & Row, 1980, pp 327-377.

Sadler LR, Tarr RW, Jungreis CA, Sekhar L: Sinus pericranii: CT and MR findings, *J Comput Assist Tomogr* 14:124-127, 1990.

Toffol GJ, Gruener G, Naheedy MH: Early-filling cerebral vein, *J Am Osteopath Assoc* 88:1007-1009, 1988.

CHAPTER 10

Posterior fossa vasculature

KEY CONCEPTS

1. The course of the basilar artery (BA) is highly variable and does not consistently delineate the belly of the pons; the anterior pontomesencephalic vein does.
2. The caudal loop of the posterior inferior cerebellar artery (PICA) can normally dip below the foramen magnum. Therefore tonsillar herniation can be diagnosed angiographically only if tonsillar branches are identified as displaced below the foramen magnum.
3. Typical displacements of major posterior fossa arteries and veins can be used to locate masses within the brainstem, fourth ventricle, vermis, or cerebellum.

I. Normal anatomy of arteries.
  A. Vertebral arteries (VAs) (Figs. 10-1 and 10-2).
    1. Origin: from subclavian arteries in 95% of cases (5% directly from aortic arch, usually left VA).
    2. Course.
      a. VAs enter transverse foramen of C6; if arch origin, C5.
      b. They pass directly superiorly to C2 where they turn laterally, then superiorly again through C1.
      c. After looping posteriorly along the atlas, each VA passes superomedially through foramen magnum.
      d. Both VAs unite in front of medulla to form BA.
    3. Branches.
      a. Extracranial: numerous small segmental spinal, meningeal, muscular branches. Abundant anastomoses exist between VA and external carotid artery branches (i.e., occipital, ascending pha-

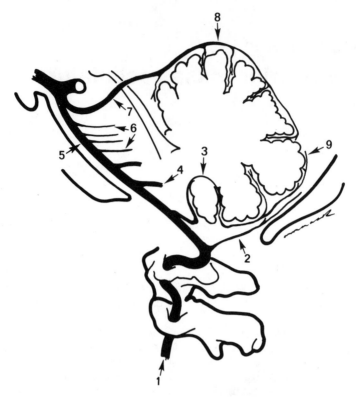

Fig. 10-1   Lateral anatomic drawing of vertebrobasilar circulation.
1. Vertebral artery
2. Posterior meningeal artery
3. Posterior inferior cerebellar artery
4. Anterior inferior cerebellar artery (cut off)
5. Basilar artery
6. Pontine perforating branches
7. Superior cerebellar artery
8. Superior vermian artery
9. Inferior vermian artery

ryngeal arteries) and provide both important sources of collateral
supply and potential routes for extracranial-to-intracranial embolization (atherosclerotic, iatrogenic).
  b. Intracranial.
     (1) Posterior meningeal artery: midline dural branch supplying
         falx cerebelli.
     (2) Anterior spinal artery: usually joins with counterpart from
         opposite side, runs in anteromedial sulcus of cord, lies 2 to
         9 mm behind vertebral bodies on lateral projection.

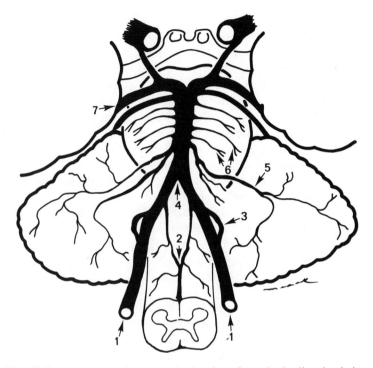

Fig. 10-2 Anteroposterior anatomic drawing of vertebrobasilar circulation.
1. Vertebral artery
2. Anterior spinal artery
3. Posterior inferior cerebellar artery
4. Basilar artery
5. Anterior inferior cerebellar artery
6. Pontine perforating branches
7. Posterior cerebral artery

(3) Posterior spinal artery: may arise from PICA; rarely visualized.

(4) Posterior inferior cerebellar artery: courses around medulla and over or across tonsil to supply it, as well as inferior vermis, choroid plexus of fourth ventricle, and inferior surface of cerebellum (Fig. 10-1).

(a) Arises 13 to 16 mm proximal to basilar artery.

(b) May arise below foramen magnum (18%).

(c) Size is highly variable and depends on size of ipsilateral anterior inferior cerebellar artery (AICA), contralateral PICA.

B. Basilar artery.

1. Origin: formed from the two VAs at medulla or lower border of pons.

2. Course: superiorly along belly of pons; may follow tortuous, wandering course in prepontine cistern and is therefore *not* a particularly good marker for belly of pons.
3. Branches.
    a. Numerous small pontine perforating branches.
    b. Anterior inferior cerebellar artery: courses backward around pons toward cerebellopontine angle and internal auditory canal meatus to supply anterior margins of cerebellar hemispheres. Typically, proximal AICA is in contact with abducens nerve and its meatal segment is anteroinferior to cranial nerves VII and VIII. Supplies cranial nerves VII and VIII and part of anterior surface of cerebellum.
    c. Superior cerebellar arteries (SCAs): arise near apex of BA and circle around brainstem in pontomesencephalic groove, just below tentorial incisura. SCAs run below oculomotor and trochlear nerves and above trigeminal nerve and supply superolateral surface of cerebellar hemispheres.
C. Normal variants.
    1. Anomalous origins of VA: from arch (5%). Hypoplasia relatively common. Aplasia extremely rare.
    2. VA may end in PICA (1%).
    3. Persistent carotid-vertebrobasilar anastomoses such as trigeminal or hypoglossal arteries have been discussed previously (see Chapters 3 and 5).
    4. VA may be fenestrated (i.e., duplicated for a variable distance).
    5. Posterior fossa arteries (SCA, AICA, PICA) can arise from internal carotid artery.

II. Normal anatomy of veins: Numerous veins are present in posterior fossa and have been described in great detail. In this era of computed tomography (CT) and magnetic resonance (MR), only three or four are of radiologic importance (Fig. 10-3), although detailed neurosurgical anatomy of tentorium, dural venous sinuses, and posterior fossa veins is important for neurosurgeons. Briefly:
A. Anterior pontomesencephalic vein (APMV).
    1. Not a single vein but a collection of tiny veins along belly of pons and mesencephalon.
    2. Usually seen a few millimeters from clivus on lateral vertebral angiograms.
B. Precentral cerebellar vein (PCV).
    1. Anteriorly convex vein that lies in front of vermis just behind roof of fourth ventricle.
    2. Should lie halfway along line (Twining's line) drawn between tuberculum sellae and torcular Herophili.

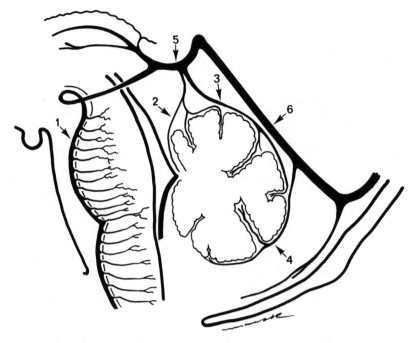

Figure 10-3   Lateral anatomic drawing of major posterior fossa veins.
1. Anterior pontomesencephalic veins
2. Precentral cerebellar vein
3. Superior vermian veins
4. Inferior vermian veins
5. Vein of Galen
6. Straight sinus

C. Superior (SVV) and inferior (IVV) vermian veins: since they outline vermis, should be paramedian on anteroposterior views. A few millimeters should separate SVVs from straight sinus on lateral images, with several millimeters also between IVVs and inner table of skull.
D. Variants, anomalies: So-called venous angiomas of posterior fossa may represent extreme anatomic varieties of tectal and white matter venous drainage and could be considered normal variants or developmental venous anomalies.
III. Pathology.
A. Vascular disease.
1. Aneurysms (see Chapter 13).
a. Less than 2% of intracranial aneurysms involve posterior fossa circulation (excluding basilar tip, which is supratentorial).

b. Location: Most arise from PICA or SCA.
c. Vertebrobasilar dolichoectasia is fusiform dilatation that can mimic intracranial mass clinically and appears on CT or MR scans as ectatic, tortuous vessel (often with slow flow) or sometimes as partially thrombosed calcified mass within foramen magnum, cerebellopontine angle cistern, or prepontine cistern. Severely ectatic basilar artery can extend through tentorial incisura and cause posterior third ventricular mass effect. Cervical VA ectasia or aneurysm is one cause of enlarged neural foramen (along with neurofibroma and hypoplastic pedicle).
2. Atherosclerotic disease.
   a. Location: commonly affects VA at its origin from arch (less severe in cervical VA segment with irregularity and stenosis of intracranial VA and BA more common).
   b. Because blood supply to brainstem and cerebellum is highly variable, clinical findings in vertebrobasilar occlusive disease are also inconstant.
3. Thrombosis and dissection: Although VA thrombosis is relatively common, both spontaneous and traumatic dissections are rare because VA is relatively protected in its cervical course through bony foramina transversaria. However, VAs are exposed from C1 to foramen magnum and positional or traumatic occlusion may occur here. Most common locations for dissections are at C6 where VA enters foramen transversarium or as it exits from C1.
4. Fibromuscular dysplasia: affects VAs less commonly than ICAs. "String-of-beads" appearance around C1-2 is classic finding.

B. Masses: Mass lesions in posterior fossa are best analyzed by compartmental approach, dividing posterior fossa into anterior (brainstem and fourth ventricle forward) and posterior (in or behind fourth ventricle) compartments. Anterior compartment can be further subdivided into intraaxial and extraaxial components, and posterior compartment can be divided into vermian (i.e., midline) and hemispheric (i.e., lateral) components. Although CT or MR scan is available for virtually all posterior fossa masses before angiography, and exceptions to this schema occur occasionally, compartmental approach works most of time (see Chapter 19).

SUGGESTED READINGS

Amarenco P, Roullet E, Goujon C, et al: Infarction in the anterior rostral cerebellum (the territory of the lateral branch of the superior cerebellar artery), *Neurology* 41:253-258, 1991.
Goulao A, Alvarez H, Monaco RG, et al: Venous anomalies and abnormalities of the posterior fossa, *Neuroradiology* 31:476-482, 1990.

Matsuno H, Rhoton AL Jr, Peace D: Microsurgical anatomy of the posterior fossa cisterns, *Neurosurgery* 23:58-80, 1988.

Matsushima T, Suzuki SO, Fukui M, et al: Microsurgical anatomy of the tentorial sinuses, *J Neurosurg* 71:923-928, 1989.

Savoiardo M, Bracchi M, Passerini A, Visciani A: The vascular territories in the cerebellum and brainstem: CT and MR study, *AJNR* 8:199-209, 1987.

Schrontz C, Dujoyny M, Ausman JI, et al: Surgical anatomy of the arteries of the posterior fossa, *J Neurosurg* 65:540-544, 1986.

CHAPTER 11

Atherosclerosis

KEY CONCEPTS

1. Atherosclerosis is the most common cause of stenotic or occlusive cerebrovascular disease.
2. Most strokes are secondary to emboli (usually from the carotid bifurcation) rather than mechanical stenosis. Between 15% and 20% may be cardiac in origin.
3. Extent of ischemia or infarct depends on the availability of collateral blood flow, the potential for which sharply decreases distal to the circle of Willis.
4. The middle cerebral artery territory is the most common location for embolic occlusion.
5. Hemodynamically significant narrowing (decreased arterial pressure) occurs when the vessel diameter is reduced by approximately 60%, although more than 90% narrowing is required to reduce flow.
6. Angiography is only about 60% accurate in determining ulceration of atherosclerotic plaques.
7. Approximately 2% of tumors are manifest as a strokelike syndrome.

I. Noninvasive imaging methods for evaluating cervicocerebral atherosclerotic disease.
   A. B-mode ultrasound, Doppler (including color-flow techniques).
   B. Ocular plethysmography.
   C. Intravenous digital subtraction angiography (IVDSA): This is not widely used because only about 80% of studies are of acceptable diagnostic quality.
   D. Vascular magnetic resonance (MR) imaging (MR angiography).
   E. Dynamic computed tomography (CT) with multiplanar reconstruction.

The significance and subsequent appropriate management of noninvasively demonstrated *asymptomatic* stenosis is unclear and beyond the scope of this book. A comparison of the efficacy of all the noninvasive techniques is also beyond our scope. When the clinical predilection is for surgical management of symptomatic patients, more precise delineation is needed and direct visualization of the vessels from the aortic arch to the middle cerebral artery bifurcation is usually required.

II. Pathology.
  A. Pathophysiology. (NOTE: No one cause of atherogenesis, no exclusive pathogenetic mechanism.)
    1. Intimal lipid deposition with overlying fibrous deposition.
    2. Smooth muscle cell proliferation in intima.
    3. Endothelial denudation and ulceration with plaque disruption.
    4. Interplaque hemorrhage.
    5. Platelet aggregation and thrombosis.
    6. Discharge of debris into vessel lumen.
    7. Lesions occur at points of hemodynamic stress; most common site in head and neck is carotid bifurcation.
  B. Pressure-flow relationships: This is a complicated subject; basics include:
    1. Hemodynamically significant stenosis lowers distal arterial pressure.
      a. Occurs with approximately 60% narrowing in vessel diameter.
      b. Flow reduction occurs only if narrowing is greater than 90%. (NOTE: Most investigators consider that high risk for stroke is present when the residual vessel lumen is 1 to 2 mm or less).
    2. "Tandem" lesions: two or more sequential stenoses in same vessel.
      a. If both are less than critically (60%) narrowed, no effect.
      b. If one is significant and other is not, more severe lesion governs flow.
      c. If both are significant, hemodynamic effect is additive with effect more pronounced as severity of stenosis increases.
      d. Most common locations for tandem lesions: carotid bifurcation/ internal carotid artery origin and carotid siphon.
III. Imaging techniques.
  A. Angiography.
    1. Intravenous digital subtraction.
      a. Advantages.
        (1) Noninvasive method.
        (2) Does not require skilled catheter manipulation.
        (3) Comparatively inexpensive.

        (4) Can be performed on both outpatients and inpatients.

   b. Disadvantages.

        (1) At most (being generous) only 80% of IVDSA studies are of diagnostic quality.

        (2) Requires large amounts of contrast material and multiple injections to profile vessels adequately.

        (3) Images degraded by:

          (a) Respiratory and patient motion.

          (b) Swallowing artifacts.

          (c) Poor cardiac output.

          (d) Vascular calcifications.

          (e) Vessel overlap.

          (f) Poorly performed injections.

          (g) Problems with mask and misregistered images.

 2. Intraarterial digital subtraction angiography (IADSA).

   a. Advantages.

        (1) With good techniques can approach cut film angiography in quality.

        (2) Small (4 or 5 Fr) catheters can be used.

        (3) Smaller amounts of contrast required.

        (4) Can be performed on both outpatients and inpatients.

        (5) Relatively nonselective techniques ("hooking" orifice, gentle hand injections) can give diagnostic-quality studies.

        (6) Multiple views (at least two each) of each vessel can be obtained quickly.

   b. Disadvantages.

        (1) Unless high resolution (e.g., 1024×1024 matrix), small vessel detail sometimes not as well delineated as on cut film angiography.

        (2) Patient motion may not permit good image subtraction.

        (3) Many current DSA systems do not acquire two planes simultaneously.

        (4) Expensive.

 3. Cut film angiography.

   a. Advantages.

        (1) Very high resolution.

        (2) Simultaneous biplanar capability usually available.

        (3) Images usually diagnostic; even if some patient motion precludes subtraction, unsubtracted films often acceptable (at least several per series).

   b. Disadvantages.

        (1) Often slower than IADSA.

        (2) Requires more selective catheterization.

(3) Pressure injection must be used.

(4) Often requires larger amounts of more concentrated contrast material than IADSA.

(5) Film cost.

(6) Technician time for manual film subtraction.

(7) Expensive.

4. Color Doppler.
   a. Advantages.
      (1) Noninvasive.
      (2) Reasonably accurate quantification of stenosis.
      (3) Velocity, flow direction, and spectral waveform can be determined.
      (4) Lower cost than arteriography.
   b. Disadvantages.
      (1) Heavily dependent on technician expertise.
      (2) Not quite as accurate as arteriography.
      (3) Occasionally difficult to differentiate very high-grade stenosis from occlusion.
      (4) Presence of distal (intracranial) solitary or tandem lesion can sometimes only be inferred and may be missed, although recent improvements in transcranial Doppler techniques have improved diagnostic accuracy.

5. MR angiography: promising but probably too early to tell which of many flow enhancement techniques will be most useful.
   a. Advantages.
      (1) Noninvasive.
      (2) Adjacent soft tissues displayed.
   b. Disadvantages.
      (1) Technical difficulties with field of view, spatial resolution, high-order motion a problem.
      (2) Expensive.
      (3) Questionable accuracy, especially if flow is slow or turbulent.

6. Dynamic CT (rapidly administered bolus of contrast material, rapid "dynamic" acquisition of multiple thin sections, multiplanar image reformatting).
   a. Advantages.
      (1) Noninvasive.
      (2) Speedy.
      (3) Less expensive than MR or catheter angiography.
      (4) Adjacent soft tissue display (much better than angiography, not quite as good as MR).
      (5) Less expensive than MR or catheter angiography but more expensive than ultrasonography.

    b. Disadvantages.

      (1) Not as accurate as catheter angiography.

      (2) Patient motion may cause image misregistration and artifactual vessel narrowing.

      (3) Mistiming of scan and contrast bolus easy.

IV. Angiographic findings in atherosclerosis.

  A. General.

    1. Vascular ectasia or tortuosity.

    2. Vascular wall calcifications.

    3. Luminal irregularities.

    4. Stenosis.

    5. Occlusion.

  B. Caveats.

    1. Angiographic diagnosis of ulceration is notoriously inaccurate (approximately 60% correlation with gross pathologic and microscopic findings).

      a. Plaques can appear smooth on angiography but ulcerated on microscopy.

      b. Angiographically irregular lesions can have intact intima.

      c. Subintimal hemorrhage can be mistaken for ulceration.

        (1) Often sharply marginated, rounded, eccentric filling defect near carotid bifurcation.

        (2) Can simulate smooth or even ulcerated atherosclerotic plaque.

        (3) Can resemble ulcer crater.

        (4) Most produce high-grade stenosis.

    2. Irregular plaque has same embolic implication as ulcerlike outpouching.

    3. Look for associated intraluminal thrombi, presence of downstream tandem lesion.

    4. Cerebral angiography per se is neither particularly sensitive nor specific; clinical correlation plays essential role in evaluation of intracranial cerebrovascular disease.

  C. Angiographic signs of stroke.

    1. Arterial occlusion.

    2. Arterial stenosis.

    3. Slow antegrade flow (contrast stasis in affected vessel[s] with persistence of arterial filling into capillary or venous phase of angiogram).

    4. Retrograde filling of occluded vessel(s) via pial collaterals.

    5. Diffuse or focal mass effect caused by edema or associated hemorrhage.

6. Vascular blush (luxury perfusion) probably results both from loss of vascular autoregulatory mechanisms within ischemic area and from increased blood flow in adjacent areas in response to acute metabolic acidosis.
7. Early draining veins (filling of a vein abnormally early in angiographic sequence), caused by arteriovenous shunting in ischemic brain.

SUGGESTED READINGS

Carroll BA: Carotid sonography, *Radiology* 178:303-313, 1991.

Creasey JL, Price RR, Presbrey T, et al: Gadolinium enhanced MR angiography, *Radiology* 175:280-283, 1990.

Edelman RR, Mattle HP, Wallner B, et al: Extracranial carotid arteries: evaluation with "black blood" MR angiography, *Radiology* 177:45-50, 1991.

Edwards JH, Kricheff II, Riles T, Imparato A: Angiographically undetected ulceration of the carotid bifurcation as a cause of embolic stroke, *Radiology* 132:369-373, 1979.

Erickson SJ, Middleton WD, Mewissen MW, et al: Color Doppler evaluation of arterial stenoses and occlusions involving the neck and thoracic inlet, *Radiographics* 9:389-406, 1989.

Foley WD, Erickson SJ: Color flow Doppler imaging, *AJR* 156:3-13, 1991.

Hadley MN, Spetzler RF, Barrow DL, et al: Management of extracranial carotid artery disease. I. Asymptomatic carotid atherosclerosis, *BNI Q* 3:17-29, 1987.

Heinz ER, Yeats AE, Djang WT: Significant extracranial carotid stenosis: detection on routine cerebral MR images, *Radiology* 170:843-848, 1989.

Jinkins JR: Dynamic CT of cranio-cervical vascular occlusive disease, *Neuroradiology* 30:105-110, 1988.

Jinkins JR: Dynamic CT of micro- and macroangiopathic states of the cerebrum, *Neuroradiology* 30:22-30, 1988.

Kandarpa K, Davids N, Gardiner GA Jr, et al: Hemodynamic evaluation of arterial stenoses by computer simulation, *Invest Radiol* 22:393-403, 1987.

Kricheff II: State of the art: arteriosclerotic ischemic cerebrovascular disease, *Radiology* 162:101-109, 1987.

Litt AW, Eidelman EM, Pinto RS, et al: Diagnosis of carotid artery stenosis: comparison of 2DFT time-of-flight MR angiography with contrast angiography in 50 patients, *AJNR* 12:149-154, 1991.

Podolak MJ, Hedlund LW, Evans AJ, Herfkens RJ: Evaluation of flow through simulated vascular stenoses with gradient echo magnetic resonance imaging, *Invest Radiol* 24:184-189, 1989.

Ruggieri PM, Laub GA, Masaryk TJ, Modic MT: Intracranial circulation: pulse-sequence considerations in three-dimensional (volume) MR angiography, *Radiology* 171:785-791, 1989.

Steinke W, Kloetzsch C, Hennerici M: Carotid artery disease assessed by color Doppler flow imaging: correlation with standard Doppler sonography and angiography, *AJNR* 11:259-266, 1990.

Stillman MJ, Ronthal M, Kleefield J, et al: Cerebral infarction: shortcomings of angiography in the evaluation of intracranial cerebrovascular disease in 25 cases, *Medicine* 66:297-308, 1987.

CHAPTER 12

Nonatheromatous causes of vascular narrowing and occlusion

KEY CONCEPTS

1. Atherosclerosis is by far the most common cause of extracranial stenosis or occlusion.
2. Common nonatheromatous causes of *cervical* internal carotid artery (ICA) or vertebral artery (VA) narrowing are reduced distal flow, fibromuscular dysplasia, traumatic or spontaneous dissection, and compression from nasopharyngeal or carotid space tumors; cervical spondylosis can also narrow the VA. Arteritis, infection, radiation angiopathy, and toxemia of pregnancy are relatively rare causes.
3. Atherosclerosis is also the most common cause of intracranial artery stenosis. Other, less common causes include idiopathic arteriopathy of childhood, neurofibromatosis, arteritis (including drug abuse), meningitis, sickle cell disease, neoplastic encasement, spasm from infection or subarachnoid hemorrhage, and use of oral contraceptives.

I. Congenital.
  A. Hypoplasia (rare).
    1. Isolated anomaly.
    2. Anencephaly.
  B. Neurocutaneous syndromes.
    1. Neurofibromatosis (renal and gastrointestinal vessels commonly affected; large cerebral arteries rarely).
      a. Supraclinoid ICA narrowing.
      b. Distal branch stenosis, occlusions.
      c. "Moya-moya" or pseudoangiomatous pattern of collateral flow.
      d. High incidence of aneurysms.

    2. Sturge-Weber syndrome (leptomeningeal angiomatosis with paucity of cortical draining veins; larger vessels rarely affected).

    3. Tuberous sclerosis.

       a. Dominant inherited disorder.

       b. Multisystem involvement.

       c. Primarily affects thoracic and abdominal aortic branches.

       d. Intracranial vascular abnormalities rare.

    4. Other, less common neurocutaneous disorders (e.g., epidermal nevus syndrome) may have associated blood vessel dysplasia and cerebral infarction.

C. Idiopathic progressive arteriopathy of childhood.

    1. Sometimes called "moya-moya" (Japanese for puff of smoke; refers to cloud of contrast material filling multiple tiny collateral vessels). This pseudoangiomatous appearance can also be caused by any slowly progressive intracranial occlusive process (e.g., neurofibromatosis, atherosclerosis, radiation therapy).

    2. Occurs in children and young adults.

    3. Cause unknown.

    4. Progressive vascular stenosis and occlusions near skull base with development of extensive pseudoangiomatous collaterals (hypertrophy of leptomeningeal, lenticulostriate, thalamoperforating, choroidal vessels, other small branches at base of brain).

D. Menkes' kinky hair syndrome.

    1. X-linked inheritance.

    2. Defective copper metabolism.

    3. Elongated tortuous vessels.

    4. Endothelial stenosis and occlusion.

E. Marfan's and Ehlers-Danlos syndromes.

    1. Usually affect extracranial vasculature.

    2. May involve cephalocervical trunks.

    3. Intracranial involvement rare.

F. Sickle cell disease.

    1. Vasa vasorum infarctions result in intimal proliferation and narrowing of parent vessel lumen.

    2. Usually affects small to medium-sized vessels.

    3. May affect large intracranial vessels (e.g., ICA).

II. Traumatic.

A. Increased intracranial presence.

    1. Vessels narrow secondary to reduced distal runoff.

    2. Lumen usually normal.

B. Blunt trauma.

    1. Direct blow, deceleration injury, chiropractic manipulation or sudden hyperextension, or lateral neck flexion.

      2. Diffusely narrowed vessel; usually spares carotid bulb and proximal ICA.

      3. Usually extends to exocranial opening of carotid canal.

      4. Often associated with:

         a. Intimal tear, subintimal dissection.

         b. Intraluminal thrombosis.

         c. Pseudoaneurysm.

         d. Intracranial emboli.

         e. Distal occlusion.

         f. Spasm.

  C. Spasm.

    1. Traumatic.

    2. Catheter induced.

    3. Subarachnoid hemorrhage.

  D. Radiation therapy.

III. Inflammatory and infectious.

  A. Nasopharyngeal infection.

  B. Sphenoid sinusitis.

  C. Basilar meningitis.

  D. Arteritis.

    1. Takayasu's (usually affects aortocervical vessels).

    2. Giant cell.

    3. Drug abuse (especially cocaine, *regardless of route of administration*).

    4. Fibromuscular dysplasia (FMD) (see below).

  E. Miscellaneous.

    1. Septic emboli.

    2. Pyogenic, fungal, or mycobacterial meningoencephalitis.

    3. Syphilis.

    4. Herpes zoster.

    5. Lupus erythematosus and other collagen-vascular disorders.

    6. Periarteritis nodosa.

    7. Sarcoid.

IV. Miscellaneous.

  A. Toxemia of pregnancy.

  B. Post partum.

  C. Oral anticoagulants.

  D. Disseminated intravascular coagulation.

  E. Drug abuse.

    1. Cocaine.

    2. Heroin.

    3. Methamphetamine.

    4. Ephedrine.

   F. Fibromuscular dysplasia.
     1. Location.
       a. Renal arteries most common.
       b. ICA next most common.
     2. Probably second most common cause (after atherosclerosis) for extracranial carotid artery and VA narrowing.
     3. Findings.
       a. Usually spares carotid bifurcation.
       b. Typically occurs near C1-2.
       c. Intracranial involvement rare.
       d. "String-of-beads" appearance or smooth tapered narrowing.
       e. Cervical pseudoaneurysm.
     4. Associated with:
       a. Hypertension (look for renal artery disease).
       b. Intracranial aneurysm.
       c. Transient ischemic attacks or stroke.
   G. "Spontaneous" dissection.
     1. Nontraumatic.
     2. Often underlying FMD, Ehlers-Danlos syndrome, cystic medial necrosis, history of chiropractic manipulation, but sometimes no cause found.
     3. May be familial.
     4. More common in younger adults.
   H. Metabolic disorders.
     1. Diabetes.
     2. Wilson's disease.
     3. Homocystinuria.
V. Neoplastic: Head and neck neoplasms may cause:
   A. Displacement.
   B. Stenosis.
   C. Vessel wall irregularities.
   D. Frank occlusion (rare).
VI. Spondylosis: Cervical spine degenerative spondylosis can cause extrinsic compression, particularly of VA.

SUGGESTED READINGS

Atkinson JLD, Sundt TM Jr, Dale AJ, et al: Radiation-associated atheromatous disease of the cervical carotid artery, *Neurosurgery* 24:171-178, 1989.

Bruno A, Adams HP Jr, Biller J, et al: Cerebral infarction due to moyamoya disease in young adults, *Stroke* 19:826-833, 1988.

Dobyns WB, Garg BP: Vascular abnormalities in epidermal nevus syndrome, *Neurology* 41:276-278, 1991.

George B, Laurian C: Impairment of vertebral artery flow caused by extrinsic lesions, *Neurosurgery* 24:206-214, 1989.

Houser OW, Mokri B, Sundt TM Jr, et al: Spontaneous cervical cephalic arterial dissection and its residuum: angiographic spectrum, *AJNR* 5:27-34, 1984.

Lewis LK, Hinshaw DB, Will AD, et al: CT and angiographic correlation of severe neurological disease in toxemia of pregnancy, *Neuroradiology* 30:59-64, 1988.

Mokri B: Traumatic and spontaneous extracranial internal carotid artery dissections, *J Neurol* 237:356-361,1990.

Mokri B, Piepgras DG, Wiebers DO, Houser OW: Familial occurrence of spontaneous dissection of the internal carotid artery, *Stroke* 18:246-251, 1987.

Osborn AG, Anderson RE: Angiographic spectrum of cervical and intracranial fibromuscular dysplasia, *Stroke* 8:617-626, 1977.

O'Sullivan RM, Robertson WD, Nugent RA, et al: Supraclinoid carotid cartery dissection following unusual trauma, *AJNR* 11:1150-1152, 1990.

Petro GR, Witwer GA, Cacayorin ED, et al: Spontaneous dissection of the cervical internal carotid artery, *AJR* 148:393-398, 1987.

Satoh S, Shibuya H, Matsushima Y, Suzuki S: Analysis of the angiographic findings in cases of childhood moyamoya disease, *Neuroradiology* 30:111-119, 1988.

Sobata E, Ohkuma H, Suzuki S: Cerebrovascular disorders assocated with von Recklinghausen's neurofibromatosis, *Neurosurgery* 22:544-549, 1988.

Theron J, Tyler JL: Takayasu's arteritis of the aortic arch, *AJNR* 8:621-626, 1987.

Wang A-M, Suojanen JN, Colucci VM, et al: Cocaine- and methamphetamine-induced acute cerebral vasospasm, *AJNR* 11:1141-1146, 1990.

Intracranial aneurysms

I. Clinicopathologic considerations.
   A. Types: saccular, fusiform, dissecting.
   B. Etiology: Most are probably degenerative lesions resulting from hemodynamic stress. Can be:
      1. Congenital-developmental.
      2. Atherosclerotic.
      3. Traumatic.
      4. Mycotic.
      5. Oncotic.
   C. Age and incidence.
      1. Incidence of 5% in autopsy series.

2. Usually become symptomatic at 40 to 60 years.
3. Uncommon in children (less than 2% of all aneurysms), rare in infants; if present, aneurysms often large and frequently located on posterior circulation.
4. Incidence increased in:
   a. FMD.
   b. Polycystic kidney disease.
   c. Aortic coarctation.
   d. Collagen diseases.
   e. Ehlers-Danlos and Marfan's syndromes.
   f. High-flow states (7% to 9% of AVMs).
   g. NF.
5. Radiographic frequency of incidental asymptomatic aneurysms of anterior circulation was 1% in recent reports.

D. Pathology: Aneurysmal sac lacks normal layers.
   1. Intima: normal or subintimal cellular proliferation.
   2. Internal elastic membrane usually absent or reduced.
   3. Muscularis: absent (ends at neck of aneurysm).
   4. Wall: may be thickened with laminated clot.
   5. Adventitia: may be infiltrated by lymphocytes and phagocytes.
   6. Lumen: thrombus often present.
   7. Parent artery: frequently has atherosclerotic changes.

E. Location (Fig. 13-1).
   1. Most congenital (berry) aneurysms arise from circle of Willis or MCA bifurcation.
      a. ACoA in 33%.
      b. ICA at PCoA origin in 33%.
      c. MCA bifurcation in 20%.
      d. Basilar tip in 5%.
      e. Posterior fossa (superior cerebellar artery, anterior and posterior inferior cerebral arteries) in 5%.
      f. Other (e.g., anterior choroidal, pericallosal) in 1% to 3%.
   2. True saccular aneurysms of vessels distal to circle of Willis are uncommon, frequently multiple, and occur in conjunction with vascular anomalies (e.g., azygous ACA, trigeminal artery). Peripheral aneurysms more often mycotic, traumatic, or associated with high-flow states such as AVM.
   3. Multiple in 15% to 20% (up to 45% multiplicity in some series); multiple aneurysms occur more often in women (2:1) and patients over 40 years of age. Female/male distribution is 11:1 if more than two aneurysms are present.

F. Presentation.
   1. Subarachnoid hemorrhage (SAH) most common. Hunt-Hess grading scale for SAH:

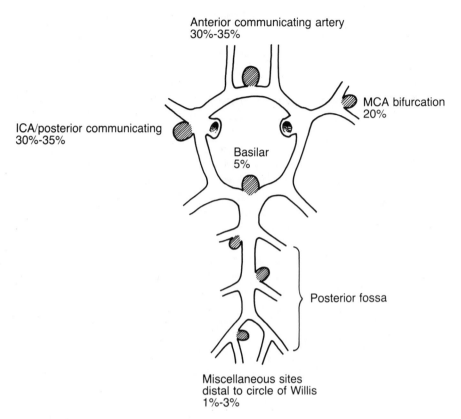

Fig. 13-1 Anatomic diagram of intracranial vasculature with common aneurysm locations noted.

    a. Grade I: asymptomatic or mild headache.
    b. Grade II: moderate to severe headache, nuchal rigidity, oculomotor palsy.
    c. Grade III: confusion, drowsiness, mild focal signs.
    d. Grade IV: stupor or hemiparesis.
    e. Grade V: coma, moribund state, extension posturing.
2. Mass effect, seizures, cranial neuropathies (especially cranial nerves II, III, IV) also common.
3. Less common: ischemic and embolic symptoms.
4. The larger the aneurysm, the more likely to rupture.
5. Increased risk of rupture with increased age.
6. Cumulative risk approximately 1% per year for unruptured aneurysms.
7. Risk of rebleeding in first 2 weeks after SAH is 20% to 50%; mor-

tality rate high (approximately 50%). Of untreated ruptured aneurysms, 50% rebleed within 6 months.

8. After rupture, roughly one third to one half die, one third survive with neurologic deficit, only one fourth to one third recover.

II. Radiology.

A. Catheter angiography is "gold standard."

1. Visualize entire intracranial circulation.

a. Cross-compression studies may be needed to demonstrate ACoA.

b. Both posterior inferior cerebellar arteries (PICAs) must be seen (either by injection of each vertebral artery separately or by reflux into contralateral vessel on single injection).

c. Oblique, submentovertex views often necessary in addition to standard anteroposterior and lateral.

d. High-quality digital subtraction or cut films required.

2. Assess for:

a. Spasm (typically maximum 1 to 2 weeks after SAH).

b. Other aneurysms. If multiple lesions are present, determine which is most likely site of rupture. Helpful signs:

(1) Largest aneurysm most likely to bleed.

(2) Adjacent mass effect from hematoma.

(3) Focal spasm.

(4) Irregularity, lobulation, apical "tit."

(5) Contrast extravasation (rare; these patients have poor prognosis).

c. Collateral circulation.

3. Normal angiogram in patients with SAH from aneurysmal rupture.

a. No abnormality found in 2% to 5% even with meticulous angiography.

b. Repeat four-vessel angiography may show abnormality in 10% to 20% of patients with initially normal angiogram.

c. Aneurysm (or cryptic vascular malformation) may have thrombosed spontaneously.

4. Angiographic appearances mimicking aneurysms.

a. Vascular loop.

(1) Delineate with multiple oblique, off-lateral views.

(2) "Double density" with loops.

b. Infundibulum at origin of PCoA (as much as 10% of cases) or, less commonly, other vessels such as anterior choroidal or lenticulostriate arteries.

(1) Smooth, funnel-shaped dilatation at vessel origin.

(2) Caused by incomplete regression of fetal vessel.

(3) Diameter 2 mm or less.

(4) Distal vessel arises from apex of infundibulum.

B. Computed tomography.
  1. Aneurysms 3 to 5 mm or larger can be seen but must be distinguished from vascular loop or ectasia.
  2. Partially or completely thrombosed aneurysms.
    a. Often have rim calcification.
    b. Partly hyperdense on non-contrast-enhanced studies.
    c. Residual lumen strongly enhanced.
    d. May have ring enhancement.
    e. May have focal mass effect.
  3. Useful for detecting SAH.
    a. High attenuation of fluid in CSF cisterns.
    b. Rough (but not total) correlation with aneurysm site.
      (1) Interhemispheric SAH common with ACoA aneurysms.
      (2) Sylvian fissure SAH common with MCA aneurysms.
      (3) Fourth ventricular clot may occur with PICA aneurysms.
      (4) Third or lateral ventricular clots with ACoA and MCA aneurysms.
C. Magnetic resonance (MR) imaging: highly variable appearance.
  1. Patent aneurysms with rapid flow.
    a. Low signal or "flow void" on both T1- and T2-weighted images.
    b. Pulsation artifact on scans without flow compensation sequences.
    c. Inhomogeneous hypointense or isointense signal may occur with turbulent flow.
    d. Paradoxical enhancement (high signal in patent aneurysms with low flow velocities).
  2. Partially thrombosed aneurysms have complex signal, often with:
    a. Flow void in residual patent lumen.
    b. Surrounding layers of multilaminated clot (bright from methemoglobin, dark from hemosiderin).
    c. Perianeurysmal hemorrhage or edema.
    d. Enlargement from repeated episodes of intramural hemorrhage.
  3. Recent studies suggest that MR angiography can detect intracranial aneurysms as small as 3 to 4 mm in diameter. Although this is promising as noninvasive screening technique, meticulous catheter angiography remains definitive diagnostic procedure.
D. Treatment: In addition to traditional surgical approaches, endovascular techniques such as balloon embolization are being used increasingly, particularly for difficult or inaccessible lesions.

SUGGESTED READINGS

Allcock JM: Aneurysms. In Newton, TH, Potts DG (eds): *Radiology of the skull and brain: angiography,* vol 4, St Louis, 1974, Mosby–Year Book, pp 2435-2489.

Atlas SW, Grossman RI, Goldberg HI, et al: Partially thrombosed giant intracranial aneurysms: correlation of MR and pathologic findings, *Radiology* 162:111-114, 1987.

Biondi A, Sciatta G, Scotti G: Intracranial aneurysms: MR imaging, *Neuroradiology* 30:214-218, 1988.

Higashida R, Halbach W, Barnwell SL, et al: Treatment of intracranial aneurysms with preservation of the parent vessel, *AJNR* 11:633-640, 1990.

Higashida RT, Halbach VV, Dowd CF, et al: Intracranial aneurysms: interventional neurovascular treatment with detachable balloons; results in 215 cases, *Radiology* 178:663-670, 1991.

Linskey ME, Sekhar LN, Hirsch W Jr, et al: Aneurysms of the intracavernous carotid artery: clinical presentation, radiographic features, and pathogenesis, *Neurosurgery* 26:71-77, 1990.

Meyer FB, Sundt TM Jr, Fode NC, et al: Cerebral aneurysms in childhood and adolescence, *J Neurosurg* 70:420-425, 1989.

Ohno K, Monma S, Suzuki R, et al: Saccular aneurysms of the distal anterior cerebral artery, *Neurosurgery* 27:907-913, 1990.

Pinto RS, Cohen WA, Kricheff II, et al: Giant intracranial aneurysms: rapid sequential computed tomography, *AJNR* 494-499, 1982.

Rhoton AL: Anatomy of saccular aneurysms, *Surg Neurol* 14:59-66, 1980.

Ross JS, Masaryk TJ, Modic MR, et al: Intracranial aneurysms: evaluation by MR angiography, *AJNR* 11:449-456, 1990.

Schubiger O, Valvanis A, Wichmann W: Growth mechanism of giant intracranial aneurysms: demonstrated by CT and MR imaging, *Neuroradiology* 29:266-271, 1987.

Sevick RJ, Tsuruda JS, Schmalbrock: Three-dimensional time-of-flight MR angiography in the evaluation of cerebral aneurysms, *J Comput Assist Tomogr* 14:874-881, 1990.

Stehbens WE: Etiology of intracranial berry aneurysms, *J Neurosurg* 70:823-831, 1989.

Todd NV, Tocher JL, Jones DA, Miller JD: Outcome following aneurysm wrapping: a 10-year-follow-up review of clipped and wrapped aneurysms, *J Neurosurg* 70:841-846, 1989.

Tsuruda JS, Halbach VV, Higashida RT, et al: MR evaluation of large intracranial aneurysms using cine low flip angle gradient–refocused imaging, *AJNR* 9:415-424, 1988.

Wiebers DO, Whisnant JP, O'Fallon WM: The natural history of unruptured intracranial aneurysms, *N Engl J Med* 304:696-698, 1981.

Wiebers DO, Whisnant JP, Sundt T, et al: The significance of unruptured intracranial aneurysms, *J Neurosurg* 66:23-29, 1987.

Wilson FMA, Jaspan T, Holland IM: Multiple cerebral aneurysms— a reappraisal, *Neuroradiology* 31:232-236, 1989.

Yamamoto Y, Asari S, Suriami N, et al: Computed tomography of the unruptured cerebral aneurysms, *J Comput Assist Tomogr* 10:21-27, 1987.

CHAPTER 14

Intracranial vascular malformations

KEY CONCEPTS

1. The four basic types of vascular malformations are:
   a. Arteriovenous malformations (AVMs)
   b. Venous malformations
   c. Capillary telangiectasias
   d. Cavernous angiomas
2. AVM is the most common symptomatic vascular malformation.
3. Venous malformation is the most common vascular malformation at autopsy.
4. Cavernous angioma is the most common vascular malformation on magnetic resonance imaging.

I. Clinicopathologic considerations.
   A. Four basic types.
      1. Arteriovenous malformations.
         a. Brain (parenchymal).
         b. Dural.
      2. Venous vascular malformations.
      3. Capillary telangiectasias.
      4. Cavernous angiomas.
   B. Parenchymal arteriovenous malformation.
      1. Congenital.
      2. Most common *symptomatic* vascular malformation.
      3. Usually solitary; 4% multiple (multiple AVMs more common in patients with Rendu-Osler-Weber or Wyburn-Mason syndromes); no sex predilection.
      4. Age at presentation: 20 to 40 years; 80% symptomatic by 50 years.

5. Location: all areas (70% to 93% supratentorial).
6. Pathology.
   a. Tortuous, tightly packed mass of enlarged arteries; dilated draining veins.
   b. No capillary bed; no normal brain within malformation.
   c. Surrounding brain often atrophic and gliotic; associated hemorrhage frequent.
   d. Calcification common.
   e. Vascular supply: pial or mixed pial-dural.
7. Associated flow-related aneurysm in 7% to 9%.
8. Presentation: subarachnoid hemorrhage, headache, seizure, neurologic deficit.
9. Risk of hemorrhage: 2% to 3% per year. (Recent data indicate that risk of hemorrhage may be as high as 4% per year and is cumulative.) Each hemorrhagic episode carries 10% to 30% risk of death and 25% risk of long-term morbidity. Size of AVM and presence or absence of hypertension have no value in predicting rupture. Incidence of hemorrhage is similar in infratentorial and supratentorial locations.
10. Dural arteriovenous malformation.
    a. Between 10% and 15% of all intracranial vascular malformations.
    b. Etiology: considered acquired, not congenital.
       (1) Traumatic.
       (2) Atherosclerotic.
       (3) Spontaneous.
    c. Common locations.
       (1) Base of skull.
       (2) Posterior fossa.
    d. Age peak 40 to 60 years.
    e. Clinical findings.
       (1) Hemorrhage rare.
       (2) Pulsatile tinnitus, exophthalmos (related to location).
    f. Theory of pathogenesis.
       (1) Thrombosis of dural sinus.
       (2) Recanalization.
       (3) Arterial fistulization.
C. Venous vascular malformation.
   1. Most common incidental vascular malformation at autopsy (2%).
   2. Sites: cerebellar and deep cerebral white matter (most commonly frontal or cerebellar).
   3. Pathology.
      a. Arteries normal; dilated medullary veins. No increase in number or size of feeding vessels.

        b. Normal intervening brain parenchyma between vessels.
4. Presentation.
        a. Usually found incidentally on computed tomography (CT) or magnetic resonance (MR).
        b. Seizure, headache; hemorrhage relatively rare.
5. Usually solitary.
6. May not be true vascular malformations; regarded by some as extreme anatomic variants or developmental venous anomalies.

D. Capillary telangiectasias.
1. Common; rarely symptomatic; usually found at autopsy (second only to venous angioma as most common vascular malformation identified at postmortem examination).
2. Sites: pons most common; cerebral cortex; spinal cord.
3. Multiple lesions common.
4. Pathology: abnormally dilated capillaries separated by normal interstitial neural tissue.
5. Central nervous system involvement in Osler-Weber-Rendu disease is rare.

E. Cavernous angiomas.
1. Most common vascular malformation seen at MR (especially with gradient echo scans).
2. Sites: anywhere.
3. Multiple in 50%; familial in 80%.
4. Age: 20 to 40 years.
5. Presentation: seizure in 60%; hemorrhage in 20% to 30%; focal or progressive neurologic deficit in 20% to 25%.
6. Pathology: endothelium-lined sinusoidal spaces without intervening neural tissue (distinguishes these from capillary telangiectasias); hemorrhage in different stages of evolution commonly present. Histologic heterogeneity common; some investigators think that cavernous angiomas and capillary telangiectasias represent extremes of single pathologic entity and propose term "cerebral capillary malformations" for this lesion spectrum.
7. Overt bleeding rate recently reported as less than 0.1% per year. Occult hemorrhages probably occur much more frequently.

II. Radiology (Table 14-1).
A. Parenchymal AVM.
1. Angiography.
        a. Tightly packed mass of enlarged feeding arteries, tortuous draining veins.
        b. AV shunting ("early draining veins"); "steal" from adjacent vessels common.

Table 14-1 Radiology of intracranial vascular malformations

Malformation	Angiography	Computed tomography	Magnetic resonance
Arteriovenous malformation			
Patent	Enlarged arteries, veins	Isodense or hyperdense on NECT	Honeycomb of flow voids
	AV shunting	Strong serpiginous enhancement on CECT	Flow-related enhancement on GRE
	Minimal mass (unless hematoma)	Hematoma may be present	Hyperintense areas of thrombi and slow flow
		Calcification in 25%	Often hemorrhage in evolution
Thrombosed	Normal	Hyperdense	Mixed signal core
	Faint blush, subtle AV shunting (if subtotal thrombosis)	Calcification frequent	Hemosiderin ring
		Some variable enhancement may be present	Gliosis, edema, atrophy of adjacent brain
Venous malformation	Arterial normal	Normal on NECT	Linear tubular flow void
	"Medusa head" of medullary veins	Stellate vessels draining into dilated transcortical vein	Flow-related enhancement on GRE
	Enlarged transcortical vein		Paradoxical enhancement if slow flow
Capillary telangiectasia	Normal	Normal, or faint blush on CECT	Hypointense
Cavernous angioma	Usually normal	Hyperdense on CECT	Hypointense-hyperintense reticulated popcornlike core
		Usually no/minimal enhancement	Low signal rim; "blooming" of low signal on GRE
		Calcification occasionally seen	Often multiple on GRE
		Usually no edema	

AV, Arteriovenous; *NECT,* nonenhanced computed tomography; *CECT,* contrast-enhanced computed tomography; *GRE,* gradient echo.

    c. Associated with aneurysm in 7% to 9% (secondary to high-flow states).

    d. Mass effect subtle unless hemorrhage is present.

    e. May be cryptic (no detectable angiographic abnormalities); partially thrombosed AVM may have only subtle blush or early draining vein.

  2. CT.

    a. Hemorrhage and associated atrophy common.

    b. Serpiginous isointense or hyperintense foci with strong enhancement following administration of contrast material.

    c. Calcification common.

  3. MR.

    a. Tightly packed honeycomb appearance; mixed signals often seen.

      (1) Serpiginous "flow voids"; absent signal in foci of calcification.

      (2) Foci of increased signal in thrombosed vessels or vessels with slow flow.

      (3) Associated hemorrhage in different stages of evolution; hemosiderin ring.

    b. Surrounding brain may have:

      (1) Atrophy.

      (2) Gliosis.

      (3) Hemorrhage.

      (4) Edema.

    c. MR angiography shows nidus well, but to date afferent arteries and venous drainage are better visualized with conventional angiography.

  4. Single photon emission computed tomography or positron emission tomography can evaluate perfusion status of adjacent brain.

B. Dural AVM and dural arteriovenous fistula (DAVF).

  1. Site of fistula or AVM best depicted with angiography.

  2. In absence of venoocclusive disease or dilated cortical veins, routine MR may be normal (role of MR angiography still debatable).

  3. Dilated cortical veins without parenchymal nidus on MR is suggestive of DAVF with venoocclusive disease. Complications are common and include subdural or parenchymal hemorrhage and venous infarction.

C. Venous malformation.

  1. Angiography.

    a. Arterial phase normal.

    b. Capillary phase normal or faint blush.

    c. Dilated medullary veins ("Medusa head") draining into en-

larged transcortical vein (pathognomonic).
2. CT.
  a. Usually normal on nonenhanced scans.
  b. Contrast-enhanced CT: stellate tangle of vessels draining into sharply defined transcortical vein that drains superficially into dural sinus or into deep subependymal veins.
  c. Usually frontal or cerebellar, near angle of ventricle.
3. MR.
  a. Linear tubular structure.
    (1) Low signal ("flow void") typical; may show flow-related enhancement on gradient echo studies.
    (2) May see paradoxical high signal if slow flow present.
  b. Hemorrhage and adjacent gliosis uncommon.
D. Capillary telangiectasias (rarely seen).
  1. Angiography: usually normal.
  2. CT: usually normal; may have faint, ill-defined hyperdensity on enhanced studies.
  3. MR: may have hypointense signal on T2-weighted image (T2WI): may have faint enhancement on T1WI with contrast.
E. Cavernous angioma.
  1. Angiography.
    a. Usually normal.
    b. Occasionally faint blush on capillary-venous phase.
  2. CT.
    a. Often hyperdense on nonenhanced CT; occasionally calcified.
    b. Enhancement varies from none or minimal to striking (uncommon).
    c. Edema usually absent but on occasion is striking.
  3. MR: complex internal structure with variable appearance. Common findings:
    a. Mixed signal mass with reticulated or popcornlike core of low- and high-signal foci.
    b. Surrounding low-signal rim (secondary to hemosiderin deposition).
    c. Gradient echo (GRE) scans show "blooming" of low signal because of magnetic susceptibility effect of hemosiderin; may demonstrate flow in residual patent vessels. *GRE scans often demonstrate multiple small lesions not visible on T2WI.*
III. Treatment options.
A. AVMs: Between 60% and 80% of patients with intracranial AVMs can be treated effectively with embolization, surgical resection, stereotactic radiation, or a combination of these methods.
  1. Endovascular (embolization).
  2. Surgical excision (often combined with embolization).

3. Stereotactic radiosurgery (usually for lesions with nidus less than 3 cm; often combined with embolization or surgery or both).
B. Venous malformation: radiosurgery or no treatment.
C. Capillary telangiectasias: no treatment.
D. Cavernous angioma: occasionally, resection of solitary or symptomatic lesion; radiosurgery.

SUGGESTED READINGS

Atlas SW, Mark AS, Fram EK, Grossman RI: Vascular intracranial lesions: applications of gradient-echo MR imaging, *Radiology* 169:455-461, 1988.

Betti O, Munari C, Rosler R: Stereotactic radiosurgery with the linear accelerator: treatment of arteriovenous malformations, *Neurosurgery* 24:311-320, 1989.

Brown RD, Weibers DO, Forbes G: The natural history of unruptured intracranial arteriovenous malformations, *J Neurosurg* 68:352-357, 1988.

DeMarco JK, Dillon WP, Halbach VV, Tsuruda JS: Dural arteriovenous fistulas: evaluation with MR imaging, *Radiology* 175:193-199, 1990.

Goulao A, Alvarex H, Monaco RG, et al: Venous anomalies and abnormalities of the posterior fossa, *Neuroradiology* 31:476-482, 1990.

Graves VB, Duff TA: Intracranial arteriovenous malformations: current imaging and treatment, *Invest Radiol* 25:952-960, 1990.

Marchal G, Bosman H, Van Fraeyenhoven L, et al: Intracranial vascular lesions: optimization and clinical evaluation of three-dimensional time-of-flight MR angiography, *Radiology* 175:443-448, 1990.

Marks MP, Lane B, Steinberg GK, Chang PJ: Vascular characteristics of intracerebral arteriovenous malformations in patients with clinical steal, *AJNR* 12:489-496, 1991.

Monaco RG, Alvarex H, Goulao A, et al: Posterior fossa arteriovenous malformations, *Neuroradiology* 31:471-475, 1990.

Nüssel F, Wegmüller H, Huber P: Comparison of magnetic resonance angiography, magnetic resonance imaging, and conventional angiography in cerebral arteriovenous malformation, *Neuroradiology* 33:56-61, 1991.

Rapacki TFX, Brantley MJ, Furlow TW Jr, et al: Heterogeneity of cerebral cavernous hemangiomas diagnosed by MR imaging, *J Comput Assist Tomogr* 14:18-25, 1990.

Rigamonti D, Johnson PC, Spetzler RF, et al: Cavernous malformation and capillary telangiectasia: a spectrum within a single pathological entity, *Neurosurgery* 28:60-64,1991.

Rigamonti D, Spetzler RF, Drayer BP, et al: Appearance of venous malformations on magnetic resonance imaging, *J Neurosurg* 69:535-539, 1988.

Robinson JR Jr, Little JR, Awad IA: The natural history of cavernous angiomas [abstract]. *J Neurosurg* 72:333A, 1990.

Seidenwurm D, Berenstein A, Hyman A, Kowalski H: Vein of Galen malformation, *AJNR* 12:347-354, 1991.

Sigal R, Krief O, Houlteville JP, et al: Occult cerebrovascular malformations: follow-up with MR imaging, *Radiology* 176:815-819, 1990.

Smith HJ, Strother CM, Kikuchi Y, et al: MR imaging in the managment of supratentorial intracranial AVMs, *AJNR* 9:225-235, 1988.

Willinsky RA, Lasjaunias P, Terbrugge K, Burrows P: Multiple cerebral arteriovenous malformations (AVMs), *Neuroradiology* 32:207-210, 1990.

Wilms G, Demaerel P, Marchal G, et al: Gadolinium-enhanced MR imaging of cerebral venous angiomas with emphasis on their drainage, *J Comp Assist Tomogr* 15:199-206, 1991.

Wilms G, Marchal G, Van Hecke P, et al: Cerebral venous angiomas, *Neuroradiology* 32:81-85, 1990.

CHAPTER 15

Stroke (including venoocclusive syndromes)

KEY CONCEPTS

1. Stroke is basically a clinical diagnosis; computed tomography (CT) is used primarily to identify hemorrhage if anticoagulation is considered. Other uses of CT or magnetic resonance (MR) are in atypical clinical presentations or to identify nonvascular causes of ischemic symptoms, such as neoplasm.
2. CT and MR findings in cerebral infarction vary with time.
3. Stroke in young persons without trauma or cardiac disease should suggest the possibility of substance abuse (e.g., cocaine, methamphetamines), birth control pills, anabolic steroids, underlying vasculopathy, and spontaneous dissection.
4. Embolic strokes occur most commonly in the middle cerebral artery; posttraumatic cerebral infarctions occur most frequently in the posterior cerebral artery distribution.

The clinical and radiologic manifestations of cerebral ischemia and infarctions vary with location, size of affected area, adequacy of collateral flow, and time.

I. Neuropathology of cerebral ischemia (quick summary—oversimplified but useful).
   A. Hierarchy of sensitivity to ischemic damage.
      1. Neurons most susceptible (some areas more vulnerable than others).
      2. Oligodendroglia least susceptible.
   B. Morphologic patterns of ischemic brain damage.
      1. Autolysis: postmortem brain tissue, brain-dead individuals; takes 12 to 24 hours to develop.
      2. Cerebral infarction: irreversible damage to all cell types in affected

area; can occur within 3 to 4 hours; often caused by emboli or local atherosclerosis.

3. Generalized or partial neuronal neurosis: neurons damaged but supporting cells intact. (Most vulnerable areas are CA1 zone of hippocampus, cerebellar Purkinje cells, small and medium-sized neurons in neostriatum, and pyramidal neurons in cortical layers 3, 4, and 6.)

4. Selective neuronal necrosis: variable time course with neuronal death in striatum within 3 hours, death of CA1 pyramidal neurons of hippocampus in 48 to 72 hours. Seen in resuscitated patients.

C. Physiology.

1. Loss of ion homeostasis (massive efflux of potassium ions and influx of sodium ions, leading to membrane depolarization) because of failure of intracellular ion pumps and influx of calcium ions.

2. Intracellular pH falls.

3. Energy metabolites (adenosine triphosphate, phosphocreatine) and substrates (glucose, glycogen) are depleted.

4. Lack of oxygen shuts down mitochondrial respiration.

5. Diglycerides and free fatty acids accumulate, leading to formation of prostaglandins, leukotrienes, and free radical intermediates.

D. Collateral blood flow, in both major vessel and microvasculature, moderates all of preceding (see Chapter 16).

II. Clinical findings.

A. Current clinical classification of cerebrovascular ischemic events.

1. Subclinical ischemia and infarction.

2. Transient ischemic attack (TIA): temporary ischemic neurologic deficit that clears completely within 24 hours.

3. Reversible ischemic neurologic deficit (RIND): term not widely used; refers to stroke that clears completely in 21 days.

4. Stroke in evolution: changing neurologic status from ischemic event.

5. Completed stroke: ischemic event resulting in permanent fixed neurologic deficit.

B. Cerebrovascular syndromes. (CAUTION: Symptoms vary widely; these are generalizations.)

1. Anterior choroidal artery (AChA) (highly variable terminal field of distribution).

a. Contralateral hemiplegia.

b. Contralateral hemianesthesia.

c. Contralateral quadratic or hemianoptic field defect (typically with sparing of macular vision).

d. Signs secondary to variable involvement of basal ganglia, hippocampus, thalamus, and mesencephalon.

2. Anterior cerebral artery (ACA) (distal to anterior communicating artery).
   a. Disordered mental state, confusion, emotional lability.
   b. Motor aphasia (if lesion on dominant side).
   c. Contralateral lower extremity hemiplegia.
3. Middle cerebral artery (MCA) syndromes vary according to site obstructed, number of branches involved, adequacy of collateral flow, and whether dominant hemisphere is involved.
   a. Complete MCA occlusion: contralateral hemiplegia, hemianesthesia, hemianopsia with global aphasia if lesion in dominant hemisphere.
   b. Coma and death may result.
   c. Precentral artery (Broca's area): contralateral lower facial and tongue weakness with motor aphasia (if dominant hemisphere involved).
   d. Central or rolandic artery: contralateral hemiplegia of variable degree.
   e. Anterior parietal artery: contralateral astereognosis, slight upper extremity weakness.
   f. Posterior parietal or angular arteries: contralateral hemianopsia, cortical-type sensory disturbances.
   g. Orbitofrontal artery: expressive aphasia.
   h. Posterior temporal artery: contralateral hemianopsia and aphasia if lesion in dominant hemisphere.
4. Posterior cerebral artery (PCA) occlusion.
   a. Thalamoperforating or thalamogeniculate arteries: thalamic pain syndrome, contralateral hemiplegia, often homonymous hemianopsia.
   b. Calcarine artery: contralateral homonymous field defect, usually with macular sparing.
   c. Variable somesthetic disturbances, motor weakness because of corticospinal tract involvement (may also be produced by PCA occlusion).
5. Vertebral artery (VA) occlusions: Clinical manifestations vary according to segment involved and adequacy of collateral flow. With total occlusion, vertigo, vomiting, coarse nystagmus, ataxia, contralateral loss of pain and temperature, and ipsilateral Horner's syndrome may be present.
6. Basilar artery (BA) occlusion (also highly variable).
   a. Total occlusion usually results in death but may cause quadriplegia or hemiplegia on one side with partial paralysis on other.
   b. Dysphagia, dysarthria, and sensory disturbances.
   c. Vertigo, vomiting, confusion, and coma.

d. "Locked-in syndrome": thrombosis of small pontine branches resulting in complete paralysis and inability to speak, with sensation often intact. Vertical eye movements can be spared and may be only means of communication with patient.

7. Stroke in young patient without trauma or underlying cardiac course should raise possibilities of:

   a. Substance abuse (e.g., cocaine by any route of administration, methamphetamines).

   b. Birth control pills (women).

   c. Anabolic steroids.

   d. Vasculopathy (e.g., fibromuscular dysplasia).

   e. Spontaneous dissection.

III. Radiology: "Stroke" is a clinical diagnosis; impact of CT and MR in management and outcome of acute cerebral ischemia is debatable. Generally accepted role of these procedures is to detect presence of acute hemorrhage before anticoagulation begins. Therefore unenhanced CT scans are usually adequate for diagnosis. If clinical history or plain CT scan findings are atypical, contrast enhancement or MR may be helpful in some cases. Approximately 1.5% of lesions with "clinically definite" stroke are nonvascular (e.g., tumors or subdural hematoma). Approximately 2% of intracranial neoplasms are first apparent as strokelike syndrome, and other diseases such as bacterial or viral cerebritis, meningoencephalitis, cysticercosis, vascular malformations, and multiple sclerosis sometimes mimic stroke clinically.

A. CT (findings depend on the infarct's age).

   1. First 24 to 48 hours.

      a. Usually normal before 12 hours, but early signs can include slight hypodensity in lentiform nucleus, slight cortical hypodensity, sulcal effacement, and loss of interface between gray and white matter.

      b. Twelve to 24 hours: poorly circumscribed focal areas of decreased attenuation in affected area; subtle mass effect (sulcal compression or effacement, ventricular displacement) often present.

      c. Enhancement following contrast administration is relatively uncommon in very early infarcts. CAUTION: Infarcted regions may become isodense with contrast material and therefore be overlooked if only enhanced scanning is performed. DOUBLE CAUTION: Some studies suggest that contrast enhancement is harmful in acute stroke (e.g., because blood-brain barrier damage is already present, permitting contrast extravasation, seizure or clinical worsening may occur).

      d. Hemorrhagic infarct in 5% to 10%.

e. Uncommon: embolic high-density (calcified) atherosclerotic plaque within vessel lumen or lesser increased density representing thrombus (e.g., "dense MCA" sign, present in 2% to 12% of stroke patients). Clot lysis may result in disappearance on subsequent scans.

2. Forty-eight to 96 hours.
   a. Focal area(s) of decreased attenuation and increasing mass effect conforming to vascular territory that involves both gray and white matter. Often wedge shaped.
   b. Increasing mass effect.
   c. Hemorrhage, if it occurs, is typically near corticomedullary junction.

3. Four to 7 days.
   a. Contrast enhancement, typically gyral, may appear as early as 3 to 4 days after ictus and persist up to 8 weeks.
   b. Edema persists.

4. Two to 8 weeks.
   a. Contrast enhancement may persist.
   b. Mass effect resolves.

5. Old infarcts.
   a. Low-attenuation areas are well delineated, represent focal encephalomalacia in affected vascular distribution.
   b. Enlargement of adjacent sulci and ventricle reflects ex vacuo hydrocephalus (i.e., secondary to loss of cerebral tissue).
   c. Calcification in old infarcts is rare. Ischemic infarcts rarely calcify; most occur in old hemorrhagic lesions.
   d. Multiple small foci of diminished density: Subclinical infarctions, subcortical arteriosclerotic encephalopathy (SAE, or Binswanger's disease), dementia, or altered mental function may be difficult to correlate with CT and MR findings (see Chapter 39). Significance of periventricular leukomalacia, multiple foci of deep white matter infarction, perivascular demyelination, and other nonspecific abnormalities is unknown. Term "lacunae" should be reserved for sharply delineated, nonenhancing, low-density lesions of white matter or basal ganglia that are 10 mm or less in diameter.

6. Embolic versus thrombolic stroke.
   a. Most clinically detectable strokes are embolic.
   b. Pial artery territory infarctions, seen as large low-attenuation areas that extend from deep brain to cortex, are most often embolic.
   c. Thrombotic infarcts are more often smaller and inhomogeneous and tend to spare cortex.

7. Miscellaneous.
   a. Most embolic strokes occur in MCA distribution.
   b. Posttraumatic cerebral infarctions almost always result from direct vascular compression caused by mass effects from hematoma, edema, or contusion that produce gross mechanical shift of brain with herniations across falx cerebri or tentorium cerebelli or both.
      (1) Found in 2% of cranial CTs performed for evaluation of trauma.
      (2) PCA distribution most commonly affected.

B. MR.
   1. Stroke is clinical diagnosis; CT is usually acceptable as screening procedure for hemorrhage.
   2. Advantages of MR over CT.
      a. MR is more sensitive in detecting subtle hemorrhage.
      b. MR may detect edema earlier because T2-weighted imaging (T2WI) is more sensitive than CT (i.e., lesions are more conspicuous). New techniques such as diffusion-weighted scans may be even more sensitive to early-onset pathophysiologic changes of acute cerebral ischemia than routine T2WI.
      c. Many strokes older than a few hours can be enhanced with gadolinium-diethylenetriaminepentaacetic acid (Gd-DTPA).
      d. Thrombosed vessels can sometimes be seen.
      e. MR can demonstrate nonvascular causes of stroke syndrome (e.g., neoplasm). Strokes tend to involve both gray and white matter (or occasionally gray matter only, with or without hemorrhage), whereas tumors infiltrate at gray-white junction or involve white matter with only partial thickness of overlying gray matter affected.
   3. Disadvantages.
      a. Cost.
      b. Longer imaging time (patient motion).
      c. Most clinical treatment protocols are based on CT studies.
   4. Findings: vary with time.
      a. Acute.
         (1) Often isointense on T1WI.
         (2) May have mild cortical low intensity outlined by subcortical edema (high signal) on T2WI.
         (3) Loss of gray matter–white matter interface.
         (4) Postcontrast scans may disclose enhanced curvilinear structures that represent cortical arterial vessels with markedly slowed circulation.
      b. Subacute.

(1) Low signal on T1WI, high signal on T2WI.

(2) Hyperintense signal sometimes seen at periphery of subacute stroke on T1WI probably represents hemorrhagic changes where blood flow is restored by recanalization or collateral supply.

  c. Chronic.

(1) Encephalomalacia seen as low-signal foci on T1WI, high on T2WI.

(2) If hemorrhage occurred, hemosiderin may be seen as subcortical low-signal foci on T2WI.

(3) Lacunar infarcts and foci of perivascular demyelination are seen as multiple deep white matter foci of increased signal on T2WI.

    5. Recent studies indicate that dynamic contrast-enhanced MR may be helpful in evaluating cerebral blood flow dynamics.

  C. Angiography (see box below and Chapter 7).

  D. Positron emission tomography, single photon emission computed tomography.

    1. Can give quantitative metabolic maps of cerebral blood flow, oxygen consumption, glucose utilization.

    2. Limited clinical utility so far.

  E. Transcranial Doppler can demonstrate reduced flow in some proximal MCA occlusions.

IV. Venous thrombotic, occlusive disease.

  A. Dural sinus thrombosis.

    1. Occurs with various clinical conditions.

      a. Dehydration.

      b. Post partum, oral contraceptive use.

      c. Hypercoagulable states.

      d. Infection (e.g., mastoiditis).

      e. Tumor (e.g., meningioma).

      f. Spontaneous.

ANGIOGRAPHIC SIGNS OF STROKE

Vessel occlusion
Retrograde flow
Slow antegrade flow
"Bare" (nonperfused) areas
Vascular blush ("luxury perfusion")
Early draining veins (nonspecific)
Mass effect (nonspecific)

---

    2. Angiography.
        a. Nonfilling of affected sinus.
        b. Intraluminal filling defects.
        c. Dilated medullary, ependymal, and superficial veins.
        d. Stasis in draining veins.
        e. Collateral venous drainage (e.g., orbit, pterygoid plexus).
    3. CT.
        a. Filling defects within sinus on contrast-enhanced scans ("empty delta" sign).
            (1) Seen in only about one third of cases.
            (2) Should be identified on several adjacent sections.
            (3) Mimics of empty delta sign: high splitting of superior sagittal sinus, variations of torcular and tentorial anatomy.
            (4) Other causes of filling defects in dural sinuses: arachnoid granulations, sinus septations.
        b. Generalized cerebral edema.
        c. Frequently associated with focal cortical venous infarcts, multiple small focal areas of edema, hemorrhage (particularly if cortical vein thrombosis also present).
        d. Enhanced scans may show apparently thickened dura (falx and tentorium) because of enlarged collateral venous channels.
    4. MR: probably best noninvasive diagnostic study findings.
        a. Early: absence of normal dural sinus "flow void" as result of thrombus (isointense on T1WI; hypointense on T2WI).
        b. Next: high signal in affected vessels caused by intraluminal clots. (CAUTION: Slow but normal blood flow can have high signal caused by flow-related enhancement.)
        c. Flow-enhancement techniques (e.g., gradient echo scans) that selectively excite only moving spins show decreased to absent signal intensity in thrombosed, nonflowing vessels, high signal in patent channels.
        d. Contrast enhancement may show high signal of dura and collateral venous channels around nonenhancing clot.
        e. MR cerebral venography may depict collateral venous drainage. Phase contrast MR permits distinction between thrombus and flowing blood.
  B. Cortical vein thrombosis.
    1. Angiography.
        a. Slow, stagnant flow in affected veins.
        b. Clots and filling defects can sometimes be seen.
        c. Collateral venous channels (e.g., medullary and subependymal veins) may be prominent.
        d. Often associated with dural sinus thrombosis.
    2. CT.

a. Multiple small hemorrhages and foci of edema.
b. Sometimes can identify coexisting sinus thrombosis.
3. MR.
a. High signal within affected vessels on T1WI.
b. High signal foci from edema and venous infarction on T2WI.
c. Hemorrhage common; findings vary with age of clot and pulse sequences used.

SUGGESTED READINGS*

Bozzao L, Bastianello S, Gantozzi LM, et al: Correlation of angiographic and sequential CT findings in patients with evolving cerebral infarction, *AJNR* 10:1215-1222, 1989.

Brant-Zawadzki M, Weinstein P, Barthowski H, Moseley M: MR imaging and spectroscopy in clinical and experimental cerebral ischemia: a review, *AJNR* 8:39-48, 1987.

Edelman RR, Mattle HP, Atkinson DJ, et al: Cerebral blood flow: Assessment with dynamic contrast-enhanced T2-weighted MR imaging at 1.5T, *Radiology* 176:211-220, 1990.

Elster AD, Moody DM: Early cerebral infarction: gadopentetate dimeglumine enhancement, *Radiology* 177:627-632, 1990.

Hazelton AE, Earnest MD: Impact of computed tomography on stroke management and outcome, *Arch Intern Med* 147:217-270, 1987.

Hecht-Leavitt C, Gomori JM, Grossman RI, et al: High-field MRI of hemorrhagic cortical infarction, *AJNR* 7:581-585, 1986.

Imakita S, Nishimura T, Yamada N, et al: Magnetic resonance imaging of cerebral infarction: time course of Gd-DTPA enhancement and CT comparison, *Neuroradiology* 30:372-378, 1988.

Kricheff II: Arteriosclerotic ischemia cerebrovascular disease, *Radiology* 162:101-109, 1987.

Kushner MJ, Zanette EM, Bastianello S, et al: Transcranial Doppler in acute hemispheric brain infarction, *Neuroradiology* 41:109-113, 1991.

Mattle HP, Wentz KU, Edelman RR, et al: Cerebral venography with MR, *Radiology* 178:453-458, 1991.

Mirvis SE, Wolf AL, Numaguchi Y, et al: Post-traumatic cerebral infarction diagnosed by CT: prevalence, origin, and outcome, *AJNR* 11:355-360, 1990.

Moody DM, Bell MA, Challa VR: Features of the cerebral vascular pattern that predict vulnerability to perfusion or oxygenation deficiency: an anatomic study, *AJNR* 11:431-439, 1990.

Moseley ME, Kucharczyk J, Mintorovitch J, et al: Diffusion-weighted MR imaging of acute stroke, *AJNR* 11:423-429, 1990.

Nabatami H, Fujimoto N, Nakamura K, et al: High intensity areas on noncontrast T1-weighted MR images in cerebral infarction, *J Comput Assist Tomogr* 14:521-526, 1990.

Nadel L, Braun IF, Kraft KA, et al: Intracranial vascular abnormalities: value of MR phase contrast imaging to distinguish thrombus from flowing blood, *AJNR* 11:1113-1140, 1991.

Plum F, Pulsinelli W: Cerebral metabolism and hypoxic-ischemic brain injury. In Asbury A, McKhann G, McDonald I (eds): *Diseases of the nervous system*, Philadelphia, 1986, Saunders, pp 1086-1100.

Ringelstein EB, Koschorke S, Holling A, et al: Computed tomographic patterns of proven embolic brain infarctions, *Ann Neurol* 26:759-765, 1989.

*Also useful are practical reviews such as the following in *MRI Decisions:* Jeff L. Creasey's discussion on differentiating tumor from infarct (March/April 1990 issue) and B.L. Dunkley and Michael Brant-Zawadzki's presentation of MR strategies for evaluating stroke syndromes (March/April 1989 issue).

Rippe DJ, Boyko OB, Spritzer CE, et al: Demonstration of dural sinus occlusion by the use of MR angiography, *AJNR* 11:199-201, 1990.

Sandercock P, Molyneaux A, Warlow C: Value of computed tomography in patients with stroke: Oxfordshire Community Stroke Project, *Br Med J* 290:193-197, 1985.

Sato A, Takahashi S, Soma Y, et al: Cerebral infarction: early detection by means of contrast-enhanced cerebral arteries at MR imaging, *Radiology* 178:433-439, 1991.

Seaman ME: Acute cocaine abuse associated with cerebral infarction, *Ann Emerg Med* 19:71-79, 1990.

Spritzer CE, Sussman SK, Blinder RA, et al: Deep venous thrombosis evaluation with limited-flip-angle, gradient-refocused MR imaging: preliminary experience, *Radiology* 166:371-375, 1988.

Tomsick TA, Brott TG, Chambers AA, et al: Hyperdense middle cerebral artery sign on CT, *AJNR* 11:473-477, 1990.

Tomura N, Inugami A, Kanno I, et al: Differentiation between cerebral embolism and thromboses on sequential CT scans, *J Comput Assist Tomogr* 14:26-31, 1990.

Tsuruda JS, Shimakawa A, Pelc NJ, Saloner B: Dural sinus occlusion: evaluation with phase-sensitive radiant-echo MR imaging, *AJNR* 12:481-488, 1991.

Virapongse C, Cazenave C, Quisling R, et al: The empty delta sign: frequency and significance in 76 cases of dural sinus thrombosis, *Radiology* 162:770-785, 1987.

Wall SD, Brant-Zawadski M, Jeffrey RB, Barnes B: High frequency CT findings within 24 hours after cerebral infarction, *Am J Radiol* 138:307-311, 1982.

Wang AM, Lin JCT, Rumbaugh CL: What is expected of CT in the evaluation of stroke? *Neuroradiology* 30:54-58, 1988.

Williams AL, Haughton VM: *Cranial computed tomography,* St Louis, 1985, Mosby–Year Book, pp 88-102.

CHAPTER 16

Patterns of collateral blood flow in occlusive cerebrovascular disease

KEY CONCEPTS

1. The circle of Willis is the most important potential source of collateral blood flow to the brain.
2. Since only 25% of persons have an intact circle of Willis, the effectiveness of this source may be anatomically limited.
3. External carotid artery (ECA) to internal carotid artery (ICA) anastomoses through the orbit and cavernous sinus are other common sources of extracranial to intracranial blood flow.
4. Small vessels over the pia and surface of the brain ("pia-arachnoid plexus") in the watershed areas interconnect the anterior cerebral, middle cerebral, and posterior cerebral artery distributions and may also supply some collateral intracranial flow.
5. Brain microvasculature circulation varies substantially, rendering some areas much more vulnerable to circulatory alterations (anoxia and hypoperfusion) than others.

I. Collateral circulation: Development of collateral blood flow depends on existence of anatomic potential for other sources of circulation, whether occlusion developed slowly or suddenly, and status of underlying cerebral vasculature.
  A. Clinical considerations: Symptoms of cerebrovascular occlusive disease vary with:
    1. Site of occlusion and area supplied by occluded vessel (see Chapter 15).
    2. Adequacy of collateral flow.
    3. Time of onset (gradual versus sudden).
    4. Preexisting status of circulatory system (e.g., when hypotension is

superimposed on already compromised vascular system as in diabetes, hypertension, aging, or atherosclerosis).

B. Anatomic considerations: Major potential sources of collateral blood flow in the face of occlusive vascular disease are:

1. Circle of Willis.
    a. By far most important source.
    b. Occlusions distal to circle of Willis have significantly reduced alternative sources of blood supply.
    c. Effectiveness limited by:
        (1) Congenitally incomplete circle of Willis. (Only 25% of brains have balanced circulation with no segment hypoplastic or absent; see Chapter 5.)
        (2) Variants that sharply limit collateralization (e.g., fetal PCA, origin of both ACAs from one ICA).
    d. If circle is intact, one vessel (such as vertebral artery [VA]) could potentially supply entire brain.

2. ECA-ICA anastomoses. (Prominent ECA-ICA communicating system exists during fetal development.)
    a. Next most important source of collateral circulation.
    b. Examples.
        (1) Ethmoidal branches of maxillary artery to ethmoidal branches of ophthalmic artery (OA) to OA to ICA.
        (2) Angular branch of facial artery to extraocular branches of OA to OA to ICA.
        (3) Superficial temporal artery to orbital branches of OA to OA to ICA.
        (4) Artery of foramen rotundum to lateral mainstem artery of ICA to ICA.
        (5) Ascending pharyngeal artery to muscular branches of VA to VA.
        (6) Occipital artery to muscular branches of VA to VA.

3. Pial-leptomeningeal anastomoses.
    a. Fine arterial and arteriolar (not capillary) plexuses in pia mater.
    b. Interconnect adjacent branches of same artery.
    c. Anastomoses between terminal branches of ACA, MCA, and PCA also occur over so-called watershed or border zone area between. This area is also most vulnerable to hypoperfusion.
    d. Can enlarge (e.g., to supply arteriovenous malformations, neoplasm, or devascularized area).
    e. In fetus and premature infant, arterial watershed is not cortical but in deep periventricular white matter adjacent to ventricles.

4. Dural collaterals.
    a. Both meningeal vessels and penetrating (transcalvarial) ECA branches.

   b. Mostly at skull base or over vertex.
   c. Usually relatively minor source of potential collateral flow.
5. Microvasculature and effects of cerebral perfusion and oxygenation deficiencies: Several distinct patterns of intraparenchymal afferent blood supply have recently been shown to exist in human brain.
   a. Some areas such as cortex, centrum semiovale, thalami, and basal ganglia have single source, whereas others (such as subcortical U fibers and external capsule) have dual or even triple supply.
   b. Patterns of vascular supply predict which areas are more vulnerable to anoxic states or hypoperfusion. Gray matter, because of its higher metabolic rate than white matter, is also more vulnerable to pure anoxia.
      (1) Cortex (anoxia, hypoperfusion at watershed).
      (2) White matter of centrum semiovale (hypoperfusion).
      (3) Basal ganglia and thalami (hypoperfusion, anoxia).
   c. Other regions are "favored" and more protected from adverse circulatory events.
      (1) Subcortical U fibers.
      (2) External capsule, claustrum, and extreme capsule.
   d. Disease states that alter status of cerebral microvasculature also are factors in determining effects of adverse circulatory events. Examples include:
      (1) Aging.
      (2) Diabetes.
      (3) Hypertension.
      (4) Atherosclerosis.

SUGGESTED READINGS

Gillilan LA: Potential collateral circulation to the human cerebral cortex, *Neurology* 24:941-948, 1974.

Moody DM, Bell MA, Challa VR: Features of the cerebral vascular pattern that predict vulnerability to perfusion or oxygenation deficiency: an anatomic study, *AJNR* 11:431-439, 1990.

Quint DJ, Boulos RS, Spera TD: Congenital absence of the cervical and petrous internal carotid artery with intercavernous anastomosis, *AJNR* 10:435-439, 1989.

Yamaki T, Tanabe S, Hashi K: Prominent development of the inferolateral trunk of the internal carotid artery as a collateral pathway to the external carotid system, *AJNR* 10:206, 1989.

CHAPTER 17

Trauma: vascular manifestations of head and neck injury

KEY CONCEPTS

1. Blunt cervical trauma can result in internal carotid artery (ICA) or vertebral artery (VA) intimal tear, pseudoaneurysm, dissection, thrombosis, or intracranial embolization.
2. Penetrating injury can result in intimal tear, laceration, occlusion, arteriovenous fistula, or false aneurysm.
3. Indirect ICA injury (e.g., deceleration type) occurs primarily at three segments where arterial mobility changes: the base of the skull (exocranial orifice of petrous carotid canal); the point at which the ICA becomes intradural; and just above the posterior communicating artery (PCoA) where the ICA is relatively fixed by the circle of Willis.
4. Carotid-cavernous fistulas can be traumatic, spontaneous, iatrogenic, or congenital in origin. Almost all are located at the horizontal or posterior (C4, C5) segments of the carotid siphon or at their junction with each other.
5. Any acutely traumatized patient with an unexplained neurologic deficit should be considered for emergency cerebral arteriography to rule out vascular injury.

I. Extracranial.
   A. Blunt trauma (including chiropractic manipulation): broad spectrum of carotid artery and less commonly VA injury including:
      1. Vasospasm without other injury.
      2. Compression, narrowing caused by:
         a. Soft tissue hematoma.
         b. Fracture or subluxation (most involve VA).
      3. Intimal tear.

105

        a. Raised intimal flap; may be accompanied by dissection, thrombosis, or distal embolization.

        b. Can occur at virtually any location.

        c. Rarely causes acute symptoms.

        d. Symptom onset varies from hours to days, occasionally even 2 to 3 weeks.

    4. Pseudoaneurysm.

        a. Typically from internal laceration or hemorrhage into vessel wall.

        b. If large, can be found on clinical examination as submucosal pharyngeal mass.

        c. Emboli can be complication of traumatic aneurysm.

    5. Thrombosis.

        a. Usually complication of intimal tear or dissection.

        b. Intraluminal filling defect or complete occlusion may result.

        c. Distal emboli a complication.

    6. Dissection.

        a. Often occurs in association with intimal tear.

        b. Usually seen as gradual long-segment tapering of affected vessels.

        c. Usually does not extend above skull base.

        d. Occlusion and distal emboli may be complications.

        e. Probably underdiagnosed in acutely injured patients. With focal neurologic deficits unexplained by computed tomographic brain scan or spinal or peripheral nerve injury, one recent series demonstrated 20% incidence of carotid dissection at angiography.

B. Rotary injury and hypertension: may stretch and compress ICA over lateral mass of atlas and axis. Intimal tear can also be caused by severe stretching of artery over transverse process of cervical vertebra because of sudden hyperextension and lateral flexion of neck to opposite side.

C. Penetrating injuries.

    1. Often intraoral (e.g., pencil or stick) in pediatric age group.

    2. Spectrum of findings includes:

        a. Vessel laceration, intimal tear.

        b. Compression from soft tissue hematoma.

        c. Intraluminal thrombus.

        d. Occlusion.

        e. Complications.

           (1) Arteriovenous fistula.

           (2) Pseudoaneurysm.

           (3) Distal embolization and stroke.

D. Deceleration injury.

    1. Typical result is ICA intimal tear at exocranial carotid canal orifice (point of transition between relative ICA fixation in petrous carotid canal and mobile cervical portion).

2. Findings.
   a. Intimal tear.
   b. Dissection (may extend into cervical or less commonly intrape-
      trous ICA).
   c. Occlusion.
   d. Complications.
      (1) Arteriovenous fistulas (carotid-jugular, carotid-cavernous)
          may develop, sometimes months or even years later.
      (2) Distal embolization.
E. "Spontaneous" dissection: Although most atherosclerotic dissections or
   dissections related to fibromuscular dysplasia occur in patients 50 years
   or older, spontaneous dissection without history of trauma or known
   vasculopathy sometimes occurs in younger patients (see Chapter 12).
   Angiographically these often appear as long, tapered eccentric stenoses
   with or without saccular pseudoaneurysm. They typically begin above
   carotid bifurcation and extend to skull base or occasionally into carotid
   canal. In 80% dissection partially or completely resolves.
F. Imaging consideration: Visualize all cephalocervical vessels from aortic
   arch to terminal intracranial branches in angiographic evaluation.
II. Intracranial.
A. Traumatic pseudoaneurysm.
   1. Etiology.
      a. Less common: skull fracture, penetrating injury.
      b. More common: shearing forces (e.g., between dural surfaces
         such as falx and ACA, tentorium and PCA).
   2. Incidence: less than 1% of intracranial aneurysms seen at operation.
   3. Location.
      a. Distal to circle of Willis.
      b. Often near dural surface.
B. Meningeal artery injury.
   1. Can result in:
      a. Epidural hematoma.
      b. Rare: pseudoaneurysm, arteriovenous fistula.
   2. Angiographic signs (uncommonly seen, since angiography is rarely
      performed in acute head trauma unless direct vascular injury is sus-
      pected).
      a. Indirect: lentiform extraaxial mass effect from epidural he-
         matoma.
      b. Direct: extravasation of contrast material along dura and middle
         meningeal artery (MMA), giving "train-track" appearance; con-
         trast material can also extravasate from lacerated vessel along
         fracture or dural tear.
C. Vessel occlusion.
   1. Etiology.

    a. "Brain death." (Massively increased intracranial pressure exceeds intraarterial pressure, resulting in cessation of cerebral perfusion; no contrast visualized beyond C2 ICA segment at angiography. Other diagnostic studies for determining brain death include dynamic radionuclide scans, contrast-enhanced computed tomography [CT] scans, xenon CT cerebral blood flow, and possibly magnetic resonance [MR] spectroscopy. NOTE: Legal criteria for establishing brain death vary.)

    b. Traumatic infarction.

      (1) Direct local vascular injury.

      (2) Secondary to brain herniations; examples:

        (a) PCA occlusion against tentorial incisura in descending transtentorial herniation.

        (b) ACA occlusion against falx in massive subfalcine herniation.

    c. Vascular dissection (intracranial less common than cervical): occurs with shearing forces at foci of transition in arterial mobility; in descending order of frequency these sites are:

      (1) Exocranial opening of petrous carotid canal (see preceding).

      (2) Point at which ICA leaves skull base and penetrates dura.

      (3) Immediately distal to PCoA origin (i.e., at point of relative stability and fixation by circle of Willis).

D. Intracranial hematomas (see Chapter 40).

  1. Usually diagnosed with CT or MR.

  2. Can also be seen on cerebral angiograms.

    a. Acute epidural hematoma.

      (1) Avascular lentiform extraaxial mass.

      (2) Rarely, arterial extravasation can be seen along MMA.

    b. Acute subdural hematoma (SDH): avascular crescentic extraaxial mass effect.

    c. Chronic SDH.

      (1) Avascular extraaxial mass.

      (2) Can be either crescentic or lentiform.

E. Carotid-cavernous fistulas: abnormal communications between carotid artery and cavernous sinus. Dural (indirect) fistulas are communications between meningeal branches of ICA or ECA and cavernous sinus. Direct fistulas are communications between intracavernous carotid artery and cavernous sinus. Symptoms caused by carotid-cavernous fistulas are related to size, duration, location, adequacy and route of venous drainage, and other factors.

  1. Etiology.

    a. Traumatic: Symptoms may appear months or even years after trauma.

    b. Vasculopathy: atherosclerotic, collagen deficiency syndrome, fibromuscular dysplasia.

    c. Iatrogenic: following endarterectomy, direct surgical trauma.

    d. Congenital: dural arteriovenous malformation.

    e. Miscellaneous: pregnancy, sinusitis, cavernous sinus thrombosis.

2. Location.

    a. Horizontal segment of intracavernous ICA in approximately 50%, posterior segment in 20%, junction of horizontal and posterior segments in 25% to 30%.

    b. ECA almost never supplies traumatic fistula but is commonly involved in spontaneous carotid-cavernous fistula.

    c. Venous drainage from engorged cavernous sinus is commonly anteriorly into orbit via superior and inferior ophthalmic veins; inferiorly through pterygoid plexus into deep face; posteriorly via petrosal sinuses into clival venous plexus and jugular veins.

3. CT.

    a. Proptosis.

    b. Enlarged superior ophthalmic vein.

    c. Enlarged (laterally bulging) cavernous sinus.

    d. Extraocular muscle engorgement.

    e. Rarely, enlargement of optic nerve sheath complex.

4. MR of dural arteriovenous fistulas at cavernous sinus.

    a. Signal void in cavernous sinus and superior ophthalmic vein.

    b. Lateral bulging of cavernous sinus wall.

    c. Proptosis.

    d. Enlarged extraocular muscles.

    e. Strong contrast enhancement of normal venous spaces of cavernous sinus; persisting signal void in high-flow areas caused by the fistula.

5. Angiography.

    a. Both ICAs and dominant VA should be studied. Selective ECA angiography should be performed for spontaneous carotid-cavernous fistulas.

    b. Most rapid filming rate available should be used.

    c. High-flow fistulas may require VA injection with simultaneous carotid artery compression on same side as fistula to demonstrate precise fistula site; double-lumen balloon catheter can be used to slow ICA flow and test tolerance to carotid artery occlusion.

    d. Collateral flow potential should be evaluated by injection of opposite ICA while carotid artery is compressed on same side as fistula.

    e. Venous drainage routes must be demonstrated.

6. Therapy.

   a. Conservative: intermittent manual carotid artery compression for several days. Low success rate, particularly with high-flow fistula.

   b. Intravascular occlusion of fistula with ICA preservation using detachable balloons is preferred treatment and is successful in nearly all cases.

   c. If b is not technically feasible, balloon trapping of ICA above and below fistula can be performed if collateral flow from contralateral carotid artery is sufficient. Success rate is 75% to 80%.

   d. Ligation or graded stenosis of CCA or cervical ICA. Cure rate is 25% to 50%. "Stump" is potential embolic source.

7. Prognosis: High-risk features indicating need for urgent treatment include:

   a. Pseudoaneurysm.

   b. Cavernous sinus varix.

   c. Venous drainage to cortical veins.

   d. Thrombosis of venous outflow pathways distant from fistula.

   e. Epistaxis.

   f. Increased intracranial pressure.

SUGGESTED READINGS

Berenstein A, Scott J, Choi IS, Persky M: Percutaneous embolization of arteriovenous fistulas of the external carotid artery, *AJNR* 7:937-942, 1986.

Davis JM, Zimmermann RA: Injury of the carotid and vertebral arteries, *Neuroradiology* 25:55-69, 1983.

Debrun G: Treatment of carotid-cavernous fistula using detachable balloon catheters, *AJNR* 4:355-356, 1983.

Fakhry SM, Jaques PF, Proctor HJ: Cervical vessel injury after blunt trauma, *J Vasc Surg* 8:501-508, 1988.

Halbach V, Hieshima GB, Higashida RT, Reicher M: Carotid cavernous fistulae: indications for urgent treatment, *AJNR* 8:627-633, 1987.

Houser OW, Mokri B, Sundt TM Jr, et al: Spontaneous cervical cephalic arterial dissection and its residuum: angiographic spectrum, *AJNR* 5:27-34, 1984.

Kato T, Tokumaru A, O'uchi T, et al: Assessment of brain death in children by means of P-31 MR spectroscopy: preliminary note, *Radiology* 179:95-99, 1991.

Komiyama M, Fu Y, Yagura H, et al: MR imaging of dural AV fistulas at the cavernous sinus, *J Comput Assist Tomogr* 14:347-401, 1990.

Mirvis SE, Wolf AL, Numaguchi Y, et al: Posttraumatic cerebral infarction diagnosed by CT: prevalence, origin, and outcome, *AJNR* 11:355-360, 1990.

Mokri B, Piepgras DG, Houser OW: Traumatic dissections of the extracranial internal carotid artery, *J Neurosurg* 68:189-197, 1988.

Morgan MK, Besser M, Johnston I, Chaseling R: Intracranial carotid artery injury in closed head trauma, *J Neurosurg* 66:192-197, 1987.

Nakstad P, Nornes H, Hange HN: Traumatic aneurysms of the pericallosal arteries, *Neuroradiology* 28:335-338, 1986.

O'Sullivan RM, Robertson WD, Nugent RA, et al: Supraclinoid carotid artery dissection following unusual trauma, *AJNR* 11:1150-1152, 1990.

Petro GR, Witwer GA, Cacayorin ED, et al: Spontaneous dissection of the cervical internal carotid artery: correlation of arteriography, CT, and pathology, *AJNR* 7:1053-1058, 1986.

Pistoia F, Johnson DW, Darby JM, et al: The role of xenon CT measurements of cerebral blood flow in the clinical determination of brain death, *AJNR* 12:97-103, 1991.

Watridge CB, Muhlbauer MS, Lowery RD: Traumatic carotid artery dissection: diagnosis and treatment, *J Neurosurg* 71:854-857, 1989.

Yamaura A, Watanabe Y, Saeki N: Dissecting aneurysms of the intracranial vertebral artery, *J Neurosurg* 72:183-188, 1990.

CHAPTER 18

Arteritis and cerebral inflammatory disease

KEY CONCEPTS

1. A variety of infectious, chemical, and mechanical agents can produce an arteritis-type pattern in the cerebral vasculature.
2. Atherosclerotic disease is the most common cause of an arteritis-like pattern of multifocal segmental vascular stenoses.
3. Most types of arteritis cannot be distinguished from one another angiographically.

I. Pathology: Arteritis is arterial wall inflammation caused by a variety of agents ranging from infectious to mechanical, chemical, and autoimmune.

II. Classification (relatively complete but not exhaustive).
   A. Infectious (viral, bacterial, mycotic) arteritis.
      1. Purulent meningitis.
      2. Tuberculous meningitis.
      3. Syphilitic meningitis (meningovascular or gummatous).
      4. Viral meningoencephalitis.
      5. Fungal meningitis.
   B. Necrotizing arteritis.
      1. Takayasu's arteritis.
      2. Temporal (giant cell) arteritis.
      3. Wegener's granulomatosis.
      4. Granulomatous angiitis.
   C. Collagen disease.
      1. Polyarteritis nodosa.
      2. Lupus erythematosus.
      3. Hypersensitivity, granulomatous allergic arteritis.

D. Miscellaneous.
 1. Sarcoidosis.
 2. Radiation arteritis.
 3. Chemical arteritis.
 4. Drug abuse arteritis.
 5. Neoplastic angiitis.
 6. Amyloid (congophilic) angiopathy.
 7. High-flow angiopathy (associated with arteriovenous malformations [AVMs] and arteriovenous fistulas).
III. Radiology: Angiographic findings are variable and nonspecific. Multiple foci of segmental stenoses and vessel occlusions are most common. Atherosclerosis is by far most common cause of arteritis-type angiographic pattern in cerebral vasculature.
 A. Radiation-induced vasculopathy.
  1. Confined to radiation ports.
  2. Histologic findings mimic accelerated focal arteriosclerosis.
  3. Angiography: multifocal stenoses of large and medium-sized intracranial vessels with scattered occlusions; smaller vessel radionecrosis may simulate diffuse cerebral arteritis.
 B. Takayasu's arteritis.
  1. Location: typically involves aorta and its major branches. Extracranial carotid and vertebral arteries are affected; intracranial vasculature is usually spared.
  2. Angiography: stenosis most common; dilatation and fusiform aneurysm also frequent.
 C. High-flow angiopathy.
  1. Etiology: high flow in afferent vessels supplying AVMs and arteriovenous fistulas.
  2. Pathology: intimal thickening and destruction, vascular thrombosis, elastic degeneration.
  3. Angiography.
   a. Ectasia and tortuosity.
   b. Aneurysm formation.
   c. Stenosis and thromboses of arterial feeders and venous drainage.
 D. Amyloid angiopathy.
  1. A cause of nontraumatic lobar hemorrhages in normointensive elderly patients.
  2. Pathology.
   a. Congophilic infiltration of vessel walls.
   b. Intimal fibrinoid change.
   c. Luminal narrowing and occlusion.
   d. Microaneurysms.
  3. Location: medium and small vessels.

4. Computed tomography and magnetic resonance.
   a. Lobar, superficial (cortical, subcortical) hemorrhages; nonspecific white matter signal hyperintensities.
   b. Clots often of different ages, multiple vascular distributions.
   c. Contrast this with hemorrhage in deep basal ganglia, brainstem, and cerebellum seen from hyperintension.
5. Angiography: findings nonspecific but include:
   a. Mass effect from associated hemorrhage.
   b. Irregular tapering of distal cortical leptomeningeal branches.
   c. Spares larger vessels.
   d. May be relatively normal.
E. Giant cell (temporal) arteritis.
   1. Internal carotid artery (ICA) involved in 25%.
   2. Location.
      a. Petrous, cavernous, and occasionally supraclinoid segments.
      b. Usually spares or only mildly affects cervical ICA.
      c. Other common locations.
         (1) Superficial temporal artery.
         (2) Vertebral artery.
         (3) Ophthalmic and posterior ciliary arteries.
   3. Angiography: nonspecific appearance.
      a. Irregular stenosis.
      b. Occlusions.
F. Neoplastic arteriopathy (see Chapter 8).
   1. Frank occlusion rare.
   2. Narrowing and encasement by mass.
   3. Gliomas (less commonly meningioma) can directly invade arterial walls.
G. Wegener's granulomatosis.
   1. Central nervous system rarely involved (diffuse vasculitis uncommon).
   2. Invasion directly from nose and paranasal sinuses can produce narrowing of ICA.
H. Granulomatous angiitis.
   1. Location.
      a. Smaller arteries and veins.
      b. Occasionally, larger intracranial arteries.
      c. Rarely affects extracranial vessels.
   2. Angiography: segmental, diffuse irregularity and narrowing of small and medium-sized arteries.
   3. May be cause of unexplained subarachnoid or intracranial hemorrhage.

I. Infectious arteritides.
   1. Caused by exudative bacterial, fungal, or tubercular meningitis.
   2. Angiography: concentric narrowing of supraclinoid ICA and proximal circle of Willis.
J. Cerebral vasculitides induced by drugs (e.g., cocaine, methamphetamines, heroin, ephedrine): Cocaine is also associated with intracranial hemorrhage, vasospasm, and occasionally ischemic cerebral infarction. Effects are independent of route of administration, amount used, or number of times used.
K. Miscellaneous: Many noninflammatory processes (e.g., sickle cell disease, fibromuscular dysplasia, neurofibromatosis) can involve intracranial vasculature and may be indistinguishable from arteritis. *Atherosclerosis is still by far most common cause of arteritis-like angiographic pattern.*

SUGGESTED READINGS

Biller J, Loftus CM, Moore SA, et al: Isolated central nervous system angiitis first presenting as spontaneous intracranial hemorrhage, *Neurosurgery* 20:310-315, 1987.

Brant-Zawadzki M, Anderson M, DeArmond SJ: Radiation-induced large intracranial vessel occlusive vasculopathy, *Am J Radiol* 134:51-55, 1980.

Faer MJ, Mead JH, Lynch RD: Cerebral granulomatous angiitis: case report and literature review, *Am J Radiol* 129:463-467, 1977.

Loes DJ, Biller J, Yuh WTC, et al: Leukoencephalopathy in cerebral amyloid angiopathy, *AJNR* 11:485-488, 1990.

Mawad ME, Hilal SK, Hichelson WJ, et al: Occlusive disease associated with cerebral arteriovenous malformations, *Radiology* 153:401-408, 1984.

Nalls G, Disher A, Daryabagi J, et al: Subcortical cerebral hemorrhages associated with cocaine abuse: CT and MR findings, *J Comput Assist Tomogr* 13:1-5, 1989.

Pear BL: Other organs and other amyloids, *Semin Roentgenol* 26:150-164, 1986.

Pile-Spellman JMD, Baker KF, Liszczak TM, et al: High-flow angiopathy: cerebral blood vessel changes in experimental chronic arteriovenous fistula, *AJNR* 7:811-815, 1986.

Vincent FM, Vincent T: Bilateral carotid siphon involvement in giant cell arteritis, *Neurosurgery* 18:773-776, 1986.

Wagle WA, Smith TW, Weiner M: Intracerebral hemorrhage caused by cerebral amyloid angiopathy: radiographic pathologic correlation, *AJNR* 5:171-176, 1984.

Wang A-M, Suojanen JN, Colucci VM, et al: Cocaine- and methamphetamine-induced acute cerebral vasospasm, *AJNR* 11:1141-1146, 1990.

Yamashita Y, Takahashi M, Bussaka H, et al: Cerebral vasculitis secondary to Wegener's granulomatosis: computed tomography and angiographic findings, *J Comput Tomogr* 10:115-120, 1986.

Yamato M, Lecky JW, Hiramatsu K, Kohda E: Takayasu arteritis: radiographic and angiographic findings in 59 patients, *Radiology* 161:329-334, 1986.

CHAPTER 19

Angiographic signs of intracranial neoplasms and brain herniations

KEY CONCEPTS

1. Direct angiographic signs of intracranial tumor are caused by increased vasculature within the lesion ("neovascularity," stain, or blush). Early (out of sequence) draining veins may be seen but are not specific signs of neoplasm.
2. Indirect angiographic signs of an intracranial mass are vessel displacements (locally represented by stretching and displacement of adjacent arterial branches or cortical veins, as well as shifts of major vessels such as the anterior cerebral artery [ACA], middle cerebral artery [MCA], and internal cerebral vein [ICV]). Decreased vasculature ("hole in the brain") may also be seen but is nonspecific, since it can be caused by any avascular lesion such as stroke, abscess, or cyst.
3. Brain herniations can be congenital (e.g., encephalocele, Chiari malformation) or acquired (secondary to an intracranial mass). Acquired herniations are divided into the following types:
   a. Subfalcine
   b. Transtentorial (descending type much more common than ascending herniation)
   c. Tonsillar
   d. Sphenoid ridge (ascending or descending)
   e. Resulting from traumatic or surgical defects in dura and calvarium

I. Neoplasms: Primary diagnosis of cerebral neoplasm is usually with computed tomography or magnetic resonance. Angiographic analysis of cerebral neoplasms is based on displacement of otherwise normal vessels and on alterations of vasculature within tumor itself.

A. Vessel displacement: Both arteries and veins may be displaced. Major vascular displacements such as anterior cerebral artery shifts are briefly summarized in Chapter 6; sylvian triangle (MCA) displacements are outlined in Chapter 7; posterior fossa tumors and their vascular manifestations are covered in Chapter 10. Arterial and venous displacements must be considered in concert for accurate angiographic localization of cerebral neoplasms. Some common tumor sites and their typical angiographic findings are summarized in Table 19-1.

B. Tumor vascularization can be decreased or increased compared with adjacent normal brain.

1. Decreased vascularization can be seen in some benign neoplasms, low-grade tumors, or neoplasms with necrosis, hemorrhage, or cyst formation. This appears as hypovascular region on late arterial or capillary phase ("hole in the brain") and may have local mass effect manifest as stretching and draping of adjacent arteries and veins. Typical examples include cystic cerebellar hemangioblastoma, cystic astrocytoma, some pituitary adenomas, and necrotic anaplastic astrocytoma. Some neoplasms such as hemangioblastoma and glioblastoma with necrosis or hemorrhage may have coexisting hypovascular and hypervascular foci.

2. Increased vasculature.

   a. Malignant tumor vasculature is often bizarre, manifest as laking and pooling of contrast material in irregular, dilated vessels (so-called neovascularity).

   b. Benign tumor vasculature in general is more regular with enlarged but otherwise normal-appearing vessels. Vascular stain or blush appearing as more or less homogeneous increased accumulation of contrast material during capillary and early venous phase is sometimes seen (e.g., with meningiomas or glomus tumors).

   c. Arteriovenous shunting, represented by early (i.e., out of sequence) appearance of draining veins, can be seen with both benign tumors (e.g., some meningiomas or glomus tumors) and malignant neoplasms (e.g., glioblastoma, anaplastic astrocytoma, vascular metastasis). Some nontumorous causes of early draining veins include infarct, contusion, epileptogenic foci, arteriovenous malformation, cerebritis, and encephalitis.

II. Brain herniations: Brain herniations are displacements of cerebral tissue into space or compartment other than one it normally occupies. Falx cerebri and tentorium cerebelli along with bony calvarial ridges divide cranial cavity into several compartments: supratentorial (with right and left hemispheres, anterior and middle fossae), infratentorial (i.e., posterior fossa), and extracranial. Extracranial herniation either is herniation of brain, meninges, or both through congenital or acquired defects in calvarial vault or skull base ·

Table 19-1   Angiographic localization of intracranial masses and brain herniations

Location of mass	Arterial displacements	Venous displacement	Comments
INTRACRANIAL MASSES—SUPRATENTORIAL			
Sellar and suprasellar (e.g., pituitary adenoma with suprasellar extension; craniopharyngioma; giant aneurysm of internal carotid artery)	Horizontal (A1 segment of ACA) elevated; Cisternal segment of AChA displaced laterally; Thalamoperforating arteries displaced posterosuperiorly; BA may be pushed back if mass is large enough	ICV may be elevated if mass is very large; APMV back if mass extends behind tuberculum sellae and clivus	A1 may be normal if mass extends superiorly through circle of Willis
Subfrontal (e.g., planum sphenoidale meningioma; esthesioneuroblastoma)	A2 may be elevated; Orbitofrontal and frontopolar branches of ACA elevated, draped over mass; Proximal ACA shift	Septal vein may be elevated or displaced	Course of A2 highly variable and should not be used as sole criterion for diagnosing subfrontal mass; "Elevation" of A2 can be normal, i.e., more apparent than real
Anterior or deep frontal (e.g., astrocytoma; hypertensive basal ganglionic hemorrhage)	Proximal ACA shift; MCA pushed back, lateral	TSV shift across midline; "alpha sign" if mass big enough	Hypertensive hemorrhages often displace lenticulostriate arteries medially
Anterior temporal (e.g., astrocytoma, trapped temporal horn)	Proximal ACA shift; Genu of MCA elevated and displaced medially; Anterior part of sylvian triangle elevated	TSV and ICV across midline; Superficial MCV may be elevated	Middle fossa meningiomas may have middle meningeal artery elevated and displaced anteromedially

Location	Arteries	Veins	Comments
Holotemporal (e.g., astrocytoma)	Square ACA shift MCA displaced medially Sylvian triangle and sylvian point elevated	TSV and ICV across midline Superficial MCV may be elevated	
Posterior frontal and anterior parietal (e.g., metastasis, astrocytoma, oligodendroglioma)	Distal ACA shift MCA and sylvian point displaced laterally	TSV and ICV across midline Venous angle (between TSV and ICV) may be compressed Subependymal veins depressed	ACA may be midline if mass is behind level of straight sinus
Posterior parietal and occipital (e.g., high–posterior convexity meningioma; astrocytoma)	Distal ACA shift MCA and sylvian triangle depressed and displaced anteriorly	ICV across midline	
Thalamic (e.g., glioblastoma)	AChA and posterior choroidal artery bowed posteriorly and superiorly Thalamoperforating branches stretched superiorly	ICV across midline	ACA may be midline
Hydrocephalus	ACA and pericallosal branches straightened and stretched MCA lateral Thalamoperforating branches straightened and stretched laterally	TSV stretched and ballooned laterally Subependymal veins elevated, stretched, and displaced laterally around enlarged ventricles	ICV midline if both lateral ventricles are symmetrically enlarged

INTRACRANIAL MASSES—POSTERIOR FOSSA

Location	Arteries	Veins	Comments
Brainstem (e.g., brainstem glioma)	BA forward PCAs (P2 segments) displaced laterally and occasionally superiorly PICA back, sometimes down	APMV forward PCV back	BA may be displaced backward if mass is exophytic

Continued.

Table 19-1   Angiographic localization of intracranial masses and brain herniations—cont'd

Location of mass	Arterial displacements	Venous displacement	Comments
INTRACRANIAL MASSES—POSTERIOR FOSSA—cont'd			
Vermis (e.g., medulloblastoma)	BA forward Vermian branches of SCA stretched superiorly PICA forward, down	PCV forward SVVs, IVVs stretched around enlarged vermis	
Cerebellar hemisphere (e.g., astrocytoma, hemangioblastoma, metastasis)	BA forward PICA forward and down; hemispheric branches bowed around mass	APMV forward PCV across midline SVVs, IVVs across midline	
Extraaxial			
Clivus meningioma	BA back; PICA back	APMV back	
Lateral (e.g., acoustic neurinoma)	Anterior inferior cerebral artery position varies; usually elevated	Petrosal vein elevated	
BRAIN HERNIATIONS			
Nasal encephalocele	Orbitofrontal ACA branches below skull base		Agenesis of corpus callosum often associated, so ACA (A2 segment) may lack its normal anteriorly convex curve and course directly superiorly
Subfalcine herniation	Various ACA and MCA shifts according to specific location of mass	ICV across midline	

	Arterial signs	Venous signs	Comments
Transalar (sphenoid wing herniations)			
Descending	Signs of large anterior fossa mass	Superficial MCV pushed back	
Ascending	Signs of large middle fossa (temporal lobe) mass	Superficial MCV elevated and displaced anteriorly	
Transtentorial			
Descending	AChA displaced medially PCoA and proximal PCA displaced inferiorly BA may be back, down	ICV across midline	PCA may be kinked or even occluded posteriorly across lip of tentorial incisura
Ascending	Signs of large posterior fossa mass Vermian branches of SCAs stretched anterosuperiorly Thalamoperforating branches of PCoA and BA anteriorly displaced	APMV anteriorly displaced PCV anteriorly, superiorly displaced	Often accompanied by signs of tonsillar herniation
Tonsillar	Signs of large posterior fossa mass effect Tonsillar branches of PICA displaced inferiorly through foramen magnum Medullary segments of PICA displaced anteriorly and inferiorly	IVVs and tonsillar veins occasionally visualized below foramen magnum	

ACA, Anterior cerebral artery; *AChA,* anterior choroidal artery; *BA,* basilar artery; *ICV,* internal cerebral vein; *APMV,* anterior pontomesencephalic vein; *MCV,* middle cerebral artery; *TSV,* thalamostriate vein; *MCV,* middle cerebral vein; *PCA,* posterior cerebral vein; *PCA,* posterior cerebral artery; *PICA,* posterior inferior cerebral artery; *PCV,* precentral cerebellar vein; *SCA,* superior cerebellar artery; *SVVs,* superior vermian veins; *IVVs,* inferior vermian veins; *PCoA,* posterior communicating artery.

or is herniation through normal foramina (e.g., tonsillar herniation through foramen magnum).

A. Congenital herniations such as encephalocele and Chiari malformations are usually diagnosed by computed tomography or magnetic resonance. If angiography is performed in such cases, presence of displaced parenchymal vessels indicates brain tissue is present in abnormal location. For example, patients with Chiari I or II have caudal displacements of tonsillar branches of posterior inferior cerebral artery below level of foramen magnum. Neurofibromatosis, another cause of congenital brain herniation, can have sphenoid wing deficiency with anterior temporal lobe and its accompanying arteries and veins displaced into orbit. Pulsatile exophthalmos is usually present.

B. Acquired herniations occur when brain tissue and its accompanying cerebral vessels are displaced out of their normal compartment into adjacent one. This occurs when intracranial mass (e.g., tumor, hematoma, or edema) is of such size that space available for expansion is insufficient to accommodate normal compartmental contents plus added volume of abnormal tissue. Acquired herniations are classified as follows.

   1. Subfalcine herniations: Medial surface of cerebral hemisphere is pushed across midline under free inferior margin of falx cerebri. Acutely occurring cerebral masses such as massive parenchymal hemorrhage, MCA infarct with edema, or subdural hematoma initially manifest their major mass effect in horizontal (i.e., subfalcine) direction. Dislocation of temporal lobe through incisura (i.e., descending herniation) typically occurs somewhat later. Angiographic manifestations of subfalcine herniation are:

      a. ACA shift (round, square, proximal, or distal depending on location of mass effect). Regardless of size or type of ACA displacement, distal pericallosal branches must return to midline under falx (see Fig. 6-4).

      b. ICV and thalamostriate vein displacement across midline.

      c. Rarely, distal ACA infarction, caused when severe transfalcial herniation compresses terminal portion of callosomarginal artery against falx.

   2. Transtentorial herniation: two types, descending and ascending.

      a. Descending transtentorial herniations are uncal, hippocampal, or both; temporal lobe is pushed medially and inferiorly over free margin of tentorial incisura. This is seen angiographically as:

         (1) Anterior choroidal artery (AChA) displacement: AChA is initially straightened and displaced medially (seen on anteroposterior views); cisternal segment is displaced inferiorly through incisura (seen on lateral views).

    (2) Posterior communicating artery and posterior cerebral artery (PCA) are also displaced inferomedially. If descending herniation is severe, PCA may be occluded distally as it is compressed against tentorial edge.

    (3) Basal vein of Rosenthal may also be displaced inferiorly.

    (4) Basilar artery may be displaced posteriorly and kinked downward.

  b. Ascending transtentorial herniation is much less common and is produced by posterior fossa masses that push superior vermis up through incisura.

    (1) PCA and superior cerebellar artery may be displaced laterally.

    (2) Superior vermian arteries and veins are displaced superiorly.

    (3) Thalamoperforating arteries may be displaced anteriorly or their normal posteriorly convex course even reversed.

3. Sphenoid ridge herniations: less common than subfalcine or tentorial herniations and occur when:

  a. Frontal lobe is forced posteroinferiorly over sphenoid ridge (i.e., descending sphenoid or transalar herniation). Supraclinoid internal carotid artery and horizontal MCA segment are displaced back and down.

  b. Temporal lobe masses elevate sylvian fissure and force anterior temporal lobe up and over greater sphenoid wing into anterior fossa (i.e., ascending sphenoid or transalar herniation). Gross elevation and anterior displacement of MCA branches and superficial middle cerebral vein are present.

4. Tonsillar herniation: Tonsils are displaced inferiorly as reflected by presence of posterior inferior cerebral artery (PICA) tonsillar branches lying below rim of foramen magnum. Since caudal medullary loop of PICA can normally be as low as C2, this finding in itself does not indicate tonsillar herniation.

5. Miscellaneous: Markedly increased intracranial pressure combined with surgically or traumatically induced dural or calvarial defects can squeeze cerebral tissue and its accompanying vessels through defect.

SUGGESTED READINGS

Mastri AR: Brain herniations. I. Pathology. In Newton TH, Potts DG (eds): *Radiology of the skull and brain,* vol 2, St Louis, 1974, Mosby–Year Book, pp 2659-2670.

Mirvis SE, Wolf Al, Numaguchi Y, et al: Post-traumatic cerebral infarction diagnosed by CT: prevalence, origin, and outcome, *AJNR* 11:355-360, 1990.

Ono M, Rhoton AL Jr, Peace D, Rodriguez RJ: Microsurgical anatomy of the tentorial incisura, *J Neurosurg* 60:365-399, 1984.

Perrett LV, Margolis MT: Brain herniations: angiography. In Newton TH, Potts DG (eds): *Radiology of the skull and brain,* vol 2, St Louis, 1974, Mosby–Year Book, pp 2671-2699.

Ropper AH: Lateral displacement of the brain and level of consciousness in patients with an acute hemispheral mass, *N Engl J Med* 314:953-958, 1986.

Rothfus WE, Goldberg AL, Tabas JH, Deeb XL: Callosomarginal infarction secondary to transfalcial herniation, *AJNR* 8:1073-1076, 1987.

Toffol GJ, Grvener G, Naheedy MH: Early-filling cerebral vein, *J Am Osteopath Assoc* 88:1007-1009, 1988.

Wickbom I: Tumor circulation. In Newton TH, Potts DG (eds): *Radiology of the skull and brain,* vol 2, St Louis, 1974, Mosby–Year Book, pp 2257-2285.

SKULL AND CRANIAL NERVES

CHAPTER 20

Base of skull and cranial nerves: normal anatomy

With H. Ric Harnsberger

KEY CONCEPTS

1. Knowing the location and contents of each foramen or fissure, canal, or fossa at the skull base allows prediction of pathologic effects by location.
2. Deep fascial compartments of the extracranial soft tissues define anatomic spread of lesions to the skull base. Understanding the normal compartmental anatomy also allows prediction of pathologic effects by location.

For a detailed discussion of skull base anatomy, cranial nerves, and fascically defined anatomic compartments of the deep face and neck, see H. Ric Harnsberger's superbly illustrated volume *Head and Neck Imaging* in the Mosby–Year Book series "Handbooks in Radiology." Abbreviated comments and references from this volume are included here as Chapters 20 and 21.

I. Normal anatomy of skull base (from inside out).
  A. Seven bones (Fig 20-1).
    1. Ethmoid.
    2. Sphenoid.
    3. Occipital.
    4. Frontal (paired).
    5. Temporal (paired).
  B. Foramina, fissures, canals, and some of their important contents (Fig. 20-2 and Table 20-1)
    1. Ethmoid: cribriform plate: cranial nerve (CN) I (olfactory).
    2. Sphenoid.
      a. Foramen ovale: CN V_3, emissary veins (from cavernous sinus to pterygoid plexus).

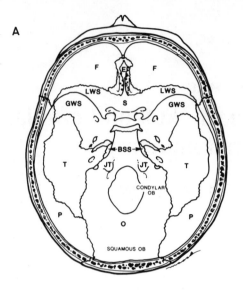

A

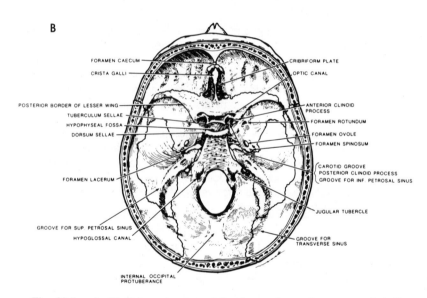

B

FORAMEN CAECUM
CRISTA GALLI
POSTERIOR BORDER OF LESSER WING
TUBERCULUM SELLAE
HYPOPHYSEAL FOSSA
DORSUM SELLAE
FORAMEN LACERUM
GROOVE FOR SUP. PETROSAL SINUS
HYPOGLOSSAL CANAL
INTERNAL OCCIPITAL PROTUBERANCE

CRIBRIFORM PLATE
OPTIC CANAL
ANTERIOR CLINOID PROCESS
FORAMEN ROTUNDUM
FORAMEN OVOLE
FORAMEN SPINOSUM
CAROTID GROOVE
POSTERIOR CLINOID PROCESS
GROOVE FOR INF. PETROSAL SINUS
JUGULAR TUBERCLE
GROOVE FOR TRANSVERSE SINUS

Fig. 20-1 **A,** Skull base drawing of five bones that make up normal skull base: paired frontal bone *(F)* and temporal bone *(T)* and unpaired ethmoid *(E)*, sphenoid *(S)*, and occipital *(O)* bones. Sphenoid bone has two distinct areas, greater wing *(GWS)* and lesser wing *(LWS)*. Occipital bone also has two areas of interest, condylar occipital bone *(OB)* and squamous occipital bone. *BSS,* Basisphenoid synchondrosis; *JT,* jugular tubercle; *P,* parietal bone. **B,** Drawing looking at skull base from endocranial viewpoint emphasizing topographic bony landmarks and apertures of skull base. Comparing **A** with this drawing allows identification of apertures by specific bone of skull base. (From Harnsberger HR: *Head and neck imaging,* Chicago, 1990, Mosby–Year Book.)

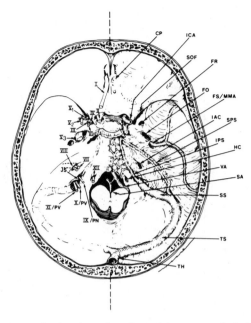

Fig. 20-2 Anatomic drawing of endocranial aspects of skull base. Right side of the figure identifies critical openings and vascular anatomy. Left side shows cranial nerves (I through XII) exiting skull base. *CP,* Cribriform plate; *ICA,* internal carotid artery; *SOF,* superior orbital fissure; *FR,* foramen rotundum; *FO,* foramen ovale; *FS/MMA,* foramen spinosum/middle meningeal artery; *IAC,* internal auditory canal; *SPS,* superior petrosal sinus; *IPS,* inferior petrosal sinus; *HC,* hypoglossal canal; *VA,* vertebral artery; *SA,* spinal artery; *SS,* sigmoid sinus; *TS,* transverse sinus; *TH,* torcular Herophili; *I,* olfactory nerve; *II,* optic nerve; *III,* oculomotor nerve; *IV,* trochlear nerve; *V_1,* ophthalmic division, trigeminal nerve; *V_2,* maxillary division, trigeminal nerve; *V_3,* mandibular division, trigeminal nerve; *VI,* abducent nerve; *VII,* facial nerve; *VIII,* vestibulocochlear nerve; *IX/PN,* vagus nerve/pars vascularis; *XI/PV,* spinal accessory nerve/pars vascularis; *XII,* hypoglossal nerve; *JS,* jugular spine. (From Harnsberger HR: *Head and neck imaging,* Chicago, 1990, Mosby–Year Book.)

    b. Foramen spinosum: middle meningeal artery.

    c. Foramen rotundum: CN V_2, emissary veins, artery of foramen rotundum.

    d. Optic canal: ophthalmic artery, optic nerve sheath complex (dura, CN II, arachnoid, cerebrospinal fluid).

    e. Superior orbital fissure: CNs III, IV, V_1, and VI, superior ophthalmic vein.

Table 20-1 Major apertures of the skull base

Aperture	Location	Fissure transmitted structure(s)	Connects
Cribriform plate	Medial floor of anterior cranial fossa	Olfactory nerve (CN I) Ethmoidal arteries (anterior and posterior)	Anterior fossa to superior nasal cavity
Optic canal	Lesser wing of sphenoid bone	Optic nerve (CN II) Ophthalmic artery Subarachnoid space, cerebrospinal fluid, and dura around optic nerve	Orbital apex to middle cranial fossa
Superior orbital fissure	Between lesser and greater sphenoid wings	CNs III, IV, V, VI Superior ophthalmic vein	Orbit to middle cranial fossa
Foramen rotundum	Middle cranial fossa floor inferior to superior orbital fissure	CN V_2 Emissary veins Artery of foramen rotundum	Meckel's cave to pterygopalatine fossa
Foramen ovale	Floor of middle cranial fossa lateral to sella	CN V_3 Emissary veins from cavernous sinus to pterygoid plexus Accessory meningeal branch of maxillary artery (when present)	Meckel's cave to nasopharyngeal masticator space (infratemporal fossa)
Foramen spinosum	Posterolateral to foramen ovale	Middle meningeal artery Recurrent (meningeal) branch of mandibular nerve	Middle cranial fossa to high masticator space (infratemporal fossa)

Foramen lacerum	Base of medial pterygoid plate at petrous apex	Meningeal branches of ascending pharyngeal artery (*not* internal carotid artery)	Not a true foramen; filled with fibrocartilage in life
Vidian canal	In sphenoid bone below and medial to foramen rotundum	Vidian artery	Foramen lacerum to pterygopalatine fossa
Carotid canal	Within petrous temporal bone	Internal carotid artery Sympathetic plexus	Carotid space to cavernous sinus
Jugular foramen	Posterolateral to carotid canal, between petrous temporal bone and occipital bone	Pars nervosa: inferior petrosal sinuses (CN IX and Jacobson's nerve) Pars vascularis: internal jugular vein, CNs X and XI, nerve of Arnold, small meningeal branches of ascending pharyngeal and occipital arteries	Posterior fossa to nasopharyngeal carotid space
Stylomastoid foramen	Behind styloid process	CN VII	Parotid space to middle ear
Hypoglossal canal	Base of occipital condyles	CN XII	Foramen magnum to nasopharyngeal carotid space
Foramen magnum	Floor of posterior fossa	Medulla and its meninges Spinal segment of CN XI Vertebral arteries and veins Anterior and posterior spinal arteries	Posterior fossa to cervical spinal canal

CN, Cranial nerve.

    f. Carotid canal: cavernous internal carotid artery.

    g. Foramen lacerum: nothing of importance.

  3. Occipital.

    a. Foramen magnum: medulla, meninges; spinal CN XI, vertebral artery and veins, anterior and posterior spinal artery.

    b. Condylar canals: emissary veins.

    c. Hypoglossal canal: CN XII.

  4. Frontal: no important apertures.

  5. Temporal.

    a. Jugular foramen: CNs IX, X, and XI; inferior petrosal sinus and internal jugular vein.

    b. Facial nerve canal: CN VII.

    c. Internal auditory canal: CN VII.

    d. Eustachian tube.

    e. Petrous carotid canal: C2 segment of internal carotid artery.

II. Normal anatomy of skull base (from outside in): In addition to following the many channels that transmit structures between cranial cavity and extraclavicular soft tissues, spread of tumors and infections often follows anatomically defined compartments demarcated by deep fascial planes. The six major spaces that abut skull base are the parapharyngeal, masticator, carotid, retropharyngeal, prevertebral, and parotid.

  A. Parapharyngeal space.

    1. Extends from submandibular space to skull base.

    2. Contains fat.

    3. Attachments encompass:

      a. Sphenoid sinus.

      b. Foramen lacerum.

  B. Masticator space.

    1. Extends from mandibular angle to skull base.

    2. Contains CN V_3, mandibular artery.

    3. Attachments encompass foramen ovale.

    4. Importance: Perineural tumor spreads along trigeminal nerve into Meckel's cave.

  C. Carotid space.

    1. Extends from aortic arch to skull base.

    2. Contains:

      a. Carotid artery.

      b. Internal jugular vein.

      c. CNs IX to XII.

      d. Cervical sympathetic chain.

      e. Lymph nodes.

    3. Attachments contain:

      a. Carotid canal.

      b. Jugular fossa.

D. Retropharyngeal space.
   1. Extends from skull base to T3.
   2. Contains fat and lymph nodes.
   3. Attachments contain clivus.
   4. Importance: provides route for infection to spread to mediastinum and skull base.
E. Prevertebral space.
   1. Extends from skull base to T3.
   2. Contains prevertebral, paraspinal, and scalene muscles; proximal brachial plexus.
   3. Attachments contain clivus.
   4. Importance: Vertebral osteomyelitis and metastases spread into this space.
F. Parotid space.
   1. Contains parotid gland, facial nerve (CN VII), retromandibular vein, external carotid and maxillary arteries, intraparotid lymph nodes.
   2. Attachments contain mastoid.
   3. Importance: Intratemporal perineural tumor spreads along CN VII.

III. Upper cranial nerves (CNs I to VI), origins to endplates (i.e., from inside out).
   A. Olfactory nerve.
      1. Anatomy: 15 to 20 nerve bundles collect fibers from olfactory mucosa in roof of nasal cavity, pierce cribriform plate, and synapse in olfactory bulb.
      2. Function: olfaction.
   B. Optic nerve (CN II) and visual pathway.
      1. Anatomy.
         a. Optic nerves: retina to chiasm.
         b. Chiasm.
         c. Optic tracts.
      2. Function: vision.
   C. Oculomotor, trochlear, and abducens nerves (CNs III, IV, and VI).
      1. Oculomotor nerve: anatomy, function.
         a. Arises from nucleus in tegmentum of midbrain.
         b. Course: ventrally through red nucleus and substantia nigra.
            (1) Exits from medial aspect of cerebral peduncle.
            (2) Courses anteriorly between posterior cerebral artery and superior cerebellar artery.
            (3) Runs under posterior communicating artery.
            (4) Enters cavernous sinus.
            (5) Most cephalad nerve in cavernous sinus (superolateral to internal carotid artery).
            (6) Exits skull through superior orbital fissure to orbit.

(7) Innervates superior, medial, and inferior rectus, levator palpebrae, and inferior oblique muscles.

(8) Parasympathetic nerves travel with CN III and control pupillary function and accommodation.

2. Trochlear nerve: anatomy, function.
   a. Arises in midbrain nucleus just caudal to CN III and ventral to aqueduct.
   b. Course.
      (1) Backward around aqueduct.
      (2) Decussates just before it emerges from dorsal midbrain to course anteriorly below free edge of tentorium.
      (3) Through dura into cavernous sinus just below oculomotor nerve.
      (4) Exits skull via superior orbital fissure into orbit.
      (5) Innervates superior oblique muscle.

3. Abducens nerve: anatomy, function.
   a. Arises from pons near midline, just anterior to fourth ventricle.
   b. Course.
      (1) Anteroinferiorly through pons.
      (2) Emerges from brainstem at pontomedullary junction.
      (3) Ascends through prepontine cistern.
      (4) Pierces dura (Dorello's canal) and runs anteriorly through cavernous sinus.
      (5) Exits skull via superior orbital fissure into orbit.
      (6) Innervates lateral rectus muscle.

D. Trigeminal nerve: has both motor and sensory components. Anatomy, function.

1. Arises from four brainstem nuclei at anterolateral aspect of fourth ventricle.
   a. Mesencephalic nucleus (proprioception from face).
   b. Main sensory nucleus (tactile sensation from face).
   c. Motor nucleus (innervation to muscles of mastication).
   d. Spinal nucleus (pain and temperature from face).

2. Course.
   a. Anteriorly through pons.
   b. Emerges from lateral pons ("root entry zone").
   c. Runs anterosuperiorly through prepontine cistern.
   d. Enters Meckel's cave (carries cerebrospinal fluid and arachnoid with it).
   e. Trigeminal (gasserian) ganglion lies in inferior part of Meckel's cave and contains cell bodies of numerous afferent sensory fibers.

    f. Trifurcates into three branches.

      (1) Ophthalmic nerve (CN V_1) exits through superior orbital fissure and in turn subdivides into lacrimal, frontal, and nasociliary nerves (innervates scalp, forehead, nose, and globe).

      (2) Maxillary nerve (CN V_2) exits through foramen rotundum, passes into pterygopalatine fossa, and runs forward into orbit through inferior orbital fissure (innervates midface and upper teeth).

      (3) Mandibular nerve (CN V_3) does not traverse cavernous sinus; runs along skull base and exits via foramen ovale to enter masticator space; subdivides into sensory branches (lower face, tongue, floor of mouth, and jaw) and motor branches (masticator nerve innervates masseter, temporalis, medial, and lateral pterygoid muscles; mylohyoid nerve supplies mylohyoid muscle and anterior belly of digastric muscle).

IV. Lower CNs (VII to XII) from origins to endplates (i.e., from inside out).

    A. Facial nerve (CN VII): anatomy, functions.

      1. Arises from:

        a. Motor nucleus in ventrolateral pontine tegmentum.

        b. Superior salivary nucleus in pons (origin of parasympathetic fibers to lacrimal, sublingual, and submandibular glands).

        c. Nucleus solitarius (taste sensation from anterior two thirds of tongue via geniculate ganglion).

      2. Course.

        a. Motor fibers loop back around CN VI nucleus (forming facial colliculus in floor of fourth ventricle) and then are joined anterolaterally by fibers from other facial nerve nuclei.

        b. Runs anterolaterally, exiting brainstem at cerebellopontine angle.

        c. Crosses cerebellopontine angle cistern to enter internal auditory canal (IAC).

        d. Runs laterally in anterosuperior quadrant of IAC.

        e. Exits IAC, runs forward in hairpin loop (through geniculate ganglion) under lateral semicircular canal, descends through facial nerve canal to exit skull via stylomastoid foramen.

        f. Parotid gland is divided into deep and superficial lobes by exocranial facial nerve.

      3. Branches.

        a. Greater superficial petrosal nerve exits at geniculate ganglion and innervates lacrimal gland.

        b. Stapedius nerve innervates stapedius muscle and prevents hyperacusis.

  c. Chorda tympani exits just before facial nerve leaves stylomastoid foramen and carries taste fibers from anterior two thirds of tongue.

  d. To muscles of facial expression, posterior belly of digastric muscle.

B. Vestibulocochlear nerve (CN VIII).
1. Anatomy.
 a. Arises from:
  (1) Dorsal and ventral cochlear nuclei in lateral aspect of inferior cerebellar peduncle (restiform body).
  (2) Nuclei receive axons from neurons with cell bodies in spiral ganglion (found in modiolus of cochlea).
 b. Course.
  (1) Runs in anteroinferior quadrant of IAC.
  (2) Courses across cerebellopontine angle cistern.
  (3) Enters brainstem at pontomedullary junction.
2. Function.
 a. Cochlear portion: hearing.
  (1) Sensory component is cochlea.
  (2) Neural component is retrocochlear acoustic pathway.
 b. Vestibular portion: balance, equilibrium.

C. Glossopharyngeal nerve (CN IX).
1. Anatomy.
 a. Arises from:
  (1) Nucleus ambiguus (motor).
  (2) Salivary nucleus (parasympathetic fibers).
  (3) Solitary nucleus (sensory).
 b. Course.
  (1) Exits lateral medulla at postolivary sulcus.
  (2) Courses across basal cistern to jugular foramen.
  (3) Exits skull through pars nervosa.
  (4) Runs in carotid space.
2. Function.
 a. Tympanic branch (Jacobson's nerve): sensory to middle ear, parasympathetic to parotid gland.
 b. Stylopharyngeus branch innervates muscle of same name.
 c. Sinus nerve supplies carotid sinus and carotid body (baroreceptors, chemoreceptors).
 d. Pharyngeal branches (afferent limb of gag reflex) are sensory to posterior oropharynx and soft palate.
 e. Lingual branch: sensation, taste (posterior one third of tongue).

D. Vagus nerve (CN X).
1. Anatomy.

      a. Arises from:
        (1) Nucleus ambiguus (motor).
        (2) Solitary nucleus (sensory).
        (3) Dorsal motor nucleus (parasympathetic).
      b. Course.
        (1) Exits lateral medulla at retroolivary sulcus.
        (2) Courses across basal cistern to jugular foramen.
        (3) Exits skull through pars vascularis.
        (4) Runs inferiorly along posterolateral aspect of carotid artery to level of:
          (a) Clavicle on right (right subclavian artery).
          (b) Aortopulmonary window on left.
    2. Function.
      a. Pharyngeal plexus: motor innervation to much of soft palate, superior and middle pharyngeal constrictors (efferent limb of gag reflex).
      b. Superior laryngeal nerve.
        (1) Internal laryngeal nerve: sensory above true vocal cords.
        (2) External laryngeal nerve: motor innervation to inferopharyngeal constrictor and cricothyroideus muscles.
      c. Recurrent laryngeal nerve: motor innervation to endolaryngeal muscles (vocal cords).
  E. Spinal accessory nerve (CN XI).
    1. Anatomy.
      a. Arises from:
        (1) Medulla (motor fibers in nucleus ambiguus).
        (2) Spinal cord (anterior horn cells of C1-5 segments).
      b. Course: Spinal segment ascends, enters skull through foramen magnum, and exits via pars vascularis of jugular fossa; it runs for short distance in carotid space, then inferiorly along sternomastoid muscle to posterior triangle of neck.
    2. Function.
      a. Spinal root innervates trapezius and sternomastoid muscles.
      b. Medullary component runs with vagus nerve and supplies endolarynx via recurrent laryngeal nerve.
  F. Hypoglossal nerve (CN XII).
    1. Anatomy.
      a. Arises from hypoglossal nucleus and paramedian floor of fourth ventricle.
      b. Course.
        (1) Runs anteriorly through medulla just lateral to medial lemniscus.

        (2) Emerges from medulla in preolivary sulcus.

        (3) Passes across medullary cistern to exit skull via hypoglossal canal.

        (4) Courses inferiorly in carotid space to level of hyoid bone, then ascends and runs forward in sublingual space of oral cavity.

  2. Function.

    a. Motor innervation to intrinsic tongue musculature.

    b. Motor innervation to extrinsic tongue musculature.

      (1) Genioglossus.

      (2) Geniohyoid.

      (3) Hyoglossus.

      (4) Styloglossus.

    c. Carries C1 root to geniohyoid and thyrohyoid muscles.

    d. C1 also combines with C2 and C3 roots to form ansa hypoglossi (innervates infrahyoid strap muscles).

SUGGESTED READINGS

Bradley WG Jr: MR of the brain stem: a practical approach, *Radiology* 179:319-332, 1991.

Harnsberger HR (guest ed): Extracranial head and neck imaging, *Semin US CT MR,* June 1986 (entire monograph).

Harnsberger HR (guest ed): Cranial nerve imaging, *Semin US CT MR,* September 1987 (entire monograph).

Harnsberger HR: *Head and neck imaging,* Chicago, 1990, Mosby–Year Book.

Laine FJ, Nadel L, Braun IF: CT and MR imaging of the central skull base. I. Techniques, embryologic development, and anatomy, *Radiographics* 10:591-602, 1990.

Lanzieri CF: MR imaging of the cranial nerves, *AJR* 154:1263-1267, 1990.

Lufkin R, Flannigan BD, Bentson JR, et al: Magnetic resonance imaging of the brain stem and cranial nerves, *Surg Radiol Anat* 8:49-66, 1986.

Mancuso AA, Harnsberger HR, Dillon WP: *Workbook for MRI and CT of the head and neck,* ed 2, Baltimore, 1989, Williams & Wilkins.

Solsberg MD, Fournier D, Potts DG: MR imaging of the excised human brainstem: a correlative neuroanatomic study, *AJNR* 11:1003-1013, 1990.

CHAPTER 21

Base of skull: pathologic anatomy

With H. Ric Harnsberger

KEY CONCEPTS

Skull base lesions can be conveniently divided into:
1. Intracranial lesions (involve the skull base from the top down). Examples are cephalocele, arachnoid cyst, and sellar and suprasellar neoplasms.
2. Lesions intrinsic to the skull base itself. Examples are osteomyelitis, fibrous dysplasia, Paget's disease, chordoma, and metastases.
3. Extracranial lesions (involve the skull base from the bottom up). Examples are infection, sinonasal tumors, and mucocele.

I. Intracranial lesions.
   A. Congenital.
      1. Cephalocele: extracranial protrusions of brain, meninges, or both through skull defect resulting from failure of mesodermal ingrowth between neural tube and overlying ectoderm.
         a. Types.
            (1) Meningocele (contains only meninges and cerebrospinal fluid [CSF]).
            (2) Encephalocele (contains both brain and meninges).
         b. Locations.
            (1) Occipital in 70%.
            (2) Frontal (nasofrontal, nasoethmoidal, nasoorbital) in 15%.
         c. Clinical findings.
            (1) Polypoid nasopharyngeal or nasion mass.
            (2) Recurrent meningitis.
            (3) CSF rhinorrhea.

      d. Radiology.

         (1) Computed tomography (CT) delineates osseous defect.

         (2) Magnetic resonance (MR) delineates soft tissue components.

    2. Arachnoid cyst.

      a. Pathology: layers of arachnoid containing CSF.

      b. Locations (most common).

         (1) Middle fossa.

         (2) Suprasellar cistern.

      c. Radiology.

         (1) CT: adjacent bone expanded and thinned; CSF density.

         (2) MR: signal intensity similar to that of CSF on all pulse sequences.

    3. Dermoid cyst.

      a. Arises from ectodermal inclusion.

      b. Location: 80% orbital, oral, or nasal; midline to paramedian.

      c. Radiologic findings vary depending on location and cyst content.

B. Vascular.

    1. Aneurysm (see Chapter 13).

      a. Locations: cavernous sinus, circle of Willis.

      b. Radiology.

         (1) CT: hyperdense, often calcified; strong enhancement in patent part of lumen; may erode bone focally.

         (2) MR: variable depending on flow and hematoma stage.

    2. Vascular malformations (see Chapter 14).

      a. Focal enlargement of vascular channels and foramina.

      b. Types affecting skull base.

         (1) Parenchymal arteriovenous malformation (AVM; rare).

         (2) Dural AVM (more common), e.g., chronic carotid-cavernous fistula.

      c. Radiology.

         (1) MR: delineates status of blood flow and adjacent brain; best for demonstrating relationship to adjacent soft tissue.

         (2) CT: bony erosion.

C. Neoplasms.

    1. Primary.

      a. Pituitary adenoma, Rathke's pouch cyst.

      b. Craniopharyngioma.

      c. Hypothalamic-opticochiasmatic glioma.

      d. Meningioma.

      e. Neural sheath tumors.

    2. Metastatic: Metastases to pituitary gland usually do not cause bone erosion because patient does not live long enough.

II. Intrinsic skull base abnormalities: Most are inflammatory, traumatic, or neoplastic in origin.

A. Infection (most are from outside in and bottom up, see III in this chapter.
   1. Osteomyelitis from:
      a. Sinus or dental infection.
      b. Deep facial space abscess.
      c. Malignant otitis externa.
   2. Mucocele or pyocele.
   3. Hypertrophic rhinosinusitis or aggressive polyposis.
B. Trauma.
   1. Fracture.
   2. Dural tear.
      a. CSF leak.
      b. Infection.
   3. Traumatic encephalocele.
C. Neoplasms.
   1. Paraganglioma (glomus jugulare).
      a. Arises from adventitia of jugular bulb along tympanic branch of cranial nerve (CN) IX (Jacobsen's nerve).
      b. Clinical findings.
         (1) CN IX, X, or XI neuropathies.
         (2) Pulsatile tinnitus.
         (3) Vascular retrotympanic mass seen if paraganglioma is jugulotympanicum type.
      c. Radiology.
         (1) CT: erosion of jugular foramen or spine; enhancing mass; calcification rare.
         (2) MR: speckled-appearing mixed signal mass.
   2. Neural sheath tumors.
      a. Schwannoma: solitary encapsulated mass *not* associated with neurofibromatosis.
      b. Neurofibroma: multiple (often plexiform) or solitary unencapsulated mass usually associated with neurofibromatosis.
      c. Location.
         (1) Any cranial nerve can be affected.
         (2) Most common in jugular foramen (CN IX, X, or XI), Meckel's cave (CN V).
      d. Radiology.
         (1) CT: smooth, scalloped expanded neural foramen, enhancing mass; calcification rare.
         (2) MR: variable but isointense on T1-weighted image (T1WI); hyperintense on T2WI most common; strong enhancement following administration of contrast material.
   3. Meningioma.
      a. Arises from leptomeninges at any site, including paranasal sinus.

    b. Locations at skull base.

        (1) Cribriform plate.

        (2) Tuberculum, diaphragm, dorsum sellae.

        (3) Sphenoid (both basisphenoid and alar).

        (4) Clivus.

        (5) Cerebellopontine angle.

        (6) Tentorium, cavernous sinus.

    c. Radiology: See Chapter 47.

        (1) Dura-based mass.

        (2) Often calcified.

        (3) Usually enhances strongly.

        (4) Hyperostosis, pneumosinus dilitans.

4. Chordoma.

    a. Arises from notochordal remnants.

    b. Location.

        (1) Between 35% and 40% are in skull base (50% sacro-coccygeal, 15% spinal).

        (2) Usually midline from sphenooccipital synchondrosis but can also be eccentric.

    c. Radiology.

        (1) CT (best for osseous detail).

            (a) Permeative, destructive mass in more than 95%.

            (b) Calcification in 50%.

            (c) Variable enhancement following administration of contrast material.

            (d) May have large nasopharyngeal and prevertebral component.

        (2) MR (soft tissue detail delineated).

            (a) Isointense or hypointense on T1WI.

            (b) Extremely hyperintense on T2WI.

5. Osteocartilaginous tumors (e.g., chondroma, osteoma, sarcoma): uncommon; partially calcified masses arising near sphenooccipital synchondrosis.

6. Primary cholesteatoma and cholesterol granuloma: erosive, expansile lesion of petrous apex and middle ear.

7. Metastases.

    a. Most common tumors affecting skull base.

    b. Source: lung, breast, prostate, or nasopharyngeal tumors (see III in this chapter).

    c. Spread.

        (1) Direct extension.

        (2) Hematogenous.

    d. Radiology.

        (1) CT: destructive, permeative, infiltrating mass.

       (2) MR: variable but typically isointense on most sequences; loss of cortical bone evidenced by low signal.

   8. Lymphoma, leukemia, myeloma, rhabdomyosarcoma (see III in this chapter).

  D. Miscellaneous, metabolic, dysplastic lesions.

    1. Fibrous dysplasia.

      a. Expands medullary cavity with fibrous tissue in various degrees of ossification.

      b. Albright's syndrome: unilateral but polyostotic fibrous dysplasia, precocious puberty.

      c. Radiology.

        (1) CT: thick, sclerotic bone ("ground glass" appearance); may have cystic components.

        (2) MR: expanded, thickened, low-signal bone.

    2. Paget's disease.

      a. Unknown etiology.

      b. Monostotic or polyostotic.

      c. Three phases.

        (1) Destructive early phase.

        (2) Combined destruction and healing in intermediate phase.

        (3) Late sclerosis.

      d. Radiology.

        (1) CT and MR show bone expansion with variable destruction and sclerosis depending on stage.

        (2) Basilar invagination may occur.

    3. Histiocytosis X.

      a. Granulomatous reticuloendotheliosis.

      b. Age: children, young adults.

      c. Radiology.

        (1) CT and MR show osteolytic lesions in skull base or calvarium.

        (2) NOTE: Histiocytosis X is one cause of thickened, enhancing infundibular or suprasellar mass in a child. Langerhans' cell histiocytes can produce similar findings in adults.

    4. Anemias and blood dyscrasias: rare.

III. Extracranial lesions involving skull base from below: Inflammation, neoplasia, and miscellaneous nonneoplastic processes such as mucocele and polyposis are most common types of abnormalities affecting skull base from bottom up.

  A. Infections.

    1. Osteomyelitis from:

      a. Sinus infection (invades directly or via naturally occurring channels to cavernous sinus).

      b. Malignant external otitis media (destructive soft tissue mass in temporal bone that can mimic neoplasm).

      c. Nasopharyngeal abscess, e.g., dental via masticator space.

  2. Fungal sinusitis (mucormycosis, aspergillosis).

      a. Multisinus, nodular, mucoperiosteal thickening with bone destruction.

      b. *Mucor* common in immunocompromised host.

      c. Aspergillosis in healthy: may present very low signal mass on MR, calcification on CT.

      d. Wegener's granulomatosis and idiopathic midline granuloma.

B. Neoplasms.

  1. Nasopharyngeal angiofibroma.

      a. Benign vascular tumor.

      b. Occurs almost exclusively in adolescent males.

      c. Originates in sphenopalatine foramen.

      d. Spreads along naturally occurring foramina and fissures.

         (1) Laterally into pterygopalatine fossa.

         (2) Superiorly into orbital apex.

         (3) Posterosuperiorly into sphenoid and cavernous sinuses.

  2. Esthesioneuroblastoma.

      a. Arises from sensory receptor cells (CN I) of olfactory mucosa.

      b. Radiology: high lateral nasal fossa mass, often extends intracranially through cribriform plate; variable signal, density, and enhancement.

  3. Nasopharyngeal tumors.

      a. Ninety-eight percent are carcinomas (80% squamous cell, 18% adenocarcinoma; latter are often from minor salivary glands).

      b. Invade skull base directly or extend perineurally (especially along trigeminal and facial nerves).

      c. Radiology: CT and MR may show:

         (1) Mass.

         (2) Bone destruction.

         (3) Obliteration of fat and mucosal planes.

         (4) Denervation atrophy of facial muscles.

         (5) Serous otitis media (from obstruction of eustachian tube orifice).

  4. Inverting papilloma.

      a. Four percent of sinonasal tumors.

      b. Lateral nasal wall origin, near junction of ethmoid and maxillary sinuses.

      c. Radiology: minimally enhancing, variably destructive mass often with associated obstructive sinusitis; can mimic malignant tumor.

  5. Miscellaneous neoplasms (e.g., lymphoma, rhabdomyosarcoma).

C. Miscellaneous nontumorous processes.
  1. Inflammatory polyposis.
    a. Radiology: CT and MR show expanded sinuses packed with well-marginated, polypoid, soft tissue masses.
    b. Usually multiple sinuses involved.
    c. Bone destruction with intracranial extension can occur.
  2. Mucocele.
    a. Accumulation of impacted mucus behind obstructed draining ostium.
    b. Most common in frontal and ethmoid sinuses.
    c. Radiology: well-delineated soft tissue mass and bone expansion; rim enhancement if infected (mucopyocele); may be hyperintense on both T1WI and T2WI.

SUGGESTED READINGS

Barkovich AJ, Vandermarck P, Edwards MSB, Cogen PH: Congenital nasal masses, *AJNR* 12:105-116, 1991.

Harnsberger HR: *Head and neck imaging,* Chicago, 1990, Mosby–Year Book.

Harnsberger HR, Osborn AG, Smoker WRK: CT in the evaluation of the normal and diseased paranasal sinuses, *Semin US CT MR* 7:68-90, 1986.

Laine FJ, Nadel L, Braun IF: CT and MR imaging of the central skull base. II. Pathologic spectrum, *Radiographics* 10:797-821, 1990.

Lanzieri CF, Shah M, Krauss D, Lavertu P: Use of gadolinium-enhanced MR imaging for differentiating mucoceles from neoplasms in the paranasal sinuses, *Radiology* 178:425-428, 1991.

Osborn AG, Harnsberger HR, Smoker WRK: Base of the skull imaging. *Semin US CT MR* 7:91-106, 1986.

Sham JST, Cheung YK, Choy D, et al: Nasopharyngeal carcinoma: CT evaluation of patterns of tumor spread, *AJNR* 12:265-270, 1991.

CHAPTER 22

"Holes in the skull": normal and abnormal

KEY CONCEPTS

1. Many normal structures can mimic abnormalities:
   a. Squamous temporal bone can be strikingly radiolucent.
   b. Vascular lakes and venous channels can appear bizarre.
   c. Emissary veins are common near the skull base and dural sinuses.
2. Differential diagnosis varies depending on the number and sites of lucent areas.

"Holes in the skull" can be single or multiple. Because differential diagnosis varies depending on number and site of lucent area(s), each group is considered separately.

I. Solitary radiolucent area.
   A. Normal.
      1. Fissures, foramina, canals, and channels (see Chapter 20).
      2. Unfused sutures.
      3. Vascular markings and emissary channels.
      4. Areas where calvarium is normally thinned.
         a. Temporal squamae.
         b. Arachnoid granulations (near dural sinus).
   B. Variants.
      1. Parietal thinning.
         a. Outer calvarial table thinned, inner intact.
         b. Often in older patients.
         c. Differential diagnosis: osteoporosis circumscripta.

2. Parietal "foramina."
   a. Typically bilateral and symmetric.
   b. Usually a few millimeters in diameter but may reach several centimeters.
   c. Differential diagnosis: burr holes, eosinophilic granuloma.
3. Sinus pericranii.
   a. Anomalous diploic or emissary venous channel between intracranial and extracranial venous circulations.
   b. Location: frontal bone most common, temporal bone least.
   c. Clinical findings: soft tissue mass under scalp that changes in size with position, Valsalva maneuver, coughing, or sneezing.
C. Congenital and developmental causes of solitary skull defects.
   1. Cephaloceles (see Chapter 21).
      a. Pathology: herniation of meninges, cerebrospinal fluid (CSF), or brain through skull defect.
      b. Location: occipital; less commonly frontal.
      c. Appearance: smooth well-marginated skull defect, usually midline, with associated soft tissue mass.
   2. Dermoid cyst (see Chapter 21).
   3. Cleidocranial dysostosis: large fontanelles, wormian bones.
   4. Neurofibromatosis: Patient may have:
      a. Absent greater sphenoid wing.
      b. Lambdoid sutural defect.
   5. Intradiploic arachnoid cyst: tiny dural defect, expanded diploic space, thinned but intact outer table.
D. Trauma and surgery.
   1. Sutural diastasis.
   2. Linear skull fracture.
   3. Leptomeningeal cyst ("growing fracture"): posttraumatic arachnoid cyst caused by herniation and subsequent enlargement of meninges and CSF into preexisting fracture. Slope of erosion is directed inward; diploic space not expanded; outer table eroded; cyst protrudes beneath scalp.
   4. Burr holes, bone flaps, craniotomy, shunt placements, and other postoperative defects.
      a. Thickening (2 to 6 mm) and contrast enhancement of underlying dura can persist for years on magnetic resonance (MR) scans.
      b. Nodular enhancement may indicate postoperative infection, recurrent or persistent neoplasm.
E. Infections: osteomyelitis.
   1. Etiology: pyogenic most common but can be fungal, syphilitic, or tubercular; often secondary to sinusitis, mastoiditis, or penetrating injury (occasionally postsurgical).

    2. Appearance: coalescent permeative destructive lesion. Sequestrum uncommon except with tuberculosis (see box below). Reactive sclerosis may occur, especially with fungal infections (e.g., actinomycosis).

F. Neoplasms, tumorlike lesions.
   1. Epidermoid tumor.
     a. Location: diploic space, both inner and outer tables involved.
     b. Appearance: well-defined, sclerotic rim, no central trabeculae.
   2. Hemangioma.
     a. Location: diploic space.
     b. Appearance: well circumscribed, lytic with "spoke-wheel" or reticulated pattern.
   3. Myeloma (solitary lesion rare).
   4. Osteogenic sarcoma.
     a. Location: diploë, both tables.
     b. Pathology: primary osteogenic sarcoma rare; more often occurs in Paget's disease or after irradiation.
     c. Appearance: destructive, poorly marginated.
   5. Lymphoma (rare primary site; diffusely infiltrating, destructive; usually no reactive sclerosis).
   6. Metastasis (solitary uncommon).
   7. Primary intracranial tumor.
     a. Can erode inner table if slow growing, superficial (e.g., oligodendroglioma, ganglioglioma, cystic astrocytoma).
     b. Rare; arachnoid cyst is more common cause of inner table erosion from intracranial mass.

G. Miscellaneous.
   1. Paget's disease.
     a. Pathology: osteoclastic resorption of trabeculae with fibrovascular connective tissue deposition.
     b. Osteoblastic, mixed patterns most common, but well-circumscribed, sharply marginated lytic defects also seen ("osteoporosis

---

DIFFERENTIAL DIAGNOSIS OF "BUTTON" SEQUESTRUM (LYTIC SKULL LESION, CENTRAL BONE REMNANT)

    Healing burr hole
    Osteomyelitis (especially tubercular)
    Radiation necrosis
    Metastasis (especially from breast)
    Eosinophilic granuloma

circumscripta"). MR shows both soft tissue and bony components (hyperintense relative to normal diploic space on T1-weighted image.)

    c. Sarcomatous degeneration in 0.9%.

  2. Fibrous dysplasia (see Chapter 23).

    a. Pathology: normal medullary space replaced by fibroosseous tissue.

    b. Craniofacial bones involved in 20%.

    c. Solitary or multiple lytic areas (monostotic six times more common than polyostotic form).

    d. With or without sclerotic regions on MR; computed tomographic appearance varies with amount of marrow replacement and mineralization.

  3. Histiocytosis.

    a. Eosinophilic granuloma.

      (1) Single or multiple.

      (2) Well circumscribed, nonsclerotic.

      (3) Appearance of "beveled" edge caused by asymmetric involvement of inner and outer tables.

    b. Hand-Schuller-Christian disease: "geographic" as well as multiple lytic lesions common.

II. Multiple radiolucent areas.

  A. Normal.

    1. Fissures, foramina, canals, and channels (see Chapter 20).

    2. Pacchionian (arachnoidal) granulations (near midline or dural venous sinus).

    3. Venous lakes and diploic channels.

  B. Metabolic.

    1. Hyperparathyroidism: stippled or "salt and pepper" pattern caused by multiple small lytic defects.

    2. Osteoporosis: age related; lytic areas represent loss of protein matrix in diploë and inner table.

  C. Neoplasm.

    1. Metastatic disease.

      a. Hematogenous from breast, lung, prostate, kidney, other primary neoplasms with osteolytic metastases.

      b. Appearance: multiple lytic defects, no reactive sclerosis.

    2. Myeloma.

SUGGESTED READINGS

Elster AD, DiPersio DA: Cranial postoperative site: assessment with contrast-enhanced MR imaging, *Radiology* 174:93-98, 1990.

Kelly JK, Denier JE, Wilner HI, et al: MR imaging of lytic changes in Paget disease of the calvarium, *J Comput Assist Tomogr* 13:27-29, 1989.

Kransdorf MJ, Moser RP Jr, Gilkey FW: Fibrous dysplasia, *Radiographics* 10:519-537, 1990.

Lanzieri CF, Som PM, Sacher M, et al: The postcraniotomy site: CT appearance, *Radiology* 159:165-170, 1986.

Sadler LR, Tarr RW, Jungreis CA, Sekhar L: Sinus pericranii: CT and MR findings, *J Comput Assist Tomogr* 14:124-127, 1990.

Weinand ME, Rangachary SS, McGregor DH, Watanabe I: Intradiploic arachnoid cysts, *J Neurosurg* 70:954-958, 1989.

CHAPTER 23

Thick skull and thin skull

KEY CONCEPTS

1. Common causes of diffuse calvarial thickening are:
   a. Normal variant
   b. Microcephaly (of any cause)
   c. Shunted hydrocephalus
   d. Long-term phenytoin (Dilantin) use
   e. Fibrous dysplasia
2. A rare cause of thick skull is blood dyscrasia.
3. Craniolacunia (lückenschädel, lacunar skull):
   a. Is a bony dysplasia of the membranous skull
   b. Is associated with Chiari type II malformation
   c. Usually disappears by 6 months of age
   d. Is *not* caused by hydrocephalus or increased intracranial pressure

---

Causes of diffuse and focal calvarial thickening and thinning are summarized in the upper box on p. 152.

I. Generalized calvarial thickening (see lower box on p. 152).
  A. Developmental.
    1. Benign hyperostosis.
      a. Location: frontal bones.
      b. Age and sex: middle-aged women.
      c. Patterns.
        (1) Nodular or diffuse.
        (2) Occasionally involves entire skull.
        (3) Usually bilateral and symmetric but can be localized and unilateral.

151

COMMON CALVARIAL ABNORMALITIES BY LOCATION

OUTER TABLE

Regional thinning
Osteoma
Cephalhematoma
Cushing's disease

INNER TABLE

Calcified subdural hematoma
Pacchionian granulations
Lacunar skull
Intracranial cyst
Slow-growing tumor
Meningioma
Hyperostosis frontalis interna

DIPLOIC SPACE

Hematologic disorders
Osteoporosis circumscripta
Long-term phenytoin administration
Mucopolysaccharidoses
Tuberous sclerosis
Cushing's disease

ALL

Acromegaly
Fibrous dysplasia
Shunted hydrocephalus
Paget's disease
Meningioma
Microcephaly

Courtesy R. Kumar.

COMMON CAUSES OF THICK SKULL

GENERALIZED

Acromegaly
Fibrous dysplasia
Shunted hydrocephalus
Hematologic disorders
Phenytoin
Microcephaly
Normal

REGIONAL

Paget's disease
Fibrous dysplasia
Hyperostosis frontalis interna

FOCAL

Osteoma
Meningioma
Fibrous dysplasia
Calcified cephalhematoma

Courtesy R. Kumar.

        (4) Spares superior sagittal sinus and adjacent venous channels.
    d. Clinical significance: none.
    e. Differential diagnosis: meningioma (crosses midline, sutures, and venous channels).
  B. Endocrine and metabolic: treated hyperparathyroidism.
    1. Associated with renal osteodystrophy.
    2. Appearance: thick, "wooly" calvarium (NOTE: Most patients with

untreated hyperparathyroidism have multiple lytic lesions that produce a mottled or "salt and pepper" pattern).
C. Hematologic disorders.
  1. Sickle cell disease.
    a. Location.
      (1) Any marrow-bearing part of calvarium.
      (2) Parietal bones most commonly affected.
      (3) Spares occipital squamae.
    b. Appearance.
      (1) Mottled diploic thickening.
      (2) "Hair on end" in advanced cases.
  2. Iron deficiency anemia and hereditary spherocytosis.
    a. Modestly thickened calvarium.
    b. "Hair on end" appearance is rare.
    c. Parietal bones most commonly affected.
D. Neoplastic disease.
  1. Osteoblastic metastases.
    a. Prostate gland and breast most common origins.
    b. Appearance: thick skull, usually not truly diffuse.
  2. Neuroblastoma.
E. Miscellaneous.
  1. Fibrous dysplasia.
    a. Location: monostotic or diffuse; craniofacial bone involvement in about 20%.
    b. Pathology: normal bone undergoes lysis and replacement by myxofibromatous tissue of low vascularity.
    c. Computed tomography (CT).
      (1) Poorly marginated medullary lesion with mixed density, inhomogeneous sclerosis (varies from "ground-glass" appearance to dense sclerosis).
      (2) Thick calvarium, expanded diploë (usually spares inner table).
      (3) Calvarial deformities with sphenoid and frontal sinus obliteration and globe displacement because of orbital deformity.
    d. Magnetic resonance (MR): diffuse low-signal changes (but not as low as with cortical bone) on T1-weighted image (T1WI), variable on T2WI.
    e. Differential diagnosis.
      (1) Paget's disease.
      (2) Metastases (often associated soft tissue mass).
      (3) Meningioma.
    f. Malignant degeneration reported rarely (0.5%).

    2. Paget's disease.
      a. Lytic and sclerotic phases.
        (1) Osteoporosis circumscripta predominates in calvarium.
        (2) Blastic phase has relatively well-delineated margins.
      b. Location: both inner and outer tables and diploë affected; soft tissue mass may be associated.
    3. Chronic (treated) hydrocephalus (postshunt).
    4. Long-term phenytoin use.
    5. Osteopetrosis.
    6. Syphilis.
    7. Trauma.
      a. Chronic calcified subdural hematomas can mimic diffuse or focal thickening.
      b. Cephalhematoma (calcification and ossification of hematoma under elevated periosteum).
    8. Osteoma (focal, does not invade diploic space).
    9. Microcephalic brain (miscellaneous causes).
   10. Dyke-Davidoff syndrome.
      a. One hemicalvarium thickened.
      b. Petrous ridge elevated.
      c. Underlying hemispheric atrophy on CT and MR.
      d. Probably caused by intrauterine vascular occlusion.
II. Diffuse calvarial thinning (see box below).
    A. Normal (especially focal areas, e.g., parietal thinning, temporal and occipital squamae).

COMMON CAUSES OF THIN SKULL

GENERALIZED	REGIONAL
Cushing's disease	Frontotemporal thinning
Hydrocephalus	Parietal thinning
Lacunar skull	Osteoporosis circumscripta
Hyperparathyroidism	Dandy-Walker syndrome
Osteogenesis imperfecta	Posterior fossa arachnoid cyst
Rickets	
Prominent (normal) convolutional markings	**FOCAL**
	Intracranial cysts (porencephalic, leptomeningeal, subarachnoid)
	Slow-growing tumor

Courtesy R. Kumar.

B. Developmental.
   1. Craniolacunia (lacunar skull, lükenschädel).
      a. Intrinsic bony dysplasia of membranous skull.
      b. Associated with Chiari type II malformation.
      c. Disappears after 6 months of age.
      d. Accompaniment, not result, of Chiari malformation.
      e. *Not* caused by hydrocephalus or increased intracranial pressure.
      f. Appearance: multiple foci of thinned, scalloped bone.
   2. Osteogenesis imperfecta.
   3. Cleidocranial dysostosis.
   4. Progeria.
C. Metabolic.
   1. Rickets.
   2. Hypophosphatemia.
D. Miscellaneous: increased (prominent) convolutional markings.
   1. Most common cause: normal variant.
   2. Can occur with chronic increased intracranial pressure.

SUGGESTED READINGS

Kransdorf MJ, Moser RP Jr, Gilkey FW: Fibrous dysplasia, *Radiographics* 10:519-537, 1990.
Kumar R: The thick and thin skull, *Radiographics*. In press.

CHAPTER 24

Intracranial calcifications: normal and abnormal

KEY CONCEPTS

1. Physiologic calcification is rare below 9 years of age. The incidence rises sharply thereafter.
2. Basal ganglia calcification is most often idiopathic, not caused by metabolic derangement.
3. Parenchymal calcification in any location other than the basal ganglia should be considered abnormal until proved otherwise.
4. Intraventricular calcification:
   a. Is normal in the glomus of the choroid plexus (can be striking)
   b. If isolated in the temporal horn, suggests neurofibromatosis
   c. Can be neoplastic (e.g., meningioma, ependymoma, choroid plexus papilloma, intraventricular oligodendroglioma)
5. Neoplasia is the most common cause of pathologic intracranial calcification in children.
6. Cerebral infarcts rarely calcify.

I. Normal: "Physiologic" calcification (i.e., calcification normally occurring in the absence of disease) is seen in variety of intracranial locations. Incidence of nonpathologic calcification increases with age; however, some calcific densities that would be considered normal in adults may be abnormal in children. For example, physiologic calcification in pineal gland and choroid plexuses is rare below 9 years of age (2%) but increases fivefold by 15 years and is common in adults.
   A. Dura and arachnoid.
      1. Falx: calcification common, usually of no significance.
      2. Tentorium.
         a. Less common than falcine calcification.

      b. When calcification present, usually at falcotentorial junction.

      c. With cellular blue nevus (Gorlin's) syndrome (rare).

   3. Petroclinoid and interclinoid ligaments: calcification normal.

   4. Arachnoid granulations.

      a. Location: parasagittal, near dural venous sinus.

      b. Number: single or multiple.

      c. Appearance: rounded calcific plaques.

   5. Dural plaques.

      a. Location: anywhere.

      b. Number: single or multiple.

      c. Appearance: dense, flat, plaquelike calcifications.

B. Pineal gland and habenula.

   1. Pineal gland.

      a. Most common normally calcified intracranial structure.

      b. Calcification uncommon under 9 years of age (only 2% have physiologically calcified pineal gland).

      c. Suspect pineal region tumor if calcification present in children less than 9 years of age.

      d. Up to 10 mm of calcification normal.

   2. Habenula.

      a. Really tela choroidea of third ventricle that calcifies.

      b. Calcification lies just above pineal recess, a few millimeters in front of pineal gland.

      c. Calcification normal in patients over 10 years of age.

      d. C-shaped, curvilinear calcification.

C. Choroid plexus.

   1. Glomus.

      a. In atria of lateral ventricles.

      b. Part of choroid plexus that most commonly calcifies.

      c. Glomus calcification can occur as early as 3 years of age but is uncommon under 9 years.

      d. Size and patterns of calcification vary widely but are usually globular and bilateral.

   2. Plexus.

      a. Calcifies less commonly than glomus.

      b. Calcification rare in third or fourth ventricle.

      c. Isolated nontumoral temporal horn choroid calcification or calcification along entire plexus suggests possibility of neurofibromatosis type 2.

D. Parenchyma: In general, parenchymal calcification in any location other than basal ganglia should be considered abnormal until proved otherwise.

   1. Basal ganglia.

      a. Usually in globus pallidus.

      b. Seen in 0.6% of computed tomographic scans.

      c. Usually bilateral and symmetric but can be unilateral.

      d. Usually idiopathic; most are unrelated to metabolic disorders such as hypoparathyroidism.

      e. Differential diagnosis.

         (1) Idiopathic.

         (2) Tuberous sclerosis.

         (3) Fahr's disease.

         (4) Toxoplasmosis.

         (5) Radiation therapy (mineralizing microangiopathy).

         (6) Disorders of calcium metabolism.

  2. Dentate nuclei.

      a. Often associated with basal ganglia calcification.

      b. Microscopic ferrous, calcific deposits often found in older persons.

      c. Differential diagnosis.

         (1) Idiopathic.

         (2) Familial (Fahr's disease).

         (3) Disorders of calcium metabolism.

  3. Blood vessels.

      a. Incidence of calcification increases with age.

      b. Most common locations: internal carotid artery, vertebrobasilar system.

II. Abnormal.

  A. Congenital and developmental.

    1. Tuberous sclerosis.

      a. Rare in children under 2 years of age.

      b. Location: 90% paraventricular, 10% parenchymal.

    2. Sturge-Weber syndrome.

      a. Calcifications appear around 2 years of age.

      b. Location.

         (1) Third or fourth cortical layer.

         (2) Found initially in posterior parietal or occipital lobe; progress anteriorly.

         (3) Occasionally bilateral or even contralateral to facial nevus flammeus.

      c. Pathology: dystrophic calcification in brain underlying meningeal angioma.

      d. Associated ipsilateral brain atrophy common.

    3. Fahr's disease (idiopathic familial cerebral ferrocalcinosis).

    4. Basal cell nevus (Gorlin's) syndrome.

      a. Spectrum.

        (1) Facial, truncal nevi.

        (2) Frontal bossing.

        (3) Odontogenic mandibular cysts.

        (4) Falx and tentorial calcification.

        (5) Increased incidence of medulloblastoma.

    b. Linear nevus sebaceus syndrome also has abnormal intracranial calcifications.

  5. Neurofibromatosis.

    a. Numerous abnormal nontumorous calcifications reported.

        (1) Choroid plexus, especially temporal horns, is sometimes calcified to unusual degree in patients with neurofibromatosis type 2.

        (2) Subependymal and basal ganglia areas less commonly affected.

        (3) Calcification in cerebellar hemispheres, surface of cerebral hemispheres (unclear whether related to hamartomas, meningoangiomatosis, glial proliferations, etc.).

    b. Neoplastic calcifications (meningiomas in neurofibromatosis type 2, tumors of glial cell origin in type 1).

B. Inflammatory.

  1. Neonatal infections: TORCH (toxoplasmosis, rubella, cytomegalovirus, herpes) syndromes caused by transplacental passage of various agents, mostly viruses during gestation.

    a. Toxoplasmosis.

        (1) One of most common causes of brain calcification in children under 1 year of age.

        (2) Calcifications typically located in:

           (a) Basal ganglia.

           (b) Cortex.

           (c) Periventricular region (less common than cytomegalovirus).

        (3) Hydranencephaly or microcephaly common.

    b. Cytomegalovirus: also common cause of intracranial calcification in neonates.

        (1) Predilection for periventricular area.

        (2) Microcephaly, ventriculomegaly, migrational disturbances (polymicrogyria) common.

        (3) Can be indistinguishable radiographically from toxoplasmosis.

    c. Herpes simplex: punctate or gyriform calcium deposits.

    d. Rubella.

        (1) Calcification in basal ganglia, brainstem, cortex, sometimes around ventricles.

(2) Microcephaly.
2. Bacterial infections.
   a. Calcification with pyogenic meningitis or abscess rare.
   b. Tuberculosis can result in several different types of intracranial calcifications (rim, globular, nodular, punctate), either single or multiple in varying locations.
      (1) Suprasellar.
      (2) Cisternal.
      (3) Basal ganglia.
      (4) Parenchymal.
      (5) Intraventricular.
3. Parasitic infections.
   a. Cysticercosis (70% have parenchymal calcifications; intraventricular or cisternal calcification less common).
   b. Echinococcosis.
   c. Coccidioidomycosis.
   d. Paragonimiasis.
C. Endocrine or metabolic.
   1. Hyperparathyroidism.
      a. Dural calcification common.
      b. Parenchymal calcification rare.
   2. Hypoparathyroidism: basal ganglia and dentate nucleus calcification. (NOTE: Most calcifications in these locations unrelated to endocrine or metabolic disorders.)
D. Vascular.
   1. Aneurysm.
      a. Calcification uncommon (5%).
      b. Location: base of brain near circle of Willis and middle fossa.
      c. Appearance: curvilinear; globular less common.
      d. Occasionally multiple (most often in females).
   2. Vascular malformations.
      a. Approximately 25% of arteriovenous malformations calcify.
      b. Cavernous angiomas frequently calcify (approximately 50%).
      c. Venous vascular malformations and developmental venous anomalies rarely calcify.
   3. Infarcts.
      a. Rarely calcify.
      b. Most calcification associated with hemorrhage, although a few ischemic strokes with subsequent calcifications have been reported.
E. Trauma.
   1. Chronic subdural hematomas sometimes calcify.
   2. Other hematomas rarely calcify.

F. Radiation therapy: calcification most common when combined with chemotherapy (e.g., methotrexate).
   1. Pathology: mineralizing microangiopathy.
   2. Locations.
     a. Basal ganglia.
     b. Gray and white matter junction.
     c. Dentate nuclei of cerebellum.
   3. Associated abnormalities: leukoencephalopathy.
G. Neoplasms: Virtually any neoplasm can calcify, although it is common in some types and rare in others. Neoplasm is most common cause of pathologic intracranial calcification in children (except possibly in areas where parasitic infestations are endemic).
   1. Astrocytoma.
     a. Between 7% and 10% of astrocytomas calcify, but since astrocytomas are most common primary central nervous system neoplasm, tumoral calcification is still more likely to be caused by astrocytoma than by oligodendroglioma.
     b. Most calcification is in low-grade astrocytomas, not anaplastic astrocytoma or glioblastoma multiforme.
   2. Oligodendroglioma.
     a. Fifty percent calcify.
     b. Oligodendrogliomas are much less frequent than astrocytomas.
     c. Mixed pathology common.
   3. Medulloblastoma: Less than 5% calcify.
   4. Ependymoma.
     a. Two thirds of infratentorial ependymomas calcify.
     b. One third of supratentorial ependymomas calcify.
   5. Craniopharyngioma.
     a. Most common neoplastic calcification in children (70% to 80% calcify).
     b. Incidence of calcification decreases with age.
     c. Location.
       (1) Both suprasellar and intrasellar in 70%.
       (2) Intrasellar in 10%.
       (3) Suprasellar only in 20%.
   6. Choroid plexus papilloma: microscopic calcification common, gross calcification relatively uncommon.
   7. Meningioma.
     a. Between 10% and 20% calcify.
     b. Hyperostosis in up to 50%.
   8. Dermoid tumor: commonly calcifies.
   9. Epidermoid tumor: usually does not calcify.
  10. Teratoma: commonly calcifies.

11. Pituitary adenoma: calcification uncommon (1% to 3%).
12. Pineal germinoma: calcification common.
13. Chordoma, chondroma, and chondrosarcoma: calcification near skull base common.
14. Lipoma.
    a. Most do not calcify.
    b. Corpus callosum lipoma may have crescentic calcification.
    c. Central nervous system lipomas are probably malformation, not true neoplasm.
15. Metastases.
    a. Calcification rare in untreated metastases (1% to 5%).
    b. Primary tumors.
       (1) Lung and breast cancer.
       (2) Chondrosarcoma and osteosarcoma.
       (3) Acinar cell tumors of pancreas.
       (4) Gastrointestinal tract cancer.
    c. Treated brain metastases can be rare cause of multiple intracranial parenchymal calcifications.

NOTE: Although calcification is seen on CT scans as high-density foci, calcified lesions of brain may have variable MR appearance. Usual finding is null effect or reduction in signal intensity; signal loss is more profound on gradient echo sequences. Uncommon finding is *hyperintense* signal on T1WI (some calcium particles with larger surface area show increased T1 relaxivity).

SUGGESTED READINGS

Burt TB, Yang PJ, Gibby W: Calcified brain metastases from ovarian cancer, *AJNR* 9:613, 1988.

Callizo JRA, Gimenez-Mas JA, Martin J, Lacas J: Calcified brain metastases from acinar-cell carcinoma of pancreas, *Neuroradiology* 31:200, 1989.

Christensen R, Pollei SR, Nerncek AA Jr: Intracerebral calcification in a child, *Invest Radiol* 22:695-697, 1987.

Grant EG, Williams AL, Schellinger D, Slovis TL: Intracranial calcifications in the infant and neonate: evaluation by sonography and CT, *Radiology* 157:63-68, 1985.

Harwood-Nash DC, Fitz CR: *Neuroradiology in infants and children*, St Louis, 1976, Mosby–Year Book, pp 142-169.

Henkelman RM, Watts JF, Kucharczyk W: High signal intensity in MR images of calcified brain tissue, *Radiology* 179:199-206, 1991.

Kapila A: Calcification in cerebral infarctions, *Radiology* 153:685-687, 1984.

Kendall B, Vavanagh N: Intracranial calcification in paediatric computed tomography, *Neuroradiology* 28:324-330, 1986.

Mayfrank L, Mohadjer M, Wullich B: Intracranial calcified deposits in neurofibromatosis type 2, *Neuroradiology* 32:33-37, 1990.

Oxonoff MB, Burrows EH: Intracranial calcification. In Newton TH and Potts DG (eds): *Radiology of the skull and brain*, vol 1, St Louis, 1976, Mosby–Year Book, pp 823-873.

CHAPTER 25

Pediatric skull and scalp: special considerations

With Richard S. Boyer

KEY CONCEPTS

1. Marrow in the clivus and calvarium of children undergoes an orderly, predictable transition from red (hematopoietic) to yellow (fatty) with age.
2. Low-signal marrow on a T1-weighted magnetic resonance image (T1WI) in older children should raise suspicion of disease (e.g., sickle cell anemia, metastases).
3. Red marrow normally enhances on a T1WI after contrast material is administered.
4. The most common nontraumatic cause of a "lump on the head" in children is a dermoid tumor.

I. Normal anatomy.
  A. Sutures.
    1. Major.
      a. Sagittal.
      b. Metopic.
      c. Lambdoid.
      d. Squamosal.
    2. Minor.
      a. Frontoethmoid.
      b. Zygomatic.
      c. Parasphenoid.
      d. Parietomastoid.
      e. Occipitomastoid.
      f. Mendosal (separates interparietal from supraoccipital portion of occipital bone).

163

   B. Fontanelles and age at closure.
     1. Anterior: 4 months to 2 years.
     2. Posterior: before 6 months.
     3. Anterolateral (pterion): 3 months.
     4. Posterolateral: before 2 years.
   C. Important synchondroses and age at closure.
     1. Frontosphenoid: 2 years.
     2. Intersphenoid: 1 year.
     3. Occipitosphenoid: 14 years or older.
     4. Exoccipital: 3 years.
   D. Cranial bone marrow and development.
     1. Tissue composition normally varies with age and anatomic location.
     2. Bone marrow in clivus and calvarium typically gives low signal on T1WI in infants less than 1 year of age.
     3. By age 15, most children have adult-type marrow (signal similar to that of subcutaneous fat).
     4. In children, active hematopoietic marrow is gradually replaced by yellow (fatty) marrow.
       a. Low-signal marrow in skull or clivus after 7 years of age is abnormal and should suggest bone marrow disease (e.g., sickle cell disease, neuroblastoma, lymphoma).
       b. Because red marrow is present in various degrees and at various locations in children, some enhancement on magnetic resonance images may occur normally up to 9 or 10 years of age.
II. Pathology.
   A. Congenital.
     1. Craniostenosis.
       a. Causes of deformities resulting from premature closure of coronal, sagittal, metopic, or lambdoid suture have been analyzed.
         (1) Cranial vault bones that fuse prematurely secondary to single suture closure act as unit (i.e., single bone plate with decreased growth potential).
         (2) Asymmetric bone deposition occurs mainly at perimeter sutures with increased bone deposition directed away from bone plate.
         (3) Sutures adjacent to prematurely fused suture compensate in growth more than noncontiguous sutures.
         (4) Enhanced symmetric bone deposition occurs along both sides of nonperimeter suture that is continuation of prematurely closed suture.
       b. Approximate incidence of craniostenosis for each suture.
         (1) Sagittal 55%.

        (2) Single coronal 10%.

        (3) Both coronals 10%.

        (4) Metopic 7%.

        (5) Lambdoid 1%.

    c. Types and causes of skull deformities.

        (1) Dolichocephaly (long head): Sagittal suture closes.

        (2) Scaphocephaly (long, narrow head): Sagittal suture closes.

        (3) Brachycephaly (short head): Coronal suture closes. (Unilateral coronal synostosis causes harlequin eye.)

        (4) Plagiocephaly (asymmetric or twisted head): Any unilateral suture closes.

        (5) Trigonocephaly (biparietal pear-shaped skull, sharply pointed skull anteriorly): Metopic suture closes.

  2. Encephaloceles (see Chapter 21).

B. Trauma: special considerations in children.

  1. Newborn skull is very elastic ("ping-pong ball" fractures).

  2. Cranial signs of nonaccidental trauma.

    a. Multiple skull fractures.

    b. Bilateral skull fractures.

    c. Fractures that cross suture lines.

    d. Subdural hematomas of differing ages.

C. Nontraumatic "lumps on the head" in children.

  1. Dermoid tumor in 61%.

    a. Most occur near or along suture lines.

    b. Most common sites are orbit and periorbital region.

    c. Associated dermal sinus tract extending intracranially through calvarial defect in 37%.

  2. Cephalohematoma deformans in 9%.

    a. Most in parietal region, do not cross suture lines.

    b. Often history of birth trauma.

    c. Differential diagnosis: fibrous dysplasia, sarcoma, meningioma, epidermoid tumor, others.

  3. Eosinophilic granuloma in 7%.

    a. Most in parietal bone but can affect any bone of calvarium.

    b. Rarely penetrate dura (usually displace it inward).

    c. Computed tomography: sharply delineated bone erosion, scalp mass (often displaces dura inward).

  4. Occult meningoceles and encephaloceles in 4%.

  5. Hamartoma in 3%.

  6. Hemangioma in 3%.

    a. Often frontonasal.

    b. May or may not involve overlying skin.

7. Fibrous dysplasia in 3%.
8. Miscellaneous (e.g., lymphangioma, plexiform neurofibroma, epidural or subgaleal abscess) in 10%.
9. Intracranial extension of extracranial mass (common with dermoid tumors) in 17% to 20%.

SUGGESTED READINGS

Dalashaw JB, Persing JA, Broaddres WK, Jane JA: Cranial vault growth in craniosynostosis, *J Neurosurg* 70:159-165, 1989.

Harwood-Nash DC, Fitz CR: *Neuroradiology in infants and children,* St. Louis, 1976, Mosby–Year Book, pp 1-169.

Meservy CJ, Towbin R, McLaurin RL, et al: Radiographic characteristics of skull fractures resulting from child abuse, *AJNR* 8:455-457, 1987.

Okada Y, Aoki S, Barkovich AJ, et al: Cranial bone marrow in children: assessment of normal development with MR imaging, *Radiology* 171:161-164, 1989.

Ruge JR, Tomita T, Naidich TP: Scalp and calvarial masses of infants and children, *Neurosurgery* 22:1037-1042, 1988.

NORMAL AND ABNORMAL DEVELOPMENT OF THE BRAIN

CHAPTER 26

Normal development of the neonatal and infant brain

KEY CONCEPTS

1. Disturbances of brain development at certain embryologic stages produce predictable defects. Examples:
   a. Three to 4 weeks gestation—anencephaly, Chiari malformation, myeloschisis
   b. Four to 8 weeks—holoprosencephalies
   c. Two to 4 months—neurocutaneous syndromes
   d. Three to 6 months—migrational disorders such as heterotopias
   e. Six months postnatal—dysmyelinating, encephaloclastic disorders
2. In general, myelination proceeds:
   a. From caudad to cephalad
   b. From central to peripheral
   c. From dorsal to ventral

The construction of the nervous system is a continuous, immensely complicated process with repeated cycles of development, modeling, and remodeling from the intrauterine period to the end of life. A complete description of neurogenesis and central nervous system modification is beyond the scope of this text. What follows are the essentials of brain embryology and myelination, particularly as they relate to morphogenetic abnormalities.

I. Brain embryology: developmental stages.
   A. Stage I: dorsal induction.
      1. Time span: 3 to 4 weeks gestation.
      2. Neural plate appears as focal ectodermal thickening overlying rod-like notochord.

      a. Neural plate invaginates, forming neural fold and then neural tube.

      b. Notochord is flanked laterally by mesodermal cells that will form future somites.

      c. Interaction with mesoderm forms dura, pia, vertebrae, and skull anlage.

      d. Regional determination.

         (1) Ectoderm overlying prechordal mesenchyme produces forebrain.

         (2) Ectoderm above chorda-mesoderm forms midbrain, hindbrain, and cervical spinal cord.

         (3) Lower cord regions arise later from tail bud.

   3. Defects.

      a. Failure to close cranially leads to anencephaly (most severe form) and cephaloceles.

      b. Chiari malformation.

      c. Myeloschisis.

 B. Stage II: ventral induction.

   1. Timing: 5 to 10 weeks.

   2. At 28 days, neural tube is enlarged rostrally.

      a. Tube constricts in two places to form three fluid-filled vesicles.

         (1) Forebrain (prosencephalon).

         (2) Midbrain (mesencephalon).

         (3) Hindbrain (rhombencephalon).

      b. Two downward bends form.

         (1) Cephalic flexure (in midbrain).

         (2) Cervical flexure (hindbrain-cord junction).

      c. First and third vesicles undergo further constrictions.

from prosencephalon

         (1) "Endbrain" (telencephalon) gives rise to cerebral hemisphere, putamen, and caudate nucleus.

         (2) "Between-brain" (diencephalon) gives rise to thalami, hypothalamus, and globus pallidus.

         (3) "Midbrain" (mesencephalon) gives rise to tectum and midbrain.

         (4) "Afterbrain" (metencephalon) gives rise to cerebellar hemispheres and vermis.

         (5) "Cord-brain" (myelencephalon) gives rise to medulla and pons.

      d. Upward bend (pontine flexure) appears between metencephalon and myelencephalon.

   3. Disturbances.

      a. Holoprosencephalies.

      b. Septooptic dysplasia.

      c. Dandy-Walker malformation.

C. Stage III: neuronal proliferation, differentiation, and histogenesis.
   1. Time: 2 to 5 months gestational age.
   2. Germinal matrix forms at 7 weeks, and migration begins at 8 weeks. (NOTE: Before 28 weeks, germinal matrix has not involuted and appears on computed tomographic scan as very high density area along lateral ventricles.)
   3. Disturbances.
      a. Macrencephaly, micrencephaly, and megalencephaly.
      b. Vascular malformations.
      c. Neurocutaneous syndromes (e.g., neurofibromatosis, Sturge-Weber syndrome).
D. Stage IV: migration.
   1. Time: 2 to 5 months gestational age.
   2. Disturbances.
      a. Schizencephaly.
      b. Agyria, pachygyria, and polymicrogyria.
      c. Neuronal heterotopias.
      d. Agenesis of corpus callosum.
E. Stage V: organization (neural organization and alignment).
   1. Time: 6 months gestational age to postnatal.
F. Stage VI: maturation and myelination.
   1. Time: 6 months gestational age to postnatal and adult.
   2. Process: myelination (see below) and further development of corpus callosum. By 9 months gestational age attains adult configurations.
   3. Disturbances.
      a. Dysmyelinating disorders.
      b. Metabolic disorders.
      c. Toxic, inflammatory, and other encephaloclastic disorders.
II. Normal brain myelination (see box, p. 172): Myelination is dynamic process that begins during fetal development and continues after birth in predictable, orderly pattern. As myelination progresses, changes in white matter maturation can be assessed with magnetic resonance imaging. Departure or delays from normal patterns can thus be detected. General features of brain myelination include progression from central to peripheral, dorsal to ventral, and caudad to cephalad. Features of normal myelination at birth and thereafter follow.
A. Birth (term infant).
   1. T1-weighted image (T1WI) (pulse repetition time [TR] = 600 msec, echo delay [TE] = 20 msec): high signal (myelination) in:
      a. Medulla.
      b. Dorsal midbrain.
      c. Inferior and superior cerebellar peduncles.
      d. Posterior limb of internal capsule.
      e. Ventrolateral thalamus.

MYELINATED AREAS AT VARIOUS AGES

1. Birth
   a. Medulla
   b. Dorsal midbrain
   c. Inferior and superior cerebellar peduncles
   d. Posterior limb of internal capsule
   e. Ventrolateral thalamus
2. One month
   a. Cerebellar white matter
   b. Corticospinal tracts
   c. Precentral and postcentral gyri
   d. Optic nerves and tracts
3. Three months
   a. Middle cerebellar peduncles
   b. Ventral brainstem
   c. Cerebellar folia
   d. Optic radiations
   e. Anterior limb of internal capsule
4. Six to 8 months
   a. Corpus callosum
   b. Most of centrum semiovale except frontal temporal
5. Twelve to 14 months: frontal temporal white matter
6. Eighteen months: like adult
7. Fifteen to 30 years: peritrigonal white matter (association tracts)

---

    2. T2-weighted image (T2WI) (TR = 3000 msec, TE = 100 to 120 msec): White matter, because it is largely unmyelinated at this age, produces higher signal than gray matter on T2WI. Low signal in myelinated areas:
      a. Dorsal midbrain.
      b. Cerebellar peduncles.
      c. Posterior limb of internal capsule.
      d. Ventrolateral thalamus.
      e. Perirolandic gyri.
B. One month.
    1. T1WI: high signal in:
      a. Deep cerebellar white matter.
      b. Corticospinal tracts.
      c. Precentral and postcentral gyri.
      d. Optic nerves and tracts.
    2. T2WI: little change.

C. Three months.
  1. T1WI: high signal in:
    a. Middle cerebellar peduncle.
    b. Ventral brainstem.
    c. Cerebellar folia.
    d. Optic radiations.
    e. Anterior limb of internal capsule.
    f. Subcortical white matter of occipital pole.
  2. T2WI: low signal in:
    a. Middle cerebellar peduncle.
    b. Anterior limb of internal capsule.
    c. Cerebellar white matter.
    d. Optic radiations.
D. Four months.
  1. T1WI: high signal in:
    a. Splenium of corpus callosum.
    b. Somewhat more rostral subcortical white matter.
  2. T2WI: not much change.
E. Six months.
  1. T1WI: high signal in:
    a. Genu of corpus callosum.
    b. More subcortical white matter in paracentral regions.
  2. T2WI: further signal decrease in centrum semiovale.
F. Eight months: nearly mature; begins to resemble adult pattern.
  1. T1WI: high signal in all but most anterior frontal white matter.
  2. T2WI.
    a. Splenium and genu of corpus callosum give uniformly low signal.
    b. Diminishing signal intensity in anterior limb of internal capsule.
G. Twelve to 14 months.
  1. T1WI: high signal in:
    a. Frontal white matter.
    b. Temporal white matter.
  2. T2WI: low signal in:
    a. Frontal white matter.
    b. Temporal white matter.
H. Eighteen months: adult pattern. (NOTE: Some areas, such as white matter dorsal and superior to ventricular trigones, have persistent high signal on T2WI and should not be considered abnormal. These association fiber tracts often do not become myelinated until second or even third decade of life. Normal area of relatively fewer white matter fibers is adjacent to frontal horns of lateral ventricles. This "cap" of high signal intensity on T2WI is also normal.) In mature brains (greater than 3 years

of age), prominent but normal areas of decreased signal intensity on T2WI occur in heavily myelinated compact fiber pathways such as anterior commissure, internal capsule, corpus callosum, and uncinate fasciculus.

III. Brain development: In addition to the preceding, new imaging modalities such as MR imaging of anisotropically restricted diffusion may prove useful in delineating both normal and abnormal myelinization as well as other disease states such as ischemic lesions.

IV. Brain metabolism: In addition to neuronal organization, cellular proliferation and differentiation, and myelination, developing brain undergoes maturational processes associated with changes in biochemical composition and metabolism. Magnetic resonance spectroscopy shows rapid, major changes in P-31 and H-1 spectra during first 3 years of life.

ACKNOWLEDGMENT

Helpful in preparing this chapter were notes from lectures I have heard Derek Harwood-Nash, Thomas P. Naidich, and A. James Barkovich give at numerous courses in which we were guest faculty.

SUGGESTED READINGS

Angevine JR Jr: Morphogenesis of the central nervous system, *BNI Q* 5:17-27, 1989.

Barkovich AJ: Normal development of the neonatal and infant brain. In *Pediatric neuroimaging*, New York, 1990, Raven Press, pp 5-34.

Bird CR, Hedberg M, Drayer BP, et al: MR assessment of myelination in infants and children, *AJNR* 10:731-740, 1989.

Curnes JT, Burger PL, Djang WT, Boyko OB: MR imaging of compact white matter pathways, *AJNR* 9:1061-1068, 1988.

Flodmark O: Radiological anatomy of the developing brain of the infant, *Riv Neuroradiol* 3(suppl 2):5-8, 1990.

Rutherford MA, Cowan FM, Manzur AY, et al: MR imaging of anisotropically restricted diffusion in the brains of neonates and infants, *J Comput Assist Tomogr* 15:188-198, 1991.

Van der Knaap MS, Valk J: Classification of congenital anomalies of the CNS, *AJNR* 9:315-326, 1988.

Van der Knaap MS, Valk J: MR imaging of the various stages of normal myelination during the first years of life, *Neuroradiology* 31:459-470, 1990.

Van der Knapp MS, van der Grond J, van Rijen PC, et al: Age-dependent changes in localized proton and phosphorus MR spectroscopy of the brain, *Radiology* 176:509-515, 1990.

CHAPTER 27

Congenital malformations: general classification

KEY CONCEPTS

1. Congenital malformations of the brain have been classified in many different ways, including categorization by the developmental stage affected (see Chapter 26). A simpler system divides congenital malformations into two major categories: disorders of organogenesis and disorders of histogenesis. (A third category, disorders of cytogenesis, is sometimes added.)

2. Disorders of organogenesis are subdivided into abnormalities of neural tube closure, disorders of diverticulation or brain cleavage, disorders of sulcation and cellular migration, disorders of size, and destructive lesions.

3. Disorders of histogenesis are represented by the neurocutaneous syndromes (e.g., tuberous sclerosis, neurofibromatosis, Sturge-Weber syndrome).

A broad spectrum of congenital central nervous system (CNS) malformations can be recognized on neuroimaging procedures such as computed tomography, magnetic resonance, and ultrasonography. These malformations are most simply divided into disorders of organogenesis and disorders of histogendisorders of diverticulation, disorders of sulcation and migration, disorders of size (microcephaly and macrocephaly), and destructive lesions such as hydrasize (microcephaly and macrocephaly), and destructive lesions such as hydranencephaly, porencephaly, and intrauterine infections.

CNS anomalies are found in approximately 1% of live births. Cerebral malformations are present in 75% of fetal deaths, and one third of major anomalies involve the CNS. An estimated 10% of intracranial anomalies are due to chromosomal anomalies, 20% to inherited factors, and 10% to adverse intrauterine environment (e.g., infection); 60% have no identifiable cause.

More than 2000 congenital cerebral malformations have been described; only the most commonly encountered are listed here.

    I. Disorders of organogenesis (altered brain development, normal histogenesis).

        A. Disorders of neural tube closure (myelomeningocele is the most common).

            1. Chiari II malformation.

            2. Cephaloceles.

            3. Agenesis of corpus callosum.

            4. Dandy-Walker complex.

            5. Cranioschisis (e.g., meningocele, encephalocele).

        B. Disorders of diverticulation or brain cleavage.

            1. Holoprosencephaly (alobar, semilobar, lobar).

            2. Septooptic dysplasia.

        C. Disorders of sulcation and cellular migration.

            1. Agyria (lissencephaly).

            2. Schizencephaly.

             3. Heterotopias.

             4. Pachygyria, polymicrogyria.

        D. Disorders of size.

            1. Microcephaly.

            2. Macrocephaly.

        E. Destructive lesions.

            1. Hydranencephaly.

            2. Porencephaly.

            3. Inflammatory diseases (rubella, cytomegalovirus infection, toxoplasmosis, herpes simplex).

            4. Hypoxia, toxicosis.

   II. Disorders of histogenesis (overall brain structure normal, but anomalous cells persist and continue to differentiate).

        A. Neurocutaneous syndromes.

            1. Neurofibromatosis.

            2. Sturge-Weber syndrome.

            3. Tuberous sclerosis.

            4. Von Hippel–Lindau disease.

        B. Vascular lesions.

        C. Congenital neoplasms.

  III. Disorders of cytogenesis.

        A. Inborn errors of metabolism.

            1. Aminoacidurias.

    2. Mucopolysaccharidoses.

    3. Lipidoses.

B. Leukodystrophies.

C. Neuronal degeneration.

D. Axonal dystrophies.

SUGGESTED READINGS

Babcock DS: Sonography of congenital malformations of the brain, *Neuroradiology* 28:428-439, 1986.

Boyer RS: MR in brain formation and malformation, *Semin US CT MR* 9:183-185, 1988.

Harwood-Nash DC, Fitz CR: *Neuroradiology in infants and children,* St Louis, 1976, Mosby–Year Book, pp 1000-1014.

Poe LB, Coleman LL, Mahwad F: Congenital central nervous system anomalies, *Radiographics* 9:801-826, 1989.

Van der Knaap MS, Valk J: Classification of congenital abnormalities of the CNS, *AJNR* 9:315-326, 1988.

CHAPTER 28

Congenital malformations: disorders of organogenesis

KEY CONCEPTS

1. Chiari I malformation (tonsillar ectopia) is not typically associated with other brain anomalies (syringohydromyelia is seen in 20% to 25%).
2. Chiari II malformations are almost always associated with some form of spinal dysraphism and meningocele or myelomeningocele.
3. A broad and varied spectrum of abnormalities in Chiari II malformations is found in the skull, dura, midbrain, cerebellum, ventricles, cisterns, brain parenchyma, spine, and cord.
4. In North American patients the most common location for cephaloceles is the occipital area.
5. Mega–cisterna magna, so-called Dandy-Walker variant, and Dandy-Walker syndrome probably represent points in the spectrum of posterior fossa cystic malformation and are not really separate entities.

I. Disorders of neural tube closure: Disorders of neural tube closure and dorsal induction are earliest CNS anomalies, occurring within third and fourth gestational weeks.
   A. Chiari malformations (I to IV) are group of unrelated anomalies initially described by Chiari. Originally three types of hindbrain malformations with hydrocephalus were delineated; later, severe cerebellar hypoplasia was added as fourth category. Chiari I and II are relatively common; Chiari III (Chiari II plus encephalocele) is very rare; Chiari IV may not exist as separate, distinct entity.
      1. Chiari I: tonsillar ectopia (deformed cerebellar tonsils displaced downward below foramen magnum into upper cervical canal). Not usually associated with other brain anomalies.

    a. Tonsillar ectopia of 3 to 4 mm is of uncertain clinical significance; greater than 5 mm often symptomatic.

    b. Associated syringohydromyelia in 20% to 25%.

    c. Mild to moderate hydrocephalus in 20% to 25%.

    d. Craniovertebral junction anomalies common.

       (1) Basilar impression in 25%.

       (2) C1 to occiput assimilation in 10%.

       (3) Klippel-Feil disease in 10%.

       (4) Incomplete ossification of C1 ring in 5%.

    e. *Not* associated with myelomeningocele.

2. Chiari II: complex malformation affecting spine, skull, dura, and hindbrain. In contrast to Chiari I, Chiari II is almost always associated with some form of spinal dysraphism and meningocele or myelomeningocele and hydrocephalus. Chiari II has high incidence of associated supratentorial anomalies. Abnormalities in Chiari II are numerous and complex; broad spectrum of radiologic findings may therefore be present in varying degrees or combinations.

    a. Skull and dural abnormalities.

       (1) Lückenschädel: dysplasia of membranous bone resulting in scalloped calvarial thinning; accompanies and is not caused by malformation; rarely persists after 6 months of age.

       (2) Low-lying torcular and transverse sinuses with small, shallow posterior fossa.

       (3) Gaping foramen magnum.

       (4) Varying degrees of falx hypoplasia or fenestration with interdigitated gyri give scalloped or serrated appearance to interhemispheric fissure.

       (5) Petrous bones and clivus may appear concave posteriorly.

       (6) Tentorial hypoplasia with wide, broad incisura; vermis and cerebellum bulge upward through tentorial notch ("cerebellar pseudotumor").

    b. Midbrain and cerebellar abnormalities.

       (1) Hindbrain dysgenesis results in downward displacement of medulla and cerebellum.

       (2) Medullary kinking in 70%.

       (3) Tectal beaking.

       (4) Anteromedial growth of cerebellum around sides of brainstem.

    c. Ventricles and cisterns.

       (1) Lateral ventricles vary in size from normal to markedly dilated and are frequently asymmetric with colpocephaly (prominent occipital horns), anterior and inferior pointing,

and concavity of frontal horns. Ventricles therefore often have scalloped appearance.

(2) Third ventricle often enlarged with deformed anterior recesses and enlarged massa intermedia.

(3) Septum pellucidum frequently absent or fenestrated.

(4) Fourth ventricle often elongated, small, and displaced caudally.

(5) Serrated, often enlarged interhemispheric fissure.

(6) Aqueductal stenosis or occlusion may be associated.

d. Parenchymal abnormalities.

(1) Microgyria and stenogyria.

(2) Gray matter heterotopias.

e. Spine and cord (see Chapter 55): Spinal dysraphism, usually myelomeningocele, is virtually always present in some form.

(1) Lumbosacral myelomeningocele in 75%, cervicothoracic in 25%.

(2) Syringohydromyelia.

(3) Tethered cord usually with lipoma.

(4) Diastematomyelia may be associated.

f. Associated anomalies: corpus callosum anomalies in 80% to 90% (usually partially absent or hypoplastic).

3. Chiari III: Chiari II with low occipital or high cervical encephalocele; very rare.

4. Chiari IV: severe cerebellar hypoplasia; very rare and may not exist as distinct, separate entity. Findings include absent or hypoplastic cerebellum, small brainstem, and large posterior fossa cerebrospinal fluid (CSF) spaces.

5. Joubert's syndrome: vermian dysgenesis and aplasia, small brainstem with profound abnormalities of medullary and oculomotor function; associated abnormalities may include polydactyly, cystic kidney disease, retinal dystrophy, and profound developmental delay.

B. Cephaloceles: protrusions of intracranial structures (meninges, CSF, brain, and ventricles—isolated or in various combinations) through skull defect.

1. Location (North America).

a. Occipital in 70%.

b. Parietal in 10% to 20%.

c. High frontal in 10%.

d. Basal in 10% (transsphenoidal and sphenopharyngeal are rarest of these).

2. Associated anomalies common.

a. Absent corpus callosum.

b. Chiari malformation.

    c. Heterotopic gray matter.

    d. Migration anomalies.

    e. Dandy-Walker syndrome.

C. Anomalies of corpus callosum: Corpus callosum develops during third and fourth months of fetal life, mostly forming from front to back (except that rostrum forms last). Agenesis may be complete or partial; if it is partial, genu is always present and splenium, rostrum, or both are absent. Callosal abnormalities are often associated (in up to 50%) with other CNS malformations such as gray matter abnormalities (heterotopias, polymicrogyria), Chiari or Dandy-Walker malformations, lipomas, cephaloceles, and interhemispheric arachnoid cysts. Classic neuroradiologic findings in corpus callosum agenesis include following.

    1. Lateral ventricles: frontal horns and bodies widely separated and parallel (not converging). Pointed, sharply angled frontal horns and bodies. Occipital horns frequently disproportionately enlarged ("colpocephaly"). Concave medial borders of lateral ventricles because of protruding longitudinal Probst bundles.

    2. Third ventricle: usually somewhat dilated and elevated with varying degree of dorsal extension and interposition between lateral ventricles. Foramen of Monro often elongated.

    3. Miscellaneous: Interhemispheric fissure (IHF) appears to be continuous with anterior third ventricle because genu is absent. In coronal views, IHF extends inferiorly between lateral ventricles to roof of third ventricle. In sagittal views, normal cingulate gyrus is absent and paramedian gyri and sulci have radial or spokelike configuration around third ventricle. Interhemispheric CSF cysts are often seen projecting superiorly between lateral ventricles. When large, these cysts may assume bizarre configurations, sometimes even obscuring underlying malformations.

    4. Associated anomalies.

        a. Cephaloceles.

        b. Lipoma.

            (1) Corpus callosum lipomas make up 30% of intracranial lipomas; half are associated with variable degrees of callosal agenesis.

            (2) Not true tumor but brain malformation.

            (3) Curvilinear calcification often present.

            (4) Prominent vessels often course through callosal lipoma.

    5. Enlarged hippocampal commissure can be seen in some cases of callosal agenesis, mimicking splenium. Splenium-like bundle of interhemispheric fiber tracts can be seen in some cases of semilobar holoprosencephaly. Prognosis varies strikingly (good in former, poor in latter).

D. Dandy-Walker complex is hindbrain congenital malformation characterized by cystic dilatation of fourth ventricle, associated with varying degrees of vermian aplasia or hypoplasia. Exact origin of Dandy-Walker complex is unknown, but theories include failure of development of anterior medullary velum (embryonic roof of fourth ventricle), atresia of outlet foramina, delayed opening of foramen of Magendie, and insult (of varying severity) to both developing cerebellar hemispheres and fourth ventricle. Cerebellar hemispheres are usually small. Radiographic features may include some or all of following.

1. Large fluid-filled fourth ventricle–cisterna magna complex.
2. Large posterior fossa with torcular lying above lambda (high tentorium).
3. Varying amounts of cerebellar and vermian hypoplasia.
4. Varying degrees of third and lateral ventricular dilatation.
5. Associated abnormalities are present in more than 60% of patients.
   a. Hydrocephalus (75%).
   b. Corpus callosum dysgenesis (20% to 25%), with or without interhemispheric cyst.
   c. Polymicrogyria and gray matter heterotopias (5% to 10%).
   d. Occipital cephaloceles (less than 5%).
   e. Polydactyly and cardiac anomalies.
6. Differential diagnosis: retrocerebellar arachnoid cyst (vermis present, displaced but normally formed fourth ventricle). Mega–cisterna magna (normally positioned torcular Herophili, normal vermis and cerebellum) is probably mild variant of Dandy-Walker complex. Ventricular or cyst shunting can lead to confusing computed tomographic or magnetic resonance (MR) findings, so preoperative studies may be necessary for correct diagnosis.
7. To emphasize: so-called Dandy-Walker variant and mega–cisterna magna probably represent points on spectrum of posterior fossa cystic malformation and are not separate entities.

II. Disorders of diverticulation and cleavage: These are also classified as disorders of ventral induction (rostral end of developing brain) and are intimately tied to development of face. Disorders of ventral induction include holoprosencephalies, septooptic dysplasia, and agenesis of septum pellucidum.

  A. Holoprosencephaly: Lateral ventricles and cerebral hemispheres arise during fourth to eighth weeks of gestation as paired diverticula from prosencephalon, forming telencephalon (cerebral hemispheres) and diencephalon (thalamus and hypothalamus). Failure to cleave prosencephalon results in failure to form separate cerebral hemispheres (i.e., holoprosencephaly). The three forms of holoprosencephaly are classified by degree of brain cleavage, although clearly spectrum exists from most severe (alobar holoprosencephaly) to mildest (lobar) form.

    1. Alobar holoprosencephaly.
       a. Most severe form.
       b. Small holosphere with central monoventricle.
       c. Fused thalami.
       d. Normal midline structures such as falx and corpus callosum are absent.
       e. Multiple craniofacial anomalies in more than 50%.
       f. Small amount of peripheral brain tissue usually present.
       g. Often associated chromosal abnormalities (trisomy 13 and trisomy 18 most common).
       h. Outcome nearly always fatal.
       i. Differential diagnosis: massive hydrocephalus (falx and interhemispheric fissure present), hydranencephaly (thalami not fused; falx present).
    2. Semilobar holoprosencephaly.
       a. Single ventricle with ocular hypotelorism and rudimentary occipital temporal horns.
       b. Thalami are fused and project into ventricular cavity.
       c. Rudimentary falx and interhemispheric fissure present.
       d. Normal facies or mild facial anomalies.
    3. Lobar holoprosencephaly.
       a. Nearly complete forebrain cleavage with shallow anterior hemispheric fissure.
       b. Well-formed ventricular system.
       c. Absent septum pellucidum.
       d. Falx present.
       e. Optic vesicles and olfactory bulbs may be hypoplastic.
  B. Septooptic dysplasia.
    1. May be mild form of lobar holoprosencephaly.
    2. Absent septum pellucidum with squared-off or boxlike appearance to frontal horns on axial images; interior pointing on coronal images.
    3. Optic nerves and chiasm small (seen on MR in only 50% of patients).
    4. Pituitary stalk may appear enlarged (two thirds have hypothalamic-pituitary dysfunction).
    5. Schizencephaly in 50%.
III. Disorders of sulcation and migration: These occur between 2 and 4 months of fetal development. Focal disturbances in neuronal migration can result in cleft brain (schizencephaly). Cortical mantle can also be too thick, too flat, or too folded, resulting in sulcal and gyral abnormalities.
  A. Schizencephaly: gray matter–lined clefts that extend through entire hemisphere from ventricle to subarachnoid space. They can be unilat-

eral or bilateral, found anywhere in cerebral hemispheres. Two types exist: type I ("closed lip," i.e., walls of the cleft are fused) and type II ("open lip," i.e., cleft walls separated or open with coexistent "hydrocephalus"). Both have full-thickness clefts through hemisphere with heterotopic gray matter (usually with polymicrogyria) lining cleft.

1. Type I: less common; often unilateral cortically lined cleft in parasylvian region, extending from hemisphere surface to ventricle; polymicrogyria or thickened cortex lining cleft. Should not be confused with postdevelopmentally acquired destructive lesions (in which defects are not lined with cortex).

2. Type II: more common; usually seen as bilaterally open, symmetric cerebral clefts lined by cortex. Most common site is sylvian fissure, extending into parietal and frontal lobe. Gray matter lining cleft is usually abnormal (polymicrogyria, pachygyria).

3. Associated anomalies: septum pellucidum absent in 80% to 90%.

B. Lissencephaly (smooth brain): widespread, although not necessarily complete, agyria. Common radiologic findings include smooth brain with absent or incomplete opercularization and thickened cortex with abnormally smooth gray-white interface. Figure-of-8 or hourglass shape of brain is due to shallow, widened sylvian fissures. Ventricular enlargement is often seen. Corpus callosum may be hypoplastic, partial, or absent. Dandy-Walker anomalies and various brainstem and cerebellar atrophies may be present as well.

C. Gray matter abnormalities such as heterotopias, megalencephaly, pachygyria, and polymicrogyria are becoming increasingly well recognized on MR scans. Signal intensity parallels that of normal gray matter, with abnormal location and configuration of disordered gray matter.

1. Neuronal heterotopias: Nodular heterotopic gray matter theoretically results from insult late in neuronal proliferation stage, allowing multiplication of neuroblasts but preventing their migration away from periventricular region. Laminar heterotopia is bandlike subcortical layer of gray matter usually lying within centrum semiovale.

2. Megalencephaly (see IV on p. 185).

3. Pachygyria: presence of a few broad, flat gyri. Agyria-pachygyria is another term used to describe lissencephaly or "smooth brain." Pachygyria can be focal or diffuse.

4. Polymicrogyria: multiple "grapelike" gyri; cortex more organized than in agyria or pachygyria. Lack of deep sulci mimics appearance of pachygyria with broad, thickened gyri. Gliotic white matter is often present in polymicrogyria but usually absent in pachygyria. Associated focal anomalous venous drainage is common and should not be mistaken for vascular malformation.

IV. Disorders of size.
  A. Microcephaly: True developmental microcephaly or microencephaly vera can occur but is uncommon. In most cases, small-sized brain is secondary to destructive or encephaloclastic disorders (e.g., infection, vascular accident).
  B. Macrocephaly: Most commonly "large head" is probably normal variant. Other causes include hydrocephalus, chronic subdural hematoma, and occasionally metabolic disorders. "Unilateral megalencephaly" is name given to hamartomatous-like overgrowth of all or part of one cerebral hemisphere with associated migrational anomalies and heterotopias. Wide spectrum of severity and extent of involvement is seen. Typically, involved hemisphere and ipsilateral ventricle are large. Cortex is thick with broad, shallow gyri. Multiple heterotopias are present. Occasionally entire hemisphere is dysplastic with no normal structures recognizable.
V. Destructive lesions.
  A. Hydranencephaly: Since this usually results from destruction of previously formed brain, midline structures such as falx cerebri are present. Thin membrane with little or no cortical remnant (usually occipital) surrounds huge, fluid-filled cavities. No recognizable ventricular structures are seen, but intact basal ganglia can usually be identified.
  B. Porencephaly: ventricular outpouchings caused by vascular or inflammatory disease, trauma, or other intrauterine insults; not lined by gray matter (contrast with schizencephaly).

SUGGESTED READINGS

Barkovich AJ: Congenital malformations of the brain. In *Pediatric neuroimaging,* New York, 1990, Raven Press, pp 77-121.

Barkovich AJ: Apparent atypical callosal dysgenesis: analysis of MR findings in six cases and their relationship to holoprosencephaly, *AJNR* 11:333-339, 1990.

Barkovich AJ, Chuang SH: Unilateral megalencephaly: correlation of MR imaging and pathologic characteristics, *AJNR* 11:523-531, 1990.

Barkovich AJ, Kjos BO, Norman D, Edwards MS: Revised classification of posterior fossa cysts and cystlike malformations based on the results of multiplanar MR imaging, *AJNR* 10:977-988, 1989.

Bird CR, Gilles FH: Type I schizencephaly: CT and neuropathologic findings, *AJNR* 8:451-454, 1987.

Byrd SE, Bohan TP, Osborn RE, Naidich TP: The CT and MR evaluation of lissencephaly, *AJNR* 9:923-927, 1988.

Kendall B, Kingsley D, Lambert SR, et al: Joubert syndrome: a clinico-radiologic study, *Neuroradiology* 21:502-506, 1990.

Naidich TP, McLone DG, Fulling KH: The Chiari II malformation. IV. The hindbrain deformity, *Neuroradiology* 25:179-197, 1983.

Naidich TP, Pudlowski RM, Naidich JB: Computed tomographic signs of the Chiari II malformation. II. Midbrain and cerebellum, *Radiology* 134:391-398, 1980.

Naidich TP, Pudlowski RM, Naidich JB: Computed tomographic signs of the Chiari II malformation. III. Ventricles and cisterns, *Radiology* 134:657-663, 1980.

Naidich TP, Pudlowski RM, Naidich JB, et al: Computed tomographic signs of the Chiari II malformation. I. Skull and partitions, *Radiology* 134:65-67, 1980.

Osborn RE, Byrd SE, Naidich TP, et al: MR of neuronal migrational disorders, *AJNR* 9:1101-1106, 1988.

Poe LB, Coleman LL, Mahmud F: Congenital central nervous system anomalies, *Radiographics* 9:801-826, 1989.

Pollei SR, Boyer RS, Crawford S, et al: Disorders of migration and sulcation, *Semin US CT MR* 9:231-246, 1988.

Smith AS, Ross JS, Blaser SI, Weinstein MA: Magnetic resonance imaging of disturbances in neuronal migration: illustration of an embryologic process, *Radiographics* 9:509-522, 1989.

Suzuki M, Takashima T, Kadoya M, et al: Pericallosal lipomas: MR features, *J Comput Assist Tomogr* 15:207-209, 1991.

Titelbaum DS, Hayward JC, Zimmerman RA: Pachygyriclike changes: topographic appearance at MR imaging and CT and correlation with neurologic studies, *Radiology* 173:663-667, 1989.

Van der Knaap MS, Valk J: Classification of congenital anomalies of the CNS, *AJNR* 9:315-326, 1988.

Wolpert SM, Scott RM, Runge VM, Kwan ESK: Difficulties in diagnosing congenital posterior fossa fluid collections after shunting procedures, *AJNR* 8:653-656, 1987.

CHAPTER 29

Congenital malformations: disorders of histogenesis and the neurocutaneous syndromes

---

KEY CONCEPTS

Neurocutaneous syndromes (phakomatoses) include:
1. Neurofibromatosis (NF)
   a. NF type 1 (von Recklinghausen's disease)
   b. NF type 2 (bilateral acoustic schwannomas)
2. Sturge-Weber syndrome
3. Tuberous sclerosis
4. Von Hippel–Lindau disease
5. Others
   a. Linear nevus sebaceus syndrome
   b. Basal cell nevus (Gorlin's) syndrome
   c. Ataxia-telangiectasia
   d. Wyburn-Mason syndrome

Dyshistogenetic disorders include such abnormalities as tuberous sclerosis (TS), neurofibromatosis (NF), von Hippel–Lindau disease (VHL), and Sturge-Weber syndrome (SWS) in addition to congenital vascular malformations (see Chapter 14) and possibly congenital neoplasms (see Chapter 49). Only the neurocutaneous syndromes are discussed in this chapter.

The neurocutaneous syndromes are congenital hereditary central nervous system (CNS) disorders that affect mainly ectodermal structures and have characteristic associated skin manifestations. Sometimes termed "phakomatoses" (Greek for a lentil-shaped object or spot), they are characterized by the presence of tumorlike malformations with blastomatous tendencies and pigment patches or angiomas in tissues of ectodermal origin, particularly the skin, peripheral nervous system, and CNS. Included in this interesting disease spectrum are NF, TS, VHL, and SWS. Miscellaneous less common phakomatoses such as basal cell nevus syndrome and ataxia-telangiectasia also occur. The manifestations of these disorders are protean; this volume summarizes only the CNS, spine, and skull abnormalities.

I. Neurofibromatosis (Table 29-1): At least eight separate forms of NF have been described, although two types, von Recklinghausen's disease (NF-1) and neurofibromatosis with bilateral acoustic schwannomas (NF-2) are generally accepted. Terms "central" and "peripheral" NF should be discarded because they are inaccurate; *both* NF-1 and NF-2 show CNS involvement. These NF disorders represent dyshistogenesis of neuroectodermal and mesodermal tissue. Inheritance is autosomal dominant with no sex predilection. Recently chromosomal loci for both NF-1 and NF-2 were pinpointed and gene responsible for NF-1 was isolated.

   A. Von Recklinghausen's disease (NF-1) seems to be associated with tumors of neurons and astrocytes.

      1. Incidence: approximately 1 in 4000 newborns affected; more than 90% of all NF cases are NF-1.

      2. Inheritance.

         a. Autosomal dominant.

         b. No sex linkage.

         c. Chromosome 17.

         d. Responsible gene has been isolated.

      3. Diagnostic criteria for NF-1 include two or more of following findings.

         a. Six or more 5 mm or larger café-au-lait spots.

         b. Either one plexiform neurofibroma or two or more neurofibromas of any type.

Table 29-1   Comparison between neurofibromatosis types 1 and 2

Type 1	Type 2
Von Recklinghausen's disease	Bilateral acoustic schwannomas
1 : 4000 (represents 90% of NF cases)	1 : 50,000 (<10% of NF cases)
Chromosome 17	Chromosome 22
Prominent skin manifestations	Minimal skin changes
Associated with tumors of neurons (hamartomas) and astrocytes (gliomas), plexiform neurofibromas, malignant nerve sheath tumors	Associated with tumors of meninges (meningiomas) and Schwann cells (cranial nerve schwannomas)
Spinal neurofibromas (often small, single)	Spinal schwannomas (often large, bilateral, multilevel)
Questionable whether spinal gliomas develop in these patients	Spinal cord ependymomas, astrocytomas

NF, Neurofibromatosis.

    c. Two or more pigmented iris hamartomas (so-called Lisch nodules).

    d. Axillary and inguinal freckling.

    e. Optic nerve glioma.

    f. First-degree relative with NF-1.

    g. Presence of characteristic bone lesion (e.g., dysplasia of greater sphenoid wing).

4. CNS manifestations occur in 15% to 20% of patients with NF-1.

    a. Optic nerve glioma (see box below).

       (1) Most common CNS tumor in NF-1.

       (2) Lesions can involve one or both optic nerves, chiasm, tracts, lateral geniculate body, and optic radiations.

       (3) Mean age of NF-1 patients with optic nerve glioma is 5 years; optic nerve glioma without NF is 12 years.

       (4) Most are histologically relatively benign (low-grade astrocytoma).

       (5) Computed tomography (CT): enlargement of optic nerve sheath complex.

       (6) Magnetic resonance (MR): lesions isointense to slightly hy-

---

OCULAR FINDINGS IN THE NEUROCUTANEOUS SYNDROMES

1. Neurofibromatosis (primarily type 1)
   a. Optic nerve glioma
   b. Lisch nodules
   c. Plexiform neurofibroma
   d. Papilledema increased intracranial pressure from central nervous system neoplasm
   e. Buphthalmos
2. Sturge-Weber syndrome
   a. Scleral telangiectasia
   b. Buphthalmos
3. Tuberous sclerosis: ocular hamartomas (retinal phakoma)
4. Von Hippel–Lindau disease
   a. Retinal hemangioblastoma
   b. Retinal detachment
   c. Vitreous hemorrhage
   d. Phthisis bulbi (microphthalmia, with or without dystrophic calcifications)
5. Wyburn-Mason syndrome: retinocephalic arteriovenous malformation

pointense on T1-weighted imaging (T1WI), mildly to strongly hyperintense on T2WI. Often seen on T2WI are other high-signal areas without mass effect in basal ganglia, internal capsule, pons, cerebral peduncles, cerebellum, and elsewhere. These may also be slightly hyperintense on T1WI and probably represent hamartomas. Enhancement after contrast administration should raise suspicion of neoplasm.

b. Nonoptic gliomas: frequency of low-grade gliomas increased in NF-1; common locations are tectal and periaqueductal regions and brainstem.

c. Nonglial neoplasms: not a feature of NF-1.

d. Vascular abnormalities: dysplastic stenosis of vessels at or near circle of Willis (see Chapter 12), intracranial and extracranial aneurysms.

e. Cranial nerve (CN) tumors: Optic nerve (CN II) neoplasms are histologically brain neoplasms and are only cranial nerve tumors associated with NF-1. Schwannomas of CNs III to XIII are feature of NF-2, not NF-1.

f. Plexiform neurofibromas: exocranial origin but often extend intracranially along natural foramina and fissures (e.g., from orbit and pterygopalatine fossa into cavernous sinus).

g. Malignant peripheral nerve sheath tumors in 5% to 10%.

h. Skull lesions.

   (1) Macrocrania frequent.

   (2) Abnormal calcifications (see Chapter 24).

   (3) Hypoplasia of greater sphenoid wing with temporal lobe herniation into orbit, pulsatile exophthalmos.

   (4) Calvarial defects (e.g., lambdoid suture).

i. Dural ectasia; can have enlarged internal auditory canals without facial or acoustic nerve masses.

5. Spine manifestations.

a. Kyphoscoliosis in one third to one half of patients.

   (1) Probably reflects primary mesodermal dysplasia.

   (2) T3 to T7 most common.

   (3) Short-segment angular deformities.

   (4) Usually mild but occasionally rapidly progressive, resulting in paraplegia.

b. Posterior vertebral body scalloping and pedicle erosion.

   (1) Usually multilevel.

   (2) Most often caused by dural ectasia.

   (3) "Dumbbell" spinal neurofibromas in 13% to 20%.

        (4) In 3%, plexiform neurofibroma is present, causing enlargement.

    c. Lateral meningoceles.

        (1) Probably caused by weakened, dysplastic meninges that protrude through enlarged intervertebral foramina (pulsion diverticula).

        (2) Thoracic most common, usually on right side; lumbosacral and cervical occur but are less common.

        (3) CT: dumbbell-shaped cerebrospinal fluid (CSF) attenuation lesion protrudes through enlarged neural foramen with adjacent thinned pedicle and scalloped vertebral body.

        (4) MR: CSF signal on all sequences.

B. NF with bilateral acoustic neurinomas (NF-2) seems to be associated with tumors of meninges and Schwann cells.

  1. Incidence: approximately 1:50,000 (much less common than NF-1).

  2. Inheritance.

    a. Autosomal dominant.

    b. No sex linkage.

    c. Chromosome 22.

  3. Diagnostic criteria are one or more of following.

    a. Bilateral CN VIII masses.

    b. First-degree relative with NF-2 and either:

        (1) Unilateral CN VIII mass *or*

        (2) Any two of following: neurofibroma, meningioma, glioma, schwannoma, or juvenile posterior subcapsular lenticular opacity.

  4. Cutaneous manifestations much less common than with NF-1; therefore NF-2 patients often older at initial diagnosis.

    a. Few small pale café-au-lait spots.

    b. Minimal or absent cutaneous neurofibromas.

    c. No Lisch nodules.

  5. CNS manifestations.

    a. Vestibulocochlear schwannomas. (NOTE: Dural ectasia without acoustic neurinomas can widen internal auditory canals in these patients).

    b. Schwannomas of other cranial nerves (CNs III to XII).

    c. Solitary or multiple meningiomas (both spinal and intracranial).

    d. Other tumors.

        (1) Questionable whether intracranial gliomas develop in patients with NF-2.

        (2) Astrocytomas of cord.

(3) Ependymomas of cord (most common intrinsic cord neoplasm in NF-2).

e. Multiple spinal schwannomas (often large, bilateral, and multilevel).

II. Sturge-Weber syndrome: also known as encephalotrigeminal angiomatosis. "Port-wine" vascular nevus flammeus in CN V distribution (part or all of face, may involve sclera), leptomeningeal venous angiomatosis, seizures, dementia, mental retardation, hemiparesis, hemianopsia, congenital glaucoma and buphthalmos ("cow-eye"), and visceral angiomas can all be features of this disease. Sporadic.

A. General.

1. Pathology: may be due to faulty development of venous drainage with resulting venous angioma confined to pial layer of leptomeninges; ipsilateral choroid plexus of lateral ventricle often also involved; 30% have ocular choroidal angioma, glaucoma; 15% have buphthalmos.

2. Intracranial lesions typically unilateral (ipsilateral to facial nerve) but can be bilateral, occasionally even contralateral.

B. Radiology: Typically sequelae of angiomatous malformation, not malformation itself, are visualized.

1. Skull films: curvilinear or gyriform calcifications, most often parietooccipital area.

2. CT.

   a. Calcification is most common finding in SWS.
      (1) Curvilinear calcifications following cerebral gyri.
      (2) Rarely seen before 2 years of age.
      (3) Usually starts in occipital lobe.
      (4) Progresses anteriorly.
      (5) Located in dystrophic cerebral cortex underlying pial angioma (possibly related to chronic hypoxia or venous infarctions), typically at second or third cortical layer.
      (6) Bilateral in up to 20%, occasionally contralateral to facial lesion.

   b. Cerebral atrophy.
      (1) Usually unilateral, ipsilateral to facial nevus.
      (2) Typically occipital but can involve entire hemisphere.

   c. Gyral enhancement following contrast media administration.

   d. Enlarged, intensely enhancing ipsilateral choroid plexus in 75% (often hyperplasia, although frank plexal angiomas have also been reported).

3. MR.

   a. Hypointensity on T2WI in areas of cortical calcification.

    b. Cerebral atrophy and miscellaneous parenchymal abnormalities.
      (1) Thickened diploë in overlying calvarium.
      (2) Widened sulci.
      (3) Some focal hyperintensities on T2WI may represent reactive gliosis of underlying white matter.
      (4) Calcifications may be effectively demonstrated with gradient echo scans.
    c. Enlarged enhancing choroid plexus in 75%.
    d. Gyral enhancement common after contrast material is administered; may be faint or striking.
    e. Collateral venous drainage may be manifested by enlarged, tortuous medullary and subependymal veins.
    f. Some reports of accelerated myelination in infants with SWS.
  4. Angiography.
    a. Arterial phase normal.
    b. Diffuse homogeneous capillary blush may be present; this is *not* angioma itself but probably represents vascular stasis and delayed venous washout because of abnormal cortical venous drainage.
    c. Paucity of superficial cortical draining veins; those present are often dysplastic, sparse, and irregular.
    d. Medullary (deep white matter) and subependymal veins enlarge to provide collateral pathways for venous drainage.
III. Tuberous sclerosis: also known as Bourneville's disease. TS is hereditary disorder with widespread potential for hamartomatous growths in multiple organ systems.
  A. General.
    1. Incidence: 1:10,000 to 50,000 patients.
    2. Inheritance.
      a. Autosomal dominant with low penetrance.
      b. No sexual or racial predilection.
    3. Clinical findings: classic triad (not always present).
      a. Adenoma sebaceum (in 90%); ash leaf spots on slit-lamp examination.
      b. Seizures (in 80% to 90%).
      c. Mental retardation (in 50% to 80%).
    4. Pathology.
      a. Subependymal hamartomas and giant cell astrocytomas: probably a spectrum of lesions.
      b. Cortical hamartomas. (Unlike subependymal hamartomas, these rarely if ever undergo neoplastic degeneration.)
      c. Ocular hamartomas ("giant drusen"): 50% of patients with TS

have retinal hamartomas; seen as calcifications at or near optic nerve head.
    d. Other lesions.
        (1) Renal: angiomyolipomas in 40% to 80%.
        (2) Cardiac: rhabdomyomas (50% of patients with cardiac myomas have TS).
        (3) Lung: cystic lymphangiomyomas and chronic fibrosis.
        (4) Liver: leiomyomas and adenomas.
        (5) Spleen and pancreas: adenomas.
        (6) Extremities: cystic bone changes and subungual fibromas.
        (7) Skull: multiple bone islands in diploic space.
        (8) Vascular: a rare cause of nonatheromatous stenosis.
  5. Radiology.
    a. CT.
        (1) Intracranial abnormalities in up to 90%.
        (2) Calcifications: increase with age (rare before 1 year of age); seen in up to 50% of patients with TS .
        (3) Malignant degeneration develops in 10% to 15% of patients with TS.
        (4) Enhancement after contrast administration should be considered indicative of neoplastic transformation.
        (5) Typical neoplasm is subependymal giant cell astrocytoma; most common near foramen of Monro.
        (6) Parenchymal hamartomas demonstrable on CT in 10% to 15%.
        (7) Ventricular dilatation (either dysplastic or secondary to foramen of Monro obstruction by giant cell astrocytoma).
    b. MR.
        (1) Subependymal nodules (signal intensity similar to that in white matter).
        (2) Cortical tubers (lesions with somewhat indistinct borders that are typically isointense or hypointense on T1WI, hyperintense on T2WI, possibly because of fibrillary gliosis or demyelination). Lesions are not enhanced.
        (3) White matter heterotopias and gliosis (signal similar to that of cortical tubers).
        (4) Giant cell astrocytoma: enhanced mass near foramen of Monro. If subependymal nodules elsewhere are enhanced, they should probably be considered malignant or at least histologically active lesions with potential to evolve.
IV. Von Hippel–Lindau disease: multisystem disease characterized by cysts, angiomas, and neoplasms of CNS and abdominal viscera.
  A. General.
    1. Inheritance.

    a. Autosomal dominance. Short arm of chromosome 3 implicated.

    b. Nearly 100% penetrance.

    c. No sex predilection.

    d. Screening recommended for at-risk family members.

2. Age at presentation: exceedingly rare before puberty. If retinal angioma, early twenties; hemangioma, early thirties; renal cell carcinoma, early to middle forties.

3. At least 25 different lesions have been described in this disorder; most important are:

    a. Retinal angiomas (50%).

    b. Cerebellar (30% to 60%), medullary, spinal (5%) hemangioblastomas.

    c. Pheochromocytoma (10%).

    d. Renal cell carcinoma (25% to 38%).

4. Clinical diagnosis of VHL if:

    a. More than one CNS hemangioblastoma is present *or*

    b. One CNS hemangioblastoma with one visceral manifestation is present *or*

    c. Patient has family history of the disease plus one manifestation.

5. CT.

    a. Cerebellar hemangioblastoma.

      (1) Between 7% and 12% of all posterior fossa tumors.

      (2) Occurs in more than half of patients with VHL.

      (3) Most occur between 20 and 50 years of age; very rare in children.

      (4) Multiple in 10%.

      (5) Solid, strongly enhancing mass in 20% to 25%.

      (6) Cystic with isodense, strongly enhancing mural nodule in 80%.

      (7) Cerebellar hemisphere vermis most common location; brainstem less common; cerebral hemisphere lesions very rare.

    b. Retinal angiomas in 5% to 20%.

6. MR.

    a. Cerebellar hemangioblastoma (craniovertebral junction is a favorite location).

      (1) Most show prolonged T1 and T2 (signal can be complex if hemorrhage has occurred).

      (2) May have large cyst with higher signal than CSF.

      (3) Nodule is enhanced strongly with contrast material (95% of lesions less than 1 cm are solid).

      (4) "Flow voids" in afferent and efferent vessels supplying lesion.

    b. Cerebral lesions.

(1) Supratentorial hemangioblastoma rare (100 reported cases).
(2) Focal areas of increased signal in white matter on T2WI have been reported; significance unknown.
c. Ocular lesions.
(1) High-signal vitreous lesions with retinal detachment.
(2) Retinal enhancement with contrast media seen in severe cases; phthisis bulbi can sometimes be identified.
d. Spinal cord lesions: in 8% to 35% in patients with VHL.
(1) Syrinxlike cyst with adjacent vessel enlargement.
(2) Isointense nodule that is strongly enhanced on T1WI after contrast material is administered.
7. Angiography.
a. One or more intensely vascular nodules.
b. Cystic component appears as larger, avascular mass effect.
8. Differential diagnosis of enhanced, cystic-appearing posterior fossa mass.
a. Adults: metastasis.
b. Adolescents: cystic astrocytoma; less commonly medulloblastoma. (Hemangioblastoma is very rare in children.)
V. Miscellaneous phakomatoses (conditions with cutaneous CNS manifestations).
A. Linear nevus sebaceus syndrome.
1. Extracranial manifestations.
a. Nevi of face, nose, scalp.
b. Malignant degeneration common (20% to 25%); basal cell carcinoma most common neoplasm.
c. Orbital abnormalities common.
(1) Aberrant lacrimal gland.
(2) Ocular colobomas.
2. Intracranial manifestations.
a. Asymmetric cerebral hemispheres (hemiatrophy or megalencephaly).
b. Unilateral ventriculomegaly, hydrocephalus, and porencephaly.
c. Heterotopic or dysplastic gray matter with sulcation abnormalities.
d. Increased incidence of cerebral neoplasms, microangioma, and leptomeningeal hemangiomas.
B. Basal cell nevus syndrome (Gorlin's syndrome).
1. Extracranial manifestations.
a. Facial truncal basal cell epitheliomas.
b. Mandibular cysts (odontogenic keratocysts) and oral and jaw tumors (ameloblastoma, squamous cell carcinoma, and fibrosarcoma).

    c. Skeletal anomalies (e.g., bifid ribs, vertebral anomalies such as spina bifida or fusion anomalies, polydactyly).
  2. Intracranial manifestations.
    a. Corpus callosum agenesis.
    b. Cerebral and choroid plexus cysts.
    c. Congenital hydrocephalus.
    d. Lamellar dural calcifications (e.g., of falx, tentorium).
    f. Neoplasms (medulloblastoma, meningioma, craniopharyngioma, and cerebellar astrocytoma).
C. Ataxia-telangiectasia.
  1. Extracranial manifestations.
    a. Cutaneous, mucosal telangiectasias.
    b. Immunodeficiencies with:
      (1) Recurrent sinopulmonary infections.
      (2) Lymphomas, leukemias.
    c. Epithelial malignancies.
  2. Intracranial manifestations.
    a. Cerebellar atrophy (of hemispheres, vermis, or both).
    b. Hemorrhage with or without occult vascular malformations.
D. Wyburn-Mason syndrome.
  1. Extracranial manifestations: dermatologic lesions in minority (range from faint cutaneous discoloration to extensive nevus of skin in trigeminal distribution; maxilla and mandible may be involved).
  2. Intracranial manifestations (primarily retinocephalic arteriovenous malformation [AVM]).
    a. Ocular: retinal or retroorbital vascular malformations, with or without pulsatile exophthalmos; optic atrophy.
    b. Parenchymal AVMs.
E. Proteus syndrome. (Probably the "elephant man" had this rather than neurofibromatosis.)
  1. Extracranial manifestations.
    a. Cutaneous verrucae.
    b. Partial gigantism.
    c. Multiple lipomas and lymphangiomas.
  2. Intracranial manifestations: macrocephaly.
F. Others: Louis-Bar syndrome, epidermal nevus syndrome, and neurocutaneous melanosis.

SUGGESTED READINGS

Altman NR, Purser RK, Post MJD: Tuberous sclerosis: characteristics at CT and MR imaging, *Radiology* 167:527-532, 1988.
Aoki S, Barkovich AJ, Nishimura K, et al: Neurofibromatosis types 1 and 2: cranial MR findings, *Radiology* 172:527-534, 1989.

Baker RS, Ross PA, Baumann RJ: Neurological complications of the epidermal nevus syndrome, *Arch Neurol* 44:227-232, 1987.

Barkovich AJ: Phakomatoses. In *Pediatric neuroimaging,* New York, 1990, Raven Press, pp 123-147.

Bell DG, King BF, Hattery RR, et al: Imaging characteristics of tuberous sclerosis, *AJR* 156:1081-1086, 1991.

Braffman BH, Bilaniuk LT, Zimmerman RA: MR of central nervous system neoplasia of the phakomatoses, *Semin Roentgenol* 25:198-217, 1990.

Chamberlain ML, Press GA, Hesselink JR: MR imaging and CT in three cases of Sturge-Weber syndrome: prospective comparison, *AJNR* 10:491-496, 1989.

Crawford SC, Boyer RS, Harnsberger HR, et al: Disorders of histogenesis: the neurocutaneous syndromes, *Semin US CT MR* 9:247-267, 1988.

Elster AD, Chen MYM: MR imaging of Sturge-Weber syndrome, *AJNR* 11:625-689, 1990.

Filling-Katz MR, Choyoke PL, Patrinas NJ, et al: Radiologic screening for von Hippel–Lindau disease: the role of Gd-DTPA enhanced MR imaging of the CNS, *J Comput Assist Tomogr* 13:743-755, 1989.

Halliday AL, Sobel RA, Martuza RL: Benign spinal nerve sheath tumors: their occurrence sporadically and in neurofibromatosis types 1 and 2, J Neurosurg 74:248-253, 1991.

Hurst RW, Newman SA, Cail WS: Multifocal intracranial MR abnormalities in neurofibromatosis, *AJNR* 9:293-296, 1988.

Martin N, Debussche C, DeBroucker T, et al: Gadolinium-DTPA enhanced MR imaging in tuberous sclerosis, *Neuroradiology* 31:492-497, 1990.

McMurdo SK Jr, Moore SG, Brant-Zawadzki M, et al: MR imaging of intracranial tuberous sclerosis, *AJNR* 8:77-82, 1987.

Nixon JR, Houser OW, Gomez MR, Okazaki H: Cerebral tuberous sclerosis: MR imaging, *Radiology* 170:869-873, 1989.

Patel U, Gupta SC: Wyburn-Mason syndrome, *Neuroradiology* 31:544-546, 1990.

Pavone L, Curatolo P, Rizzo R, et al: Epidermal nevus syndrome, *Neurology* 41:266-271, 1991.

Poe LB, Coleman LL, Mahmud F: Congenital central nervous system anomalies, *Radiographics* 9:801-826, 1989.

Rhodes RE, Friedman HS, Hatten HP Jr, et al: Contrast-enhanced MR imaging of neurocutaneous melanosis, *AJNR* 12:380-382, 1991.

Sarwar M, Schafer ME: Brain malformations in linear nevus sebaceus syndrome: an MR study, *J Comput Assist Tomogr* 12:338-340, 1987.

Sato Y, Waziri M, Smith W, et al: Hippel-Lindau disease: MR imaging, *Radiology* 166:241-246, 1988.

Schultz SM, Twickler DM, Wheeler DE, Hogan TD: Ameloblastoma associated with basal cell nevus (Gorlin) syndrome: CT findings, *J Comput Assist Tomogr* 11:901-904, 1987.

Stirnae GK, Solomon MA, Newton TH: CT and MR of angiomatous malformations of the choroid plexus in patients with Sturge-Weber disease, *AJNR* 7:623-627, 1986.

Wasenko JJ, Rosembloom SA, Duchesneau PM, et al: The Sturge-Weber syndrome: comparison of MR and CT characteristics, *AJNR* 11:131-134, 1990.

VENTRICLES, CISTERNS, AND SUBARACHNOID SPACES

CHAPTER 30

Ventricles, cisterns, and subarachnoid spaces: normal anatomy

KEY CONCEPTS

1. Each cerebrospinal fluid (CSF) cistern has characteristic vascular and neural contents.
2. The foramen of Monro is a Y-shaped structure with an arm of the Y extending to each lateral ventricle and the base of the Y connected to the third ventricle.
3. Cavum septi pellucidi is a normal structure that appears during intrauterine development. It is part of the ventricular system and usually communicates with it.
4. Cavum vergae does not exist in the absence of a cavum septi pellucidi.
5. Cavum velum interpositum is a subarachnoid space above the third ventricle and below the corpus callosum.

CSF is produced by the choroid plexus and normally circulates from the cerebral ventricles to the subarachnoid spaces of the brain and spinal cord. Via absorption from tufts of arachnoid villi that project into the lacunae alongside the superior sagittal sinus, CSF is circulated into the cardiovascular system. The ventricular system and cisternal anatomy are particularly well delineated on multiplanar magnetic resonance (MR) scans.

I. Ventricles (Fig. 30-1).
   A. Fourth ventricle.
      1. Gross anatomy: Borders of the fourth ventricle are:
         a. Anterior: pons and medulla. Nuclei of cranial nerves (CNs) V through XII lie beneath or just below floor of fourth ventricle.
         b. Posterior: superior and inferior medullary vela and vermis.

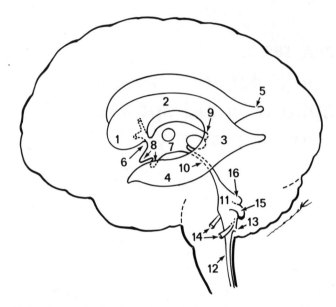

Fig. 30-1 Anatomic drawing of ventricular system (view is from lateral, slightly cephalad aspect).

1. Frontal horn, lateral ventricle
2. Body, lateral ventricle
3. Atrium, lateral ventricle
4. Temporal horn, lateral ventricle
5. Occipital horn, lateral ventricle
6. Foramen of Monro
7. Body, third ventricle
8. Optic and infundibular recesses, third ventricle
9. Suprapineal recess, third ventricle
10. Aqueduct
11. Body, fourth ventricle
12. Obex
13. Foramen of Magendie
14. Lateral recesses of fourth ventricle with foramen of Luschka
15. Posterior superior recesses, fourth ventricle (cap cerebellar tonsils)
16. Fastigium, fourth ventricle

    c. Lateral: superior and inferior cerebellar peduncles.
    d. Inferior: posterosuperior recesses cap cerebellar tonsils.
  2. Fourth ventricle communicates:
    a. Superiorly with third ventricle via aqueduct of Sylvius.
    b. Inferiorly via obex with central canal of medulla and spinal cord.

      c. Posteroinferiorly with cisterna magna via foramen of Magendie.

      d. Posterolaterally with medullary and cerebellopontine angle (CPA) cisterns via lateral recesses and foramen of Luschka. Choroid plexus from fourth ventricle extends around medulla via these recesses into adjacent CPA cisterns.

   3. Radiology.

      a. On sagittal MR scans, midpoint of line drawn between tuberculum sellae and torcular should intersect middle of fourth ventricle.

      b. On coronal MR scans, fourth ventricle looks like elongated rhomboid.

      c. On axial computed tomographic (CT) and MR scans, fourth ventricle looks like kidney bean turned on its side.

      d. CSF flow is mainly out through foramina of Luschka and Magendie.

B. Cerebral aqueduct (of Sylvius).

   1. Gross anatomy.

      a. Borders.

         (1) Anteriorly: periaqueductal gray matter of midbrain (tegmentum).

         (2) Posteriorly: tectum (quadrigeminal plate).

      b. Communicates:

         (1) Anterosuperiorly with third ventricle.

         (2) Posteroinferiorly with fourth ventricle.

   2. Radiology.

      a. On sagittal MR, has concavity that curves downward and forward toward floor of third ventricle.

      b. Flow void on MR scans without flow compensation represents area of high-velocity signal loss.

C. Third ventricle.

   1. Gross anatomy.

      a. Borders.

         (1) Lateral: thalami.

         (2) Anterior: anterior commissure and lamina terminalis.

         (3) Inferior: hypothalamus, infundibulum, optic chiasm, and mammillary bodies.

         (4) Posterior: pineal gland.

         (5) Superior: fornix, tela choroidea or velum interpositum, internal cerebral veins, and choroid plexus (transverse fissure).

      b. Communicates:

         (1) Posteroinferiorly with fourth ventricle via aqueduct.

         (2) Anterosuperiorly with lateral ventricle via foramen of Monro.

      c. Recesses.
        (1) Optic recess: V-shaped recess over optic chiasm.
        (2) Infundibular recess: shallower V-shaped recess bordered inferiorly by infundibular stalk and posteriorly by tuber cinereum of hypothalamus.
        (3) Suprapineal recess: tail-like posterior elongation above pineal gland.
      d. Projections into third ventricle.
        (1) By massa intermedia (interthalamic adhesion).
        (2) By infundibulum and optic chiasm below.
        (3) By anterior and posterior commissures in front and behind.
    2. Radiology.
      a. On sagittal MR or reformatted CT, elongated, complex curved shape with upward, backward, and downward arc.
      b. On axial scans, narrow CSF-filled cleft between thalami.
D. Interventricular foramina (of Monro): Y-shaped paramedian passage joining third ventricle to lateral ventricles.
    1. Gross anatomy.
      a. Borders.
        (1) Anterior: pillars (columns) of fornix and septum pellucidum.
        (2) Posterior: choroid plexus.
    2. Radiology: short Y-shaped CSF structure.
E. Lateral ventricles: complex C-shaped structures with frontal horn, body, trigone or atrium, and occipital and temporal horns. Relatively symmetric, paired lateral ventricles diverge from midline as they pass posteriorly.
    1. Gross anatomy.
      a. Borders (vary according to part of ventricle).
        (1) Superior: mostly corpus callosum.
        (2) Lateral: caudate nucleus.
        (3) Medial: septum pelliculum anteriorly, then fornix.
        (4) Inferior: choroid plexus, stria terminalis (between border of caudate nucleus and thalamus), thalamus, then hippocampus as it forms floor of temporal horn.
      b. Communicates inferiorly with third ventricle.
    2. Radiology.
      a. On sagittal MR scans, C-shaped CSF structure curving around thalamus.
      b. On axial MR and CT scans frontal horns are separated by septum pellucidum. Posteriorly, lateral ventricles diverge and pass into temporal and occipital lobes.

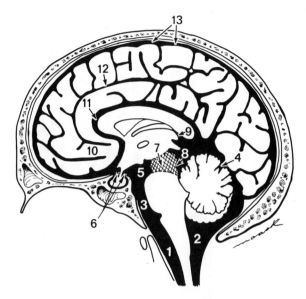

Fig. 30-2 Anatomic drawing of intracranial subarachnoid spaces and cisterns (in black). Wings of ambient cisterns (cross-hatched area) curve around mesencephalon and connect quadrigeminal to basal cisterns.

1. Medullary cistern
2. Cisterna magna
3. Pontine cistern
4. Superior cerebellar cistern
5. Interpeduncular cistern
6. Chiasmatic (suprasellar) cistern
7. Ambient cistern
8. Quadrigeminal plate cistern
9. Velum interpositum
10. Cistern of lamina terminalis
11. Pericallosal cistern
12. Cingulate sulcus
13. Convexity subarachnoid space

    c. On coronal CT and MR scans frontal horns are shaped somewhat like inverted triangles and body is more flattened; temporal horns look like **C** on its side.

3. Normal variations.

    a. Asymmetric size common.

    b. Coarcted or coapted parts of ventricles, particularly frontal and occipital horns, also common.

    c. Cavum septi pellucidi: nearly always present in fetus; potentially

Table 30-1 Major subarachnoid cisterns and their contents

Cistern	Location	Contents
POSTERIOR FOSSA CISTERNS		
Medullary cistern	Anterior to medulla	Vertebral arteries; anterior, posterior spinal arteries; CN XII
Cisterna magna	Posterior to medulla and clivus	Posterior inferior cerebellar artery; inferior cerebellar veins; CNs IX, X, XI
Pontine cistern	Between pons and clivus	Vertebrobasilar arteries; origins of anterior inferior cerebellar and superior cerebellar arteries; anterior pontomesencephalic venous plexus; CN VI
Cerebellopontine angle cistern	Between petrous temporal bone, cerebellum, pons, and tentorium	Anterior inferior cerebellar artery; sometimes superior petrosal veins; CNs V, VII, VIII
Superior cerebellar cistern	Between tentorium and vermis, cerebellar hemispheres; connects with quadrigeminal cistern anterosuperiorly	Superior cerebellar artery; superior vermian veins
SUPRASELLAR (BASAL) CISTERNS		
Interpeduncular cistern	Between cerebral peduncles	Basilar artery; origins of thalamoperforating and posterior choroidal arteries; CN III

Cistern	Location	Contents
Chiasmatic (suprasellar) cistern	Above sella	Distal internal carotid artery; origins of anterior and middle cerebral arteries; posterior communicating artery; anterior choroidal artery; proximal basal vein of Rosenthal; optic tracts, chiasm, CN II; hypothalamus infundibulum, mammillary bodies; anterior recesses of third ventricle
MESENCEPHALIC CISTERNS		
Ambient cistern	Around midbrain; connects suprasellar, pontine, and quadrigeminal cisterns	Posterior cerebral artery; basilar artery; superior cerebellar artery; CN IV; mesencephalic veins
Quadrigeminal cistern	Behind pineal and quadrigeminal plate; connects ambient and superior cerebellar cisterns	Pineal gland; posterior third ventricle; posterior choroidal artery; vein of Galen and basal vein of Rosenthal
Velum interpositum	Above third ventricle; below corpus callosum and fornix; anterior continuation of quadrigeminal cistern	Internal cerebral veins; branches of anterior and posterior choroidal arteries
LATERAL SUPERIOR CISTERNS		
Sylvian fissure	Between insula and opercula; connects medially with suprasellar cistern	Middle cerebral artery and its branches; superficial middle cerebral vein
Convexity subarachnoid spaces	Over surface of of hemispheres	Cortical arteries; veins

CN, Cranial nerve.

       CSF-filled space that can persist into adulthood and communicates with lateral ventricle.

    d. Cavum vergae: posterior extension of cavum septi pellucidi below corpus callosum and above fornix. Never seen in absence of cavum septi pellucidi.

    e. Cavum velum interpositum: anterior continuation of quadrigeminal cistern above third ventricle.

II. Subarachnoid cisterns (Fig. 30-2): These all interconnect. Via foramina of Luschka and Magendie, fourth ventricle communicates with subarachnoid space. Division of subarachnoid space into individual cisterns with their locations and contents is summarized in Table 30-1.

SUGGESTED READINGS

Amundsen P, Newton TH: Subarachnoid cisterns. In Newton TH, Potts DG (eds): *Radiology of the skull and brain, ventricles and cisterns,* St Louis, 1978, Mosby–Year Book, pp 3588-3711.

Jinkins JR: The cisternal ventricle, *AJNR* 9:111-113, 1988.

Malko JA, Hoffman JC Jr, Green RC: MR measurement of intracranial CSF volume in 41 elderly normal volunteers, *AJNR* 12:371-374, 1991.

Matsuno H, Rhoton AL Jr, Peace D: Microsurgical anatomy of the posterior fossa cisterns, *Neurosurgery* 23:58-80, 1988.

Pappas CTE, Sonntag VKH, Spetzler RF: Surgical anatomy of the anterior aspect of the third ventricle, *BNI Q* 6:2-10, 1990.

CHAPTER 31

Ventricles, cisterns, and subarachnoid spaces: abnormalities of ventricular shape, configuration, and position

KEY CONCEPTS

1. Congenital causes of misshapen or malpositioned ventricles include the holoprosencephalies, schizencephaly ("cleft brain"), agenesis of the corpus callosum, Chiari II malformation, and Dandy-Walker syndrome.
2. Abnormal configuration or deformation of the ventricles can also be seen with porencephaly, ventricular diverticula in severe obstructive hydrocephalus, heterotopic gray matter or subependymal hamartomas, Huntington's disease, and other conditions.
3. A nearby tumor, hematoma, or other intracranial mass can produce focal deformation of the ventricles; a remote mass effect with brain herniation is another cause of abnormal ventricular configuration or position.

I. Congenital and developmental: Some of these anomalies are considered in detail in Chapter 28. A brief summary that focuses on these abnormalities as they affect the ventricles follows.
   A. Holoprosencephaly: complex spectrum of congenital anomalies characterized by absent or partial cleavage and differentiation of the embryonic prosencephalon. There are three general types:
      1. Alobar: most severe form; large monoventricular cavity with dorsal cyst. No falx or interhemispheric fissure; fused thalami; multiple craniofacial anomalies such as cyclopia and cebocephaly. No corpus callosum or septum pellucidum.
      2. Semilobar: monoventricle more differentiated with partial formation of interhemispheric fissure. Rudimentary temporal and occipital horns often present. Thalami partially separated so that a small third

209

ventricle can sometimes be identified. Septum pellucidum and corpus callosum absent. NOTE: Enlarged hippocampal commissure can mimic corpus callosum splenium (see Chapter 28).

3. Lobar: further differentiation and hemispherization. Thalami separate. Some formation of falx, although anterior falx may be dysplastic. Corpus callosum usually absent; septum pellucidum absent.

B. Septooptic dysplasia.
1. Consists of:
   a. Hypoplasia of optic nerves.
   b. Absent or hypoplastic septum pellucidum.
   c. Hypothalamic-pituitary dysfunction commonly associated.
2. Computed tomography (CT) and magnetic resonance (MR).
   a. Absent or hypoplastic septum pellucidum.
   b. Frontal horns appear squared off or boxlike.
   c. Schizencephaly in 50%.
   d. Dysplastic ventricular dilatation with cerebral white matter hypoplasia may represent mild form of lobar holoprosencephaly.

C. Schizencephaly: full-thickness clefts extending from ventricle to brain surface and lined by gray matter, typically in region of sylvian fissure. May be unilateral or bilateral, symmetric or asymmetric; clefts can be open or closed ("open" or "closed" lip). Frequent gray matter heterotopias and foci of pachygyria and polymicrogyria shown clearly with MR.

D. Porencephaly: True porencephalic (literally "hole-in-the-brain") cysts are enclosed areas of encephalomalacic brain secondary to hemorrhage or infarction and should not be lined with ependyma even though they appear to be connected to the ventricles. Entrapment of cerebrospinal fluid (CSF) leads to mass effect. Polyporencephaly with isolated areas of bands and adhesions leading to compartmentalization of the ventricles results from severe brain infection, either ventriculitis or meningoencephalitis.

E. Corpus callosum agenesis: separated, parallel lateral ventricles with high-riding third ventricle. Twenty-five percent of children with corpus callosum agenesis have associated interhemispheric cysts that connect with third ventricle.

F. Chiari II malformation: ventricles often asymmetric with pointed or scalloped appearance. Fourth ventricle may be small, elongated, and low lying.

G. Dandy-Walker syndrome: fourth ventricle open posteriorly to large retrocerebellar cystic space. Cyst may herniate upward through tentorium, giving keyhole configuration. Trapped fourth ventricle and posterior fossa arachnoid cysts may also have this appearance. In both instances vermis is present, whereas it is absent in Dandy-Walker syndrome. Corpus callosum agenesis is frequently associated with Dandy-Walker malformation.

H. Dandy-Walker "variant": really not separate entity; belongs to spectrum of Dandy-Walker malformation. Hypoplasia of inferior vermis only with posterior slitlike space from fourth ventricle to cisterna magna.

I. Ventricular diverticula appear as CSF-containing outpouchings in cases of severe hydrocephalus. Medial atrial wall of lateral ventricle is common location.

J. Heterotopias and hamartomas can deform ventricular walls.

K. Huntington's disease is generalized degenerative process involving multiple structures, including basal ganglia, cerebral cortex, and thalamus. Although generalized cerebral atrophy can be seen, most characteristic CT or MR finding is focal caudate nucleus atrophy resulting in flat or outwardly convex margins of frontal horns.

II. Acquired: Focal mass effects — regardless of etiology — can deform or displace portions of ventricular system. In addition to focal deformations produced by such lesions as tumors and hematomas, generalized displacements of cerebral tissue (with accompanying CSF spaces) from one compartment to another occur.

A. Subfalcine herniation: Third and lateral ventricles are shifted under falx cerebri. Compression of ipsilateral lateral ventricle is typical. When herniation is severe, dilatation of contralateral ventricle occurs because of functional obstruction at foramen of Monro.

B. Descending or ascending transtentorial herniations: Herniation of cerebellar vermis upward through incisura can compress and displace cerebral aqueduct and posterior third ventricle. Sufficiently severe descending herniation can kink and depress aqueduct and medulla inferiorly. Unilateral descending herniation can also displace fourth ventricle away from side of mass as temporal lobe herniates into ipsilateral cerebellopontine angle cistern.

SUGGESTED READINGS

Barkovich AJ: Congenital malformations of the brain. In *Pediatric neuroimaging,* New York, 1990, Raven Press, pp 77-121.

Barkovich AJ, Kjos BO, Norman D, Edwards MS: Revised classification of posterior fossa cysts and cystlike malformations based on the results of multiplanar MR imaging, *AJNR* 10:977-988, 1989.

Barkovich AJ, Newton TH: MR of aqueductal stenosis: evidence of a broad spectrum of tectal distortion, *AJNR* 10:471-476, 1989.

Barkovich AJ, Norman D: MR imaging of schizencephaly, *AJNR* 9:297-302, 1988.

Chuang S, Harwood-Nash D: Tumors and cysts, *Neuroradiology* 28:463-475, 1986.

Manelfe C et al: Neuroradiology study of holoprosencephalies, *J Neuroradiol* 9:15-45, 1989.

Wolfson BJ, Faerber EN, Truex RC Jr: The "keyhole": a sign of herniation of a trapped fourth ventricle and other posterior fossa cysts, *AJNR* 8:473-477, 1987.

McGahan JP, Nyberg DA, Mack LA: Sonography of facial features of alobar and semilobar holoprosencephaly, *AJR* 154:143-148, 1990.

Sherman JL, Camponovo E, Citrin CM: MR imaging of CSF-like choroidal fissure and parenchymal cysts of the brain, *AJNR* 11:939-945, 1991.

CHAPTER 32

Ventricles: abnormalities of size

KEY CONCEPTS

1. Ventricular enlargement has four general causes: physiologic (caused by the normal aging process), obstructive (intraventricular or extraventricular), atrophic (reflecting parenchymal loss caused by a variety of insults), and possibly cerebrospinal fluid (CSF) overproduction (from choroid plexus papilloma, although this is debatable).
2. CSF flow phenomena can be depicted on magnetic resonance (MR) scans without flow compensation and cause striking variability in signal intensity in both normal and pathologic states.
3. Small ventricles are generally an unreliable indicator of intracranial pressure (ICP). Increased ICP is more accurately reflected by the appearance of the subarachnoid spaces and CSF cisterns.
4. Computed tomography (CT) may reveal the presence of hydrocephalus but not the cause. MR without and with contrast enhancement often delineates both the site and the nature of obstructive lesions. The periaqueductal area, posterior third ventricle, fourth ventricle, and cervical spinal cord should be carefully examined in cases of unexplained hydrocephalus.

I. Small ventricles.
  A. Normal: Some authors have attempted to define excessively small ventricles on CT, suggesting a bifrontal cerebral index less than 22%. This ratio of maximum width of anterior horns divided by transverse inner skull diameter at same level is usually about 30%. However, presence of small ventricles with otherwise normal-appearing CSF spaces probably represents part of normal spectrum. Normally ventricles increase slightly in size until 60 years of age, with relatively rapid enlargement thereafter.

B. Postshunt: Chronic overdrainage, also known as shunt dependency or slit-ventricle syndrome, is combination of chronic recurrent symptoms of increased ICP and partial or total collapse of shunted ventricles. CT or MR scans show shunted, slitlike ventricles.

C. Increased ICP: Ventricular size correlates relatively poorly with ICP. Since small ventricles can be normal, better indicator of increased ICP is effacement of subarachnoid spaces. Scans in patients with pseudotumor cerebri or benign intracranial hypertension are usually normal.

D. Pseudotumor cerebri: ventricles normal; subarachnoid spaces may appear slightly prominent but do not differ significantly from normal. Role of CT and MR is primarily to exclude other diseases with presentations similar to idiopathic intracranial hypertension (pseudotumor cerebri).

II. Ventricular enlargement: can be physiologic, atrophic, obstructive, or due to CSF overproduction. Term "hydrocephalus" is usually reserved for dynamic processes resulting from CSF flow blockage or CSF overproduction. Intraventricular obstructive hydrocephalus (IVOH, or noncommunicating hydrocephalus) refers to obstruction of CSF flow anywhere from lateral ventricles to fourth ventricular outlet foramina. Extraventricular obstructive hydrocephalus (EVOH, or communicating hydrocephalus) refers to obstruction distal to ventricular system. MR has improved accuracy of diagnosis in patients with hydrocephalus because of its ability to show small obstructing lesions not depicted by CT, delineate ventricular anatomy more precisely, and elucidate CSF flow phenomena in both normal and hydrocephalic states. CSF flow is related to cardiac systole. On non-flow-compensated T2-weighted MR scans, flow-related signal dropout causes striking heterogeneity in intensity of CSF. Hypointensity is most pronounced where large CSF volume moves through small space such as cerebral aqueduct, third and fourth ventricles, or foramen of Magendie. This is most apparent during time at which systemic arterial pulse wave is transmitted to brain. Presence of CSF flow void sign is useful indicator of ventricular pathway patency but cannot reliably be used to distinguish patients with brain atrophy from those with EVOH. Absence of CSF flow void sign may indicate obstruction but must be correlated with other signs and technical factors (such as cardiac gating) to be interpreted correctly.

A. Normal.
1. Slight physiologic increase in ventricular size normally occurs with age (see preceding).
2. Premature infants also often have mildly enlarged ventricles.

B. Congenital.
1. Occlusion at foramen of Monro is usually acquired (see "Infection"). Congenital atresia is extremely rare.
2. Aqueductal stenosis: On CT or MR, lateral and third ventricles are enlarged whereas fourth ventricle is normal. CAUTION: MR imaging

should be performed in all such cases to rule out periaqueductal, posterior third ventricular, or posterior fossa obstructing lesion.

   3. Chiari II and Dandy-Walker malformations may have associated hydrocephalus. Enlarged ventricles without evidence of abnormal CSF dynamics may simply reflect dysplasia associated with malformation.

   4. Colpocephaly: Occipital horns are disproportionately large compared with remainder of ventricular system. This frequently occurs with other abnormalities such as corpus callosum agenesis.

C. Vascular and metabolic.

   1. Atrophic enlargement of lateral ventricles has variety of causes, including aging, multiinfarct dementia, posttraumatic or postinflammatory encephalomalacia, alcoholism or drug abuse, long-term steroid use, radiation therapy and chemotherapy, and deprivational states. CT shows proportionate sulcal-cisternal and ventricular enlargement. Temporal horns may be slightly enlarged but are typically less prominent than those seen with either EVOH or IVOH.

   2. With subarachnoid or intraventricular hemorrhage, obstructive hydrocephalus may occur within few hours.

D. Infection.

   1. Ependymitis or ventriculitis can produce IVOH (e.g., foramen of Monro obstruction). Look for associated ependymal enhancement.

   2. With meningitis, ventricular enlargement can occur either as result of arachnoid block (EVOH or communicating hydrocephalus) or, later, from encephalomalacia (atrophic, or ex vacuo, changes). Encystment of ventricle or part of it when its CSF outlets are occluded because of ependymal reaction after intraventricular hemorrhage or infection is uncommon but clinically important. "Trapped fourth ventricle" occurs with isolated obstruction of central aqueduct and fourth ventricular outlet foramina. Isolated fourth ventricle should be distinguished from posterior fossa cysts and cystic tumors. In former, fourth ventricle is compressed and displaced, whereas with entrapment an enlarged rounded CSF space is present in usual location of fourth ventricle. With cystic astrocytomas, foci of contrast enhancement can often be identified.

E. Neoplasms and related conditions.

   1. Colloid cyst: These typically appear as well-delineated high-attenuation or high-signal lesions at foramen of Monro (see Chapter 33). Lateral ventricles are enlarged; third and fourth ventricles are usually normal.

   2. Intraventricular tumors: Choroid plexus papilloma can have panventricular enlargement. Some authors ascribe this to overproduction of CSF, whereas others believe it is secondary to intraventricular hem-

orrhage from neoplasm. NOTE: Intraventricular or paraventricular neoplasms can produce focal obstruction ("entrapment") of ventricular segment. Other intraventricular or paraventricular neoplasms can produce IVOH (see Chapter 33). Increased signal around ventricles on T2-weighted MR scans reflects transependymal CSF flow.

3. Extraventricular tumors of sufficient size can also produce IVOH (e.g., large pituitary adenoma with foramen of Monro obstruction).

F. Miscellaneous: Focal enlargement of part or all of ventricle can occur with inflammatory or neoplastic entrapment (see preceding). Focal parenchymal loss from surgery, trauma, infarction, or miscellaneous abnormalities such as Pick's or Huntington's disease can result in segmental ventricular enlargement. Cerebral hemiatrophy, or Dyke-Davidoff-Masson syndrome, can be congenital or acquired and is characterized on CT by unilateral loss of brain substance (enlarged lateral ventricle and sulci), thickened calvarium, overdevelopment of ipsilateral paranasal sinuses, and elevation of petrous ridge.

SUGGESTED READINGS

Bradley WG Jr, Kortman KE, Burgoyne B: Flowing cerebrospinal fluid in normal and hydrocephalic states: appearance on MR images, *Radiology* 159:611-616, 1986.

Bradley WG Jr, Whittemore AR, Kortman KE, et al: Marked cerebrospinal fluid void: indicator of successful shunt in patients with suspected normal pressure hydrocephalus, *Radiology* 178:459-466, 1991.

Britton J, Marsh H, Kendall B, Kingsley D: MRI and hydrocephalus in childhood, *Neuroradiology* 30:310-314, 1988.

Citrin CM, Sherman JL, Gangarosa RE, Scanlon D: Physiology of the CSF flow-void sign, *AJNR* 7:1021-1024, 1986.

El Gammal T, Allen MB Jr, Brooks BS, Mark EK: MR evaluation of hydrocephalus, *AJNR* 8:591-597, 1987.

Enzmann DR, Pelc NJ: Normal patterns of intracranial and spinal cerebrospinal fluid defined with phase-contrast cine MR imaging, *Radiology* 178:467-474, 1991.

Jack CR Jr: Brain and cerebrospinal fluid volume: measurement with MR imaging, *Radiology* 178:22-24, 1991.

Jinkins JR: Clinical manifestations of hydrocephalus caused by impingement of the corpus callosum on the falx, *AJNR* 12:331-340, 1991.

Kohn MI, Tanna NK, Herman GT, et al: Analysis of brain and cerebrospinal fluid volumes with MR imaging, *Radiology* 178:115-122, 1991.

Sherman JL, Citrin CM, Bowen BJ, Gangarosa RE: MR demonstration of altered cerebrospinal fluid flow by obstructing lesions, *AJNR* 7:571-579, 1986.

Sherman JL, Citrin CM, Gangarosa RE, Bowen BJ: The MR appearance of CSF flow in patients with ventriculomegaly, *AJNR* 7:1025-1031, 1986.

Silbergleit R, Junck L, Gebarski SS, Hatfield MK: Idiopathic intracranial hypertension (pseudotumor cerebri): MR imaging, *Radiology* 170:207-209, 1989.

CHAPTER 33

Ventricles, cisterns, and subarachnoid spaces: intraventricular masses

KEY CONCEPTS

1. The most common intraventricular mass is a choroid plexus cyst.
2. Colloid cysts are rare in children.
3. Only 1% of meningiomas are intraventricular.
4. Most supratentorial ependymomas are extraventricular.

I. Congenital or developmental.
  A. Neuroepithelial cysts: Autopsy studies commonly show presence of neuroepithelial inclusions throughout neuraxis in all age groups. Most inclusions are small and asymptomatic. Neuroepithelial inclusion cysts can occur anywhere along neuraxis; they may be intraparenchymal, intraventricular, extraaxial, or even occasionally intraosseous. Most cysts arise from choroid plexus, commonly in atrium of lateral ventricle, or from ependyma of third ventricle adjacent to foramen of Monro.
    1. Colloid cyst.
      a. Origin: controversial but thought to arise from primitive neuroepithelium of tela choroidea.
      b. Considered congenital lesion but rarely seen in children.
      c. Location: anterior part of third ventricle, typically at foramen of Monro.
      d. Pathology: homogeneous-appearing amorphous eosinophilic substance ("colloid") lined with cuboidal cylindrical cells and outer layer of connective tissue that includes vessels.
      e. Contents: variable (mucoid materials, cholesterol, fat, cerebrospinal fluid [CSF], desquamated cells).
      f. CT: variable.

(1) Non-contrast-enhanced CT: isodense or hyperdense most common but can occasionally be hypodense.

(2) Contrast-enhanced CT: usually no enhancement, but occasionally thin rim of peripheral enhancement discernible.

(3) Hydrocephalus common (moderate symmetric enlargement of lateral ventricle).

(4) Splaying of posterior frontal horns around cyst is typical.

g. MR: highly variable; more heterogeneous than on CT.

(1) Hyperintensity on T1-weighted imaging (T1WI) correlates with high cholesterol content.

(2) Marked T2 shortening often present in central part of cyst.

2. Choroid plexus cysts.

   a. Most common intraventricular mass (seen in approximately 1% of fetal ultrasound scans but common in all ages).

   b. Usually small, asymptomatic, incidentally seen (up to 50% of some autopsy series).

   c. Reported association with trisomy 18 and trisomy 21.

   d. May occur anywhere, but typical location is glomera of lateral ventricles.

   e. MR: cystic collection within choroid plexus glomus; signal similar to CSF (can be slightly hyperintense).

3. Ependymal (neuroepithelial) cyst.

   a. Density and signal similar to CSF; cyst wall easily seen on MR.

   b. Can be found in any ventricle, typically in third ventricle or atria of lateral ventricle.

   c. Differential diagnosis: cysticercosis cysts (usually multiple, associated with parenchymal or cisternal cysts; may change position), epidermoid tumors (usually extraaxial but may occur in fourth ventricle or temporal horns; surface irregular or frondlike; signal on MR similar to that of CSF), *Echinococcus* cysts (intraventricular location exceedingly rare).

B. Disorders of histogenesis.

1. Tuberous sclerosis (see Chapter 29).

   a. Paraventricular foci of gemistocytic astrocytes form characteristic subependymal nodules that frequently calcify.

   b. Giant cell astrocytoma develops in 10%, typically adjacent to foramen of Monro. Any tuber that shows enhancement with contrast media should be considered neoplastic until proved otherwise.

2. Sturge-Weber disease (see Chapter 29): ipsilateral choroid plexus enlargement in 70%.

C. Disorders of organogenesis: heterotopic gray matter (abnormality of cellular migration).
1. Subependymal neuronal and glial nodules.
2. Isodense on CT, isointense with gray matter on MR.
3. Frequently associated with other congenital anomalies.
II. Vascular.
A. Vascular malformations.
1. Arteriovenous malformations (see Chapter 14).
a. Dilated arterial feeders, draining veins, and venous varices may project into ventricles.
b. Sometimes arise in choroid plexus.
B. Hematoma.
1. Congenital: Germinal plate hemorrhage in premature infant can produce intraventricular clot.
2. Trauma: choroid plexus and intraventricular hemorrhage.
3. Hypertension: Basal ganglionic hemorrhage can dissect into ventricles.
III. Inflammatory.
A. Cysticercosis.
1. Central nervous system (CNS) involvement in 60% to 90%.
2. Can be parenchymal, meningobasal, spinal, or intraventricular.
3. Intraventricular cysts in 25% to 50% of patients.
4. CT and MR.
a. Fourth ventricle most commonly affected, although can occur anywhere.
b. Striking cyst mobility may be present.
c. Mural nodule can be identified on MR; cyst wall hyperintense on T2-weighted image; cyst contents generally similar to CSF.
d. Mass effect, obstructive hydrocephalus, and pericystic ependymal inflammatory reaction may be present.
e. Basilar meningeal enhancement may occur.
f. May appear as low-density-signal, ring-enhancing lesion on either CT or MR.
B. Trapped (isolated) ventricle.
1. Can occur anywhere; typically fourth ventricle.
2. Focal enlargement of affected ventricle sac.
3. MR can demonstrate slight differences in trapped fluid signal and subtle changes of associated ventriculitis.
IV. Neoplasms: Ten percent of CNS neoplasms are partly or completely intraventricular. In a recent series, most common lateral ventricular neoplasms were choroid plexus papillomas and meningiomas, followed by subependymomas, subependymal giant cell astrocytomas, and metastasis or lymphoma. Histologic findings:

A. Primary.
   1. Astrocytoma.
      a. Most common intraventricular location is frontal horn. Cystic cerebellar astrocytomas in children may be seen as fourth ventricular masses.
      b. Giant cell astrocytomas are typically located at foramen of Monro, usually associated with tuberous sclerosis. Another tumor that occurs at this location is pilocytic astrocytoma.
      c. Oligodendrogliomas may be purely intraventricular.
   2. Meningioma.
      a. One percent of meningiomas are intraventricular.
      b. Atrium of lateral ventricle most common location.
      c. Frequently calcified.
   3. Ependymoma and subependymoma.
      a. Infratentorial ependymomas typically arise in and expand fourth ventricle. Often partially calcified, cystic, with heterogeneous MR signal and enhancement.
      b. Supratentorial ependymomas most often occur outside ventricles; when intraventricular, atrium or frontal horn of lateral ventricles is most common site.
      c. Subependymomas in older patients: body of lateral ventricle (frontal horn), fourth ventricle.
   4. Craniopharyngioma: Rarely, craniopharyngioma can arise entirely within third ventricle.
   5. Medulloblastoma.
      a. Hyperdense fourth ventricular mass on nonenhanced CT; strong, uniform enhancement.
      b. MR: isointense or hypointense on T1WI; usually enhanced strongly.
      c. Calcification, hemorrhage, and cyst formation may occur but are rare.
   6. Choroid plexus papilloma (CPP) and carcinoma.
      a. First decade of life (lateral ventricular tumor in child younger than 5 years of age is usually CPP).
      b. Atrium of lateral ventricle most common location.
      c. Isodense or hyperdense on nonenhanced CT; strong, uniform enhancement after contrast media administration.
      d. MR: mixed isointense and hypointense, strong enhancement.
      e. Nonobstructive hydrocephalus (from overproduction of CSF?) common.
      f. Carcinomas uncommon (1 in 10 choroid plexus neoplasms); tend to show adjacent parenchymal invasion with surrounding edema.
   7. Epidermoid tumor.

   a. Typically extraaxial; often found in cerebellopontine angle;
      when intraventricular, usually seen within fourth ventricle.
   b. Rarely calcify.
   c. Low attenuation on CT.
   d. MR signal intensity usually similar to CSF.
8. Dermoid tumor.
   a. Fourth ventricle or midline extraaxial location, often suprasellar.
   b. Low attenuation on CT, fat signal on MR most common.
   c. Occasionally calcify; usually no enhancement.
   d. Ruptured cyst may produce striking fluid and fat levels in ventri-
      cles.
9. Primitive neuroectodermal tumor.
   a. Body of lateral ventricle, frontal horn.
   b. Age: less than 5 years.
   c. Appearance: often bulky mass, partially calcified; cysts and
      hemorrhage common; patchy contrast enhancement.
V. Differential diagnosis (see boxes below and opposite).

COMMON LATERAL VENTRICULAR MASSES

FORAMEN OF MONRO

Adult: colloid cyst, metastasis
Child: subependymal giant cell astrocytoma, pilocytic astrocytoma

TRIGONE AND ATRIUM

Adult or child: choroid plexus and neuroepithelial (noncolloidal) cysts
Child less than 5 years: choroid plexus papilloma
Older child: ependymoma
Adult: meningioma

BODY OF LATERAL VENTRICLE

Child less than 5 years: choroid plexus papilloma, primitive neuroectodermal
   tumor, teratoma
Older child: ependymoma, pilocytic astrocytoma
Adult: subependymoma, glioblastoma, lymphoma, metastasis, neuroepithelial
   (noncolloidal) cyst

ANY LOCATION

Cysticercosis cyst

COMMON THIRD VENTRICULAR MASSES

FORAMEN OF MONRO

Adult: colloid cyst, metastases
Child: subependymal giant cell astrocytoma, pilocytic astrocytoma, neurofibromatosis

ANTERIOR RECESSES AND INFERIOR THIRD VENTRICLE (INTRINSIC OR EXTRINSIC)

Adult: pituitary adenoma, lymphoma, metastasis, aneurysm, meningioma
Child: germinoma, histiocytosis X, glioma, craniopharyngioma

BODY OF THIRD VENTRICLE

Child: choroid plexus papilloma
Adult: glioma

POSTERIOR THIRD VENTRICLE

Child: pineal tumor, glioma, vascular malformation
Adult: pineal tumor, vertebrobasilar ectasia or aneurysm

ANYWHERE

Cysticercosis cyst, ependymal cyst

COMMON FOURTH VENTRICULAR MASSES

BODY

Child: ependymoma, medulloblastoma, astrocytoma (from brainstem or cerebellum), cysticercosis
Adult: dermoid or epidermoid tumor, cysticercosis, metastases

LATERAL RECESSES

Child: ependymoma
Adult: choroid plexus papilloma

INFERIOR FOURTH VENTRICLE AND OBEX

Child: glioma
Adult: subependymoma, metastases

SUGGESTED READINGS

Barloon TJ, Yuh WTC, Knepper LE, et al: Cerebral ventriculitis: MR findings, *J Comput Assist Tomogr* 14:272-275, 1990.

Ciricillo SF, Davis RL, Wilson CB: Neuroepithelial cysts of the posterior fossa, *J Neurosurg* 72:302-305, 1990.

Czervionke LF, Daniels DL, Meyer GA, et al: Neuroepithelial cysts of the lateral ventricles: MR appearance, *AJNR* 8:609-613, 1987.

Jelenik J, Smirniotopoulos JG, Parisi JE, Kanzer M: Lateral ventricular neoplasms of the brain, *AJNR* 11:567-574, 1990.

Maeder PP, Holtas SL, Basibuyuk LN: Colloid cysts of the third ventricle, *AJNR* 11:575-581, 1990.

Ostlere SJ, Irving HC, Wilford RJ: Fetal choroid plexus cysts: a report of 100 cases, *Radiology* 175:753-755, 1990.

Teitelbaum GP, Otto RJ, Lin M, et al: MR imaging of neurocysticercosis, *AJNR* 10:709-718, 1989.

CHAPTER 34

Ventricles, cisterns, and subarachnoid spaces: ependymal enhancement

KEY CONCEPTS

1. Subtle ependymal abnormalities may be more easily detected on contrast-enhanced computed tomography (CT) than T2-weighted scan (T2WI) unless magnetic resonance (MR) contrast material is used and T1-weighted studies (T1WI) are performed.
2. The major differential diagnosis of abnormal ependymal enhancement is inflammatory versus neoplastic disease.

Contrast enhancement of the ventricular ependyma on CT or MR is a nonspecific finding. Although some normal structures within or adjacent to the ventricles may superficially resemble abnormal ependymal enhancement, they are easily distinguished. With ependymal enhancement, the major differential diagnosis is typically between inflammatory and neoplastic disease.

I. Normal.
  A. Vascular structures: Enhancement around lateral margins of lateral ventricles can be normal (e.g., lateral atrial, caudate, and thalamostriate veins); enhancement of occipital horns is not. Normal enhancement is patchy or discontinuous; complete contiguous ependymal enhancement after administration of contrast material is abnormal.
    1. Subependymal veins on contrast-enhanced CT and MR (particularly if flow compensation is used) may give appearance of segmental ependymal enhancement.
    2. Choroid plexus, particularly in temporal horns and fourth ventricle, may superficially resemble ependymal enhancement.
  B. Periventricular: Mild subependymal and periventricular increased MR

signal on T2WI can normally be seen in elderly patients; continuous linear or nodular enhancement on T1WI after contrast material is administered is abnormal.

II. Abnormal.
  A. Vascular malformations.
    1. Arteriovenous malformations: Periventricular arteries and veins may become engorged. Flow void on MR is common.
    2. Venous angioma: "Medusa head" of medullary subependymal veins with enlarged transcortical draining vein can appear as enhancing lesion (typically at frontal horn or margin of lateral ventricle) on CT, flow void on MR, or area of increased signal on contrast-enhanced scans with flow compensation techniques develop.
    3. Dural sinus occlusion and cortical vein thrombosis may enlarge subependymal veins as collateral venous drainage pathways.
    4. Sturge-Weber syndrome: Paucity of normal cortical venous drainage under leptomeningeal angioma may lead to enlarged medullary and subependymal veins.
  B. Inflammatory.
    1. Ventriculitis, ependymitis (e.g., after shunt placement, meningitis, intrathecal chemotherapy).
    2. Meningitis or abscess rupture into ventricles can produce ventriculitis and ependymal enhancement as complication.
    3. Inflammatory cyst with rupture.
  C. Neoplastic: Subtle ependymal or subependymal disease may be more easily seen on contrast-enhanced CT than routine nonenhanced MR, since T2 lengthening typically produced may be indistinguishable from cerebrospinal fluid (CSF) signal on T2WI. Subtle ependymal enhancement can be detected on contrast-enhanced T1WI. Wide variety of disseminated meningeal malignant neoplasms, including metastatic carcinoma, lymphoma, and primary brain tumor, may have subependymal involvement. Periventricular tumor spread is manifest on both CT and MR as areas of either diffuse or nodular contrast enhancement surrounding part or all of ventricular system. Relatively high percentage of patients with proven disseminated meningeal neoplasms have no abnormalities visible on contrast-enhanced CT scans. Although MR with contrast material is more sensitive for ependymal and leptomeningeal disease, it too can be falsely negative (a recent series showed 36% sensitivity for proven leptomeningeal metastases).
    1. Primary intracranial tumors that can spread along ependymal surfaces.
      a. Pineal neoplasms (typically germinoma or pineoblastoma).
      b. Medulloblastoma, primitive neuroectodermal tumors.

c. Ependymoma.

d. Astrocytoma (high-grade astrocytoma or glioblastoma multiforme; rarely oligodendroglioma).

e. Choroid plexus tumors.

f. Lymphoma.

2. Metastatic tumors.

   a. Most commonly from breast, lung, or melanoma.

   b. Retinoblastoma (more commonly sulcal or cisternal enhancement).

3. Lymphoma, leukemia: Central nervous system involvement with lymphoma and leukemia is common, yet CT and MR abnormalities in these patients are relatively infrequent. Ventricular enhancement may also be related to shunt tube placement and intrathecal chemotherapy.

III. Differential diagnosis (see box below).

DIFFERENTIAL DIAGNOSIS OF EPENDYMAL AND SUBEPENDYMAL ENHANCEMENT

1. Normal (never complete contiguous enhancement)
2. Vascular
   a. Afferent and efferent vessels with vascular malformation
   b. Collateral venous drainage (dural sinus or cortical vein occlusion; Sturge-Weber syndrome)
3. Inflammatory
   a. Chemical ventriculitis (e.g. from shunt placement, intrathecal chemotherapy)
   b. Meningitis, abscess rupture
   c. Inflammatory cyst rupture
4. Primary intracranial neoplasm
   a. Pineal tumors (germinoma, pineoblastoma)
   b. Medulloblastoma
   c. Ependymoma
   d. Astrocytoma (malignant, glioblastoma)
   e. Choroid plexus neoplasm
   f. Lymphoma
5. Metastatic (extracranial primary)
   a. Retinoblastoma, ocular melanoma (more often leptomeningeal metastases)
   b. Extracranial: most commonly breast, lung, melanoma

SUGGESTED READINGS

Barloon TJ, Yuh WTC, Knepper LE, et al: Cerebral ventriculitis: MR findings, *J Comput Assist Tomogr* 14:272-275, 1990.

Hudgins PA, Davis PC, Hoffman JC Jr: Gadopentetate dimeglumine–enhanced MR imaging in children following surgery for brain tumor: spectrum of meningeal findings, *AJNR* 12:301-307, 1991.

Murray PA, Harnett AN, Thompson J, et al: Periventricular enhancement: a non-pathognomonic sign of intracerebral tumors, *Br J Radiol* 62:1075-1078, 1989.

Rippe DJ, Borko OB, Friedman HS, et al: Gd-DTPA-enhanced MR imaging of leptomeningeal spread of primary intracranial CNS tumor in children, *AJNR* 11:329-332, 1990.

Yousem DM, Patrone PM, Grossman RI: Leptomeningeal metastases: MR evaluation, *J Comput Assist Tomogr* 14:255-261, 1990.

CHAPTER 35

Ventricles, cisterns, and subarachnoid spaces: meningeal disease processes

---

KEY CONCEPTS

1. *Any* process that causes meningeal irritation can cause meningeal enhancement.
2. The differential diagnosis of meningeal enhancement on computed tomography (CT) and magnetic resonance (MR) includes:
   a. Normal
   b. Inflammatory disease
   c. Leptomeningeal metastases
   d. Benign meningeal fibrosis (e.g., postoperative)
   e. Trauma
3. If possible, cisternal and leptomeningeal enhancement should be distinguished from gyral enhancement because the differential diagnoses for these two findings are distinct.

Contrast enhancement of the meninges is a nonspecific finding. When abnormal, the basal and peritentorial cisterns (see Chapter 30) appear filled by intensely enhancing leptomeninges; this can superficially resemble subarachnoid hemorrhage as seen on noncontrast CT scans. Less frequently the sylvian cisterns, interhemispheric fissure, posterior fossa cisterns, and superficial sulci are affected. Leptomeningeal enhancement should be distinguished from gyral enhancement. Although these two processes may occasionally be associated, their differential diagnostic spectra are usually quite different. With leptomeningeal enhancement the differential diagnosis is usually a normal or inflammatory-reactive condition versus neoplastic disease.

I. Normal.
  A. Dura and meninges.
    1. Dural structures such as falx and tentorium normally appear slightly

more dense than adjacent brain or cerebrospinal fluid (CSF) on non-contrast CT scans.

2. Obliquely sectioned but normal dural structures (such as tentorium) and their venous tributaries can sometimes appear bizarre on contrast-enhanced CT scans.

3. Enhancement of dura (e.g., falx, tentorium, lateral cavernous sinus walls) is normal on both CT and MR.

4. Some enhancement of leptomeninges on contrast-enhanced MR scans is normal. Leptomeningeal enhancement should be:
   a. Thin (less than 1 mm).
   b. Smooth and linear.
   c. Discontinuous (focal; occurs in short segments).
   d. Of minimal intensity, most striking at vertex and anterior temporal lobe, little around sides and base of brain (exception: cavernous sinus).
   e. Somewhat less intense than cavernous sinus signal.

5. Abnormal leptomeningeal enhancement.
   a. Thick.
   b. Focal nodularity.
   c. Continuous.
   d. Base of brain.
   e. As bright as or brighter than cavernous sinus.

B. Vessels.

1. Arteries and veins within cisterns and subarachnoid spaces are normally slightly more dense than CSF on noncontrast CT scans.

2. If CT scans are obtained too quickly after contrast administration, strong intravascular enhancement can mimic leptomeningeal disease. In such questionable cases, careful examination of basal cisterns (including interpeduncular fossa) discloses normal CSF around strikingly enhanced vessels.

3. Contrast enhancement in small vessels with slow flow can mimic leptomeningeal enhancement on MR scans if T1-weighted imaging (T1WI) is performed with flow compensation.

II. Subarachnoid hemorrhage (SAH) and trauma (see Chapters 13 and 45).

A. Acute SAH.

1. CSF cisterns appear opacified on nonenhanced CT (approximately 66 Hounsfield units for 100% blood).

2. May be difficult to see on MR, since blood in acute SAH has relaxation times similar to those of normal brain.

3. Intensity of blood on T1WI typically increases with time because of conversion to methemoglobin.

B. Subacute SAH.

1. Cisternal enhancement can occur up to several weeks after SAH,

possibly representing initial inflammatory response or increased vascular permeability caused by arachnoiditis.

    2. Increased intensity of CSF on MR probably represents methemoglobin formation with T1 shortening.

  C. Chronic SAH.

    1. Rarely, superficial pial siderosis is caused by repeated episodes of SAH and can be manifest as abnormal contrast enhancement of leptomeninges.

    2. Superficial and subependymal siderosis appears as hypointense foci in ventricular and subpial regions on MR scans. This hemosiderin effect is most striking on T2-weighted studies and gradient echo scans.

  D. Previous trauma: Meningeal or parenchymal enhancement adjacent to resolving hematoma can occur; chronic subdural hematoma or effusion can have associated fibrous membrane that is enhanced by contrast material.

III. Inflammatory disease (see Chapter 37).

  A. Bacterial meningitis.

    1. General: Density may be increased in basal cisterns, interhemispheric fissure, and other subarachnoid spaces because of meningeal hypervascularity and fibrinous or hemorrhagic exudate. Contrast enhancement may be striking; coexisting gyral and ependymal enhancement can also occur if underlying cerebritis or ventriculitis is present. Contrast-enhanced MR is superior to CT in evaluation of patients with suspected meningitis; precontrast studies are needed to delineate hemorrhagic conditions such as infarction.

    2. Meningovascular syphilis is characterized by widespread lymphocytic infiltration of meninges and perivascular spaces with arteritis but is most often seen as multifocal ischemic infarcts.

  B. Granulomatous meningitis.

    1. Tuberculous meningitis may obliterate basilar cisterns with thick fibrinous exudate that is isodense and isointense with brain on both CT and MR; striking enhancement occurs after contrast material is administered. Hydrocephalus, parenchymal tuberculomas, and infarcts secondary to arterial narrowing and stenosis can be associated conditions.

    2. Fungal meningitis can be indistinguishable from bacterial or tuberculous meningitis.

    3. Neurosarcoidosis has protean manifestations. Between 1% and 5% of patients with systemic sarcoidosis have clinical evidence of central nervous system (CNS) involvement; 14% to 16% prevalence is seen at autopsy. Hydrocephalus is most common abnormality. Sarcoid can also cause a focal or diffuse granulomatous meningoen-

cephalitis with predilection for pituitary infundibulum, optic chiasm, and cranial nerves. Parenchymal enhancing masses sometimes are seen, particularly at base of brain. Extraaxial masses mimicking meningioma have been reported, as has gyral enhancement with nodular and linear enhancing foci extending from cortex into deep white matter along Virchow-Robin spaces. On MR, most sarcoid deposits are hyperintense on T2WI and are typically subfrontal meningeal or hypothalamic-suprasellar lesions. Leptomeningeal sarcoidosis is strongly enhanced by contrast material.

C. Viral meningitis: Herpes simplex encephalitis can have minimal contrast enhancement in meningeal pattern, but patchy, widespread, low-attenuation, parenchymal foci are most characteristic early findings, particularly in children. In adults with herpes simplex encephalitis, temporal lobes are most commonly affected.

D. Rheumatoid pachymeningitis.
   1. Extraarticular features of rheumatoid arthritis are common, but CNS involvement is rare.
   2. Meningeal involvement is more common than parenchymal disease, but both have been reported.
   3. Leptomeningeal enhancement on CT has been attributed to increased vascularity resulting from associated inflammatory reaction.
   4. Focal granulomatous masses in dura, subdural spaces, and leptomeninges can be seen, mimicking meningioma.

E. Miscellaneous.
   1. Histiocytosis X can cause diffuse or nodular leptomeningeal enhancement.
   2. Diffuse benign leptomeningeal thickening or fibrosis commonly follows craniotomy, shunt placement, intrathecal chemotherapy, and other invasive procedures. This probably represents form of chemical meningitis and does not necessarily indicate tumor or infection.
   3. Idiopathic hypertrophic cranial pachymeningitis is rare disease manifest as dural thickening along falx and tentorium. Dural sinus occlusion and cranial nerve palsies may be present.

IV. Infarction: Mild enhancement of meninges adjacent to subacute infarction has been reported.

V. Neoplastic disease: Clinical diagnosis of disseminated meningeal malignant neoplasms is often difficult. Imaging studies are frequently normal or nonspecific. Recent study reports that leptomeningeal metastases may be so subtle or inapparent as to be overlooked with MR imaging even with contrast enhancement.

A. Meningioma may have dural thickening and prominent enhancement far beyond area of focal tumor.

B. Primary brain tumors such as medulloblastoma (posterior fossa primi-

DIFFERENTIAL DIAGNOSIS: MENINGEAL ENHANCEMENT

1. Normal
   a. Thin
   b. Smooth
   c. Discontinuous
   d. Mostly near vertex
   e. Not as intense as cavernous sinus
2. Hemorrhage
   a. Subacute subarachnoid hemorrhage
   b. Pial siderosis or fibrosis
3. Infection or inflammation
   a. Bacterial meningitis (including syphilis)
   b. Granulomatous meningitis
      (1) Tuberculous
      (2) Fungal
      (3) Sarcoid
   c. Viral (uncommon)
   d. Rheumatoid
   e. Benign leptomeningeal fibrosis
      (1) Surgery
      (2) Shunt
      (3) Chemotherapy
   f. Miscellaneous
      (1) Histiocytosis X
      (2) Idiopathic hypertrophic cranial pachymeningitis
4. Infarction: mild meningeal enhancement overlying area of subacute infarction
5. Neoplasm
   a. Primary meningeal neoplasm: meningioma
   b. Primary central nervous system tumors with potential for leptomeningeal spread
      (1) Malignant astrocytoma
      (2) Pineal tumors
      (3) Medulloblastoma
      (4) Ependymoma
      (5) Choroid plexus neoplasm
      (6) Lymphoma
   c. Orbital tumors with leptomeningeal spread
      (1) Reticuloblastoma
      (2) Ocular melanoma
   d. Metastatic extracranial tumors (lung, breast, melanoma, lymphoproliferative malignancies most common)
   e. Paraneoplastic syndrome

tive neuroectodermal tumor), ependymoma, astrocytoma (in brain or even spinal cord), choroid plexus tumors, and primary CNS lymphoma can all seed subarachnoid space. Pineal tumors (germ cell line neoplasm such as germinoma, embryonal cell carcinoma, teratocarcinoma, and pineal parenchymal tumors such as pineoblastoma) can have CSF dissemination. Retinoblastoma and ocular melanoma also have a predilection for cisternal spread.

C. Carcinomas (e.g., breast, lung, gastric) can have following findings indicative of leptomeningeal metastases:
   1. Sulcal-cisternal enhancement.
   2. Ependymal-subependymal enhancement.
   3. Abnormal tentorial enhancement. (Some authors distinguish between *lepto*meningeal [i.e., pia-arachnoid metastasis] and *pachy*-meningeal [i.e., dural carcinomatosis]. Latter is usually associated with adjacent calvarial metastases.)
   4. Communicating hydrocephalus.

D. Lymphoproliferative malignancies (e.g., lymphoma, leukemia) can have leptomeningeal enhancement on MR or CT. Both are often normal even in presence of CSF cytologic evidence of neoplasm.

E. Dural carcinomatosis can mimic subacute or chronic subdural hematoma on CT with mass effect and sulcal effacement. MR is helpful in making this differentiation (intermediate, not high, signal intensity; enhancement after administration of contrast material). Skull metastases can have adjacent meningeal enhancement.

VI. Differential diagnosis of meningeal thickening and enhancement (see box, p. 231).

SUGGESTED READINGS

Allison DJ, Marano GD: Computed tomography of rheumatoid pachymeningitis, *AJNR* 6:976-977, 1985.

Burke JW, Podrasky AE, Bradley WG Jr: Meninges: benign postoperative enhancement on MR images, *Radiology* 174:99-102, 1990.

Chaeres DW, Bryan RN: Acute subarachnoid hemorrhage: in vitro comparison of MR and CT, *AJNR* 7:223-228, 1986.

Chang KH, Han MH, Roh JK, et al: Gd-DTPA-enhanced MR imaging in intracranial tuberculosis, *Neuroradiology* 32:19-25, 1990.

Chang KH, Han MH, Roh JK, et al: Gd-DTPA-enhanced MR imaging of the brain in patients with meningitis, *AJNR* 11:69-76, 1990.

Davis PC, Friedman NC, Fry SM, et al: Leptomeningeal metastasis: MR imaging, *Radiology* 163:449-454, 1987.

Destian S, Heier LA, Zimmerman RD, et al: Differentiation between meningeal fibrosis and chronic subdural hematoma after ventricular shunting, *AJNR* 10:1021-1026, 1989.

Gomori JM, Grossman RI, Goldberg HI, et al: High-field spin-echo MR imaging of superficial and subependymal siderosis secondary to neonatal intraventricular hemorrhage, *Neuroradiology* 29:339-342, 1987.

Hayes WS, Sherman JL, Stern BJ, et al: MR and CT evaluation of intracranial sarcoidosis, *AJNR* 8:841-847, 1987.

Holland BA, Perret LV, Mills CM: Meningovascular syphilis: CT and MR findings, *Radiology* 158:439-442, 1986.

Hudgins PA, Davis PC, Hoffman JC Jr: Gadopentetate diglumine–enhanced MR imaging in children following surgery for brain tumor: spectrum of meningeal findings, *AJNR* 12:301-307, 1991.

Kramer ED, Rafto S, Packer RJ, Zimmerman RA: Comparison of myelography with CT follow-up versus gadolinium MRI for subarachnoid metastatic disease in children, *Neurology* 41:46-50, 1991.

Martin N, Masson C, Henin D, et al: Hypertrophic cranial pachymeningitis, *AJNR* 10:477-484, 1989.

Noorbehesht B, Engmann DR, Sullender W, et al: Neonatal herpes simplex encephalitis: correlation of clinical and CT findings, *Radiology* 162:813-819, 1987.

Phillips ME, Tyals TJ, Kambhu SA, Yuh WTC: Neoplastic vs. inflammatory meningeal enhancement with Gd-DTPA, *J Comput Assist Tomogr* 14:536-541, 1990.

Rippe DJ, Boyko OB, Friedman HS, et al: Gd-DTPA-enhanced MR imaging of leptomeningeal spread of primary intracranial CNS tumor in children, *AJNR* 11:329-332, 1990.

Rodesch G, Van Bogaert P, Mavroudakis N, et al: Neuroradiologic findings in leptomeningeal carcinomatosis: the value interest of gadolinium-enhanced MRI, *Neuroradiology* 32:26-32, 1990.

Rokumaru A, O'uchi T, Eguchi T, et al: Prominent meningeal enhancement adjacent to meningioma on Gd-DTPA-enhanced MR images: histopathologic correlation, *Radiology* 175:431-433, 1990.

Sherman JL, Stern BJ: Sarcoidosis of the CNS, *AJNR* 11:915-923, 1990.

Sze G, Soletsky S, Bronen R, Krol G: MR imaging of the cranial meninges with emphasis on contrast enhancement and meningeal carcinomatosis, *AJNR* 10:965-975, 1989.

CHAPTER 36

Ventricles, cisterns, and subarachnoid spaces: extraaxial collections and masses

KEY CONCEPTS

1. Arachnoid cysts occur most commonly in the middle fossa, followed by the posterior fossa (retrocerebellar), suprasellar cistern, quadrigeminal cistern, and convexity.
2. A prominent frontal subarachnoid space can be normal in infants but must be distinguished from external hydrocephalus, atrophy, and subdural effusions.

Pathologic processes external to the brain but inside the calvarial vault can reflect prominence or enlargement of otherwise normal spaces (e.g., increased subarachnoid space secondary to brain atrophy), abnormal collections of fluid (e.g., arachnoid cysts and subdural hematoma), or abnormal tissue (e.g., meningioma and dural metastases).

I. Congenital and developmental.
   A. Normal anatomic variants.
      1. Mega–cisterna magna (see Chapter 28).
      2. In infancy, subarachnoid spaces may appear prominent. In absence of increased or decreased occipitofrontal head circumference, coexisting ventricular dilation, or arrested head growth after insult, this is probably normal.
   B. Abnormal.
      1. External hydrocephalus: widened subarachnoid space, particularly frontal or frontoparietal and interhemispheric fissure with minimal or no ventricular enlargement in infant with rapidly increasing occipitofrontal head circumference. May be difficult to distinguish

from chronic subdural hematoma on computed tomography (CT); magnetic resonance (MR) may be helpful.

2. Cerebral atrophy: uniformly prominent sulci (without disproportionate bifrontal subarachnoid space widening) combined with proportionate dilatation of ventricles and basal cisterns; often history of arrested head growth, microcephaly, or central nervous system (CNS) insult such as hypoxic-ischemic episode.

3. Arachnoid cysts.
   a. Congenital intraarachnoid cerebrospinal fluid (CSF) collections.
   b. One percent of all atraumatic intracranial mass lesions.
   c. Between 60% and 90% occur in pediatric age group, most under 10 years of age.
   d. Can be asymptomatic but may cause neurologic deficit by compressing brain or obstructing CSF flow.
   e. Arise within and expand CSF cistern. Specific location in descending order of frequency: middle fossa and sylvian fissure (50%), vermian (retrocerebellar) cistern (25%), suprasellar cistern (10%), cerebellopontine angle and quadrigeminal plate cistern (5% to 10% each), and cerebral sulci and convexity (5%).
   f. Radiology: noncalcified smoothly demarcated extraparenchymal mass that does not enhance and parallels CSF signal on MR, density on CT.
   g. Differential diagnosis: low-density tumor such as epidermoid tumor or cystic astrocytoma, old infarct, chronic subdural hygroma (MR is helpful in such cases). Specific differentiation must be made between posterior fossa (suprasellar) arachnoid cyst (PFAC) and dilated third ventricle, between interhemispheric arachnoid cyst and porencephaly, and between posterior fossa arachnoid cyst and Dandy-Walker malformation. (PFACs are clearly separate from vallecula and fourth ventricle, which may be compressed but is of normal configuration; with Dandy-Walker malformation, cyst appears as extension of fourth ventricle.)

II. Vascular and traumatic.
   A. Arteriovenous malformations (AVMs) and aneurysms.
      1. Enlarged dural sinuses from high-flow AVMs can appear as extraaxial mass and even cause obstructive hydrocephalus. Radiographic findings include flow voids on MR and slight hyperdensity on CT with strong, uniform enhancement following rapid infusion of contrast media.
      2. Subarachnoid hemorrhage from ruptured aneurysm, AVM, or trauma (see Chapters 13 and 41).
      3. Giant aneurysm and venous varix can occur as extraaxial mass.

B. Traumatic (for more extensive discussion, see Chapters 17 and 42).
1. Acute subdural or epidural hematoma: Typical subdural hematomas are linear or crescentic and extensive, whereas classic epidural clot is biconvex or lentiform and relatively focal. This distinction is not absolute. Most hematomas are hyperdense on nonenhanced CT; occasionally extremely anemic patients or patients with coagulation disorders (such as disseminated intravascular coagulation) have acute isodense hematomas.
2. Chronic epidural or subdural hematomas and effusions: variable signal but often hyperintense on both Tl- and T2-weighted MR scans.
3. Calcified chronic subdural hematomas have high attenuation on CT and typically conform to inner table of calvarium.
4. Subdural drains and shunts.
C. Atrophic conditions: diffuse prominence of subarachnoid spaces and cisterns with proportionate enlargement of ventricles. Long list of causes, some of which are:
1. Hypoxic-ischemic insult.
2. Trauma (e.g., repeated nonaccidental trauma).
3. Infection (e.g., meningitis).
4. Radiation therapy and chemotherapy.
5. Steroids.
6. Dehydration.
7. Deprivational states and malnutrition.
8. Neurodegenerative diseases.
D. Miscellaneous extraaxial masses.
1. Extramedullary hematopoiesis.
a. Hematopoietic tissue located in subdural space is rare but can occur with disorders such as myeloproliferative disorders and toxic or tumoral bone destruction.
b. Multiple, hyperdense, homogeneously enhancing extraaxial masses on CT.
c. Differential diagnosis: multiple meningiomas, multiple subdural hematomas.
2. Sarcoid: Twenty percent of patients with CNS involvement have isolated dural thickening.
III. Infection (see Chapter 36).
A. Focal abnormalities.
1. Subdural empyema.
2. Subdural effusions.
B. Diffuse abnormalities.
1. Meningitis.
2. Syphilis with hypertrophic pachymeningitis.
3. Idiopathic hypertrophic pachymeningitis.

IV. Neoplastic.
  A. Primary tumors: meningiomas (focal, en plaque; meningiomatosis; see Chapter 47).
  B. Metastatic tumors (see Chapter 50).
    1. Prostate, lung, renal, and breast carcinoma can all have isodense or hyperdense meningeal metastases on nonenhanced CT and isointense but enhancing meningeal mass on MR. Five percent of these tumors metastasize to calvarium; of these, 15% extend into subdural space. Subdural and epidural tumor extensions can appear similar to hematomas; however, tumors are enhanced uniformly and are often associated with destructive calvarial changes.
    2. Metastatic neuroblastoma can involve calvarium or orbit and adjacent epidural and epicranial tissues. In such cases dural boundary is almost always intact, although it may be so attenuated that dura-based masses simulate intracerebral lesions.
    3. Leptomeningeal infiltrate with lymphoma or leukemia is common, but CT is relatively ineffective in demonstrating CSF involvement. When infiltrate is present, isodense or slightly hyperdense dura-based masses with moderate homogeneous enhancement are seen. MR is more sensitive but still may fail to delineate documented CSF spread.
    4. Plasmacytoma: may rarely arise from dura; may mimic meningioma.

SUGGESTED READINGS

Boyko OB, Cooper DF, Grossman CB: Contrast-enhanced CT of acute isodense subdural hematoma, *AJNR* 12:341-343, 1991.

Chuang S, Harwood-Nash D: Tumors and cysts, *Neuroradiology* 28:463-475, 1986.

Harsh GR, Edwards MSB, Wilson CG: Intracranial arachnoid cysts in children, *J Neurosurg* 64:835-842, 1986.

Heier LA, Zimmerman RD, Amster JL, et al: Magnetic resonance imaging of arachnoid cysts, *Clin Imaging* 13:281-291, 1989.

Kolawole TM, Patel PJ, Mahdi AH: Arachnoid cysts: computed tomography findings on CT, *CT: J Comput Tomogr* 11:156-159, 1987.

Martin N, Masson C, Henin D, et al: Hypertrophic cranial pachymeningitis, *AJNR* 10:477-484, 1989.

Maytal J, Alvarez LA, Elkins CM, Shinnar S: External hydrocephalus: radiologic spectrum and differentiation from cerebral atrophy, *AJNR* 8:271-278, 1987.

Sze G, Soletsky S, Broman R, Krol G: MR imaging of the cranial meninges with emphasis on contrast enhancement and meningeal carcinomatosis, *AJNR* 10:965-975, 1989.

ABNORMALITIES OF BRAIN PARENCHYMA

CHAPTER 37

Central nervous system infection and inflammatory disease

KEY CONCEPTS

1. Common congenital central nervous system (CNS) infections comprise toxoplasmosis, rubella, cytomegalovirus, and herpes simplex (TORCH syndrome). Sometimes syphilis is also included.
2. CNS complications of human immunodeficiency virus (HIV) include:
   a. Diffuse cerebral atrophy
   b. White matter disease (HIV encephalopathy, progressive multifocal leukoencephalopathy)
   c. Tumors
      (1) Scalp: Kaposi's sarcoma
      (2) Brain: primary lymphoma
   d. Infection: toxoplasmosis most common

I. Congenital infections: as a group sometimes called TORCH (for toxoplasmosis, rubella, cytomegalovirus, herpes). Other, less common types of intrauterine infection include syphilis, varicella, listeriosis, hepatitis B, and human parvovirus. Manifestations depend on fetal age at time of insult; infection during first two trimesters generally leads to congenital malformations, whereas third-trimester infections result in destructive (encephaloclastic) lesions. Fetal infections are acquired primarily by transplacental passage (mostly viruses) or through amniotic fluid (mostly bacteria).

A. Cytomegalovirus (CMV).

   1. Incidence: Now that maternal rubella is relatively well controlled, CMV is most common maternal viral infection (13% of all pregnancies). CMV is isolated from urine in 1% of asymptomatic newborns.

  2. Pathology: Predilection for rapidly growing cells of germinal matrix leads to periventricular calcification.
  3. Associated abnormalities: polymicrogyria (secondary to late second-trimester migrational disturbances), chorioretinitis, microphthalmia, hepatosplenomegaly, anemia, thrombocytopenia.
  4. Computed tomography (CT).
     a. Microcephaly.
     b. Ventriculomegaly (ex vacuo type of hydrocephalus).
     c. Periventricular calcification.
     d. Parenchymal infarctions.
     e. Polymicrogyria common.
  5. Magnetic resonance (MR).
     a. Microcephaly and marked ventriculomegaly.
     b. Periventricular hyperintense foci on T2-weighted image (T2WI).
  6. Ultrasonography (intrauterine) may show:
     a. Bilateral periventricular calcifications (hypoechoic periventricular ringlike zones).
     b. Widespread cerebral necrosis.
     c. Multiple organ system abnormalities.
B. Toxoplasmosis.
  1. Incidence: up to 1% of pregnancies.
  2. Pathology: *Toxoplasma gondii* oocytes with diffuse inflammatory infiltration of meninges, brain, and ependyma.
  3. Associated abnormalities: can cause hydranencephaly if second-trimester infection occurs.
  4. CT.
     a. Microcephaly.
     b. Calcification in basal ganglia, cortex, and periventricular region.
     c. Atrophy, encephalomalacia, and porencephaly.
     d. Ventricular dilatation.
C. Herpes simplex (type 2).
  1. Incidence: 1 in 2000 to 5000 births; brain involvement in 30%.
  2. Pathology: visceral disease or meningoencephalitis.
  3. CT.
     a. Very early: can be normal.
     b. Intermediate in course: progressive low-attenuation foci (white matter edema), high-attenuation gray matter; lesions typically bilateral and symmetric.
     c. Late: atrophy, punctate and gyriform calcification.
  4. MR: gray matter involvement important early sign; loss of gray-white contrast on both T1WI and T2WI; nonhemorrhagic low signal (magnetic susceptibility effect) in residual cortex has been reported.

D. Rubella.
  1. In first two trimesters most commonly causes malformations.
  2. In third trimester causes hydrocephalus, microcephaly, microphthalmia, and atrophy with calcification (periventricular, basal ganglia, brainstem, cortex).
II. Acquired infections.
  A. Parenchymal.
    1. Encephalitis.
      a. Agents: usually viral or toxic (e.g., herpes).
      b. Herpes encephalitis.
        (1) Thirty percent of cases are pediatric.
        (2) Most common cause of nonepidemic fatal encephalitis in United States.
        (3) Pathology: fulminant, necrotizing, hemorrhagic meningoencephalitis.
        (4) Location: preference for temporal lobe; bilateral in 20% to 50%.
        (5) CT: may be normal early, then low-attenuation areas without focal enhancement; hemorrhage in 50%; gyral enhancement late.
        (6) MR: cortical edema (hypointense on T1WI, hyperintense on T2WI) and hemorrhage; often temporal (insula), then frontal; parietal lobes can also be affected.
      c. Subacute sclerosing panencephalitis (SSPE).
        (1) Primarily disease of children between 5 and 12 years of age.
        (2) Probably caused by reactivation of measles virus (long latent period).
        (3) Pathology: both gray and white matter affected (gray matter with gliosis and perivascular lymphocytic infiltration; white matter with gliosis and demyelination).
        (4) CT: nonspecific. Early: edema. Intermediate: multifocal low-density areas in periventricular and subcortical white matter followed by generalized atrophy in advanced cases.
        (5) MR: hyperintense white matter changes on T2WI.
      d. Reye's syndrome.
        (1) ? Toxic (effect of salicylates combined with virus?).
        (2) Disease of children.
        (3) Liver failure; CNS changes nonspecific (normal or diffuse cerebral edema).
      e. Acute disseminated encephalomyelitis.
        (1) Primarily disease of children.
        (2) Onset 1 to 2 weeks after initial infection.

        (3) Probably autoimmune-mediated demyelination.

        (4) CT: bilateral, confluent, low-attenuation changes in subcortical white matter.

        (5) MR: prolonged T2 of white matter of both hemispheres and cerebellum; bilateral, often extensive, relatively symmetric.

        (6) Differential diagnosis: multiple sclerosis.

  2. Abscess.

    a. Etiology.

        (1) Hematogenous (cardiac, pulmonary, drug abuse).

        (2) Direct extension (temporal bone, sinuses).

        (3) Trauma (direct penetrating, postsurgical, comminuted fracture).

    b. Early cerebritis stage (onset to 4 days).

        (1) Pathology: focal or multifocal inflammatory process with edema, hyperemia, perivascular inflammatory infiltrate, petechial hemorrhage, and necrosis.

        (2) CT: low-attenuation mass effect with or without patchy or gyriform enhancement.

        (3) MR: ill-defined regions of prolonged T1 and T2 relaxation with some mass effect, usually some patchy enhancement following contrast media administration.

    c. Late cerebritis stage (between 4 and 10 days).

        (1) Affected brain undergoes necrosis with formation of granulation tissue rim.

        (2) CT and MR: ring enhancing lesion with mass effect and edema. (Presence of ring lesion does not necessarily indicate mature, encapsulated abscess.) Delayed scans may show accumulation of contrast media within center of lesion.

    d. Abscess (early capsule stage).

        (1) Pathology: cavity of necrotic tissue and pus or caseous material surrounded by collagenous capsule.

        (2) CT and MR: thin-walled, smooth, well-defined, ring enhancing lesions (can persist long after clinical resolution).

    e. Abscess (late capsule stage): thicker wall, decreased edema and mass effect.

    f. Granulomatous abscess.

        (1) Tuberculoma.

        (2) Sarcoid.

        (3) Fungal.

        (4) Parasitic (e.g., cysticercosis).

B. Ventriculitis and ependymitis.

  1. Ependymal inflammation, usually secondary to rupture of periventricular abscess.

2. Differential diagnosis: ependymal metastases, prominent subependymal veins.
C. Meningitis.
  1. Anatomy of meninges (Table 37-1).
  2. Common organisms: vary with age of patient.
    a. Neonate: *Escherichia coli,* group B streptococci.
    b. Children: *Haemophilus influenzae, Streptococcus pneumoniae, Neisseria meningitidis.*
    c. Adults: *N. meningitidis, S. pneumoniae,* other streptococci.
  3. Pathology of leptomeningitis.
    a. Etiology.
      (1) Most commonly hematogenous from remote site.
      (2) Less commonly by direct extension (temporal bone, sinuses).
      (3) Agents: numerous.
      (4) Spreads along pia of vessels within Virchow-Robin spaces.
    b. Stages.
      (1) Early: pial vessel congestion, endothelial swelling, inflammatory infiltrate of vessel wall.
      (2) Midphase: vessel wall necrosis and thrombosis, which can lead to cortical infarction, cerebritis, and nidus for abscess development.
      (3) Later: exudate in basal cisterns and sulci.
      (4) Still later: thickened fibrotic leptomeninges.
  4. Radiology.
    a. CT and MR: may be normal in early stages; abnormalities include:
      (1) Basal cisterns and sulci poorly visualized on CT (isodense exudate on non-contrast-enhanced T1WI).

Table 37-1   Meningeal anatomy

Meninx	Layer	Space formed
Pachymeninx →	Dura mater	Epidural (between inner table of skull and dura)
		Subdural (between dura and arachnoid)
Leptomeninx	Arachnoid	Subarachnoid (between arachnoid and pia)
	Pia mater	Subpial (not a true space because pia is tightly adherent to cortex)

          (2) Focal or generalized cerebral edema.

          (3) Focal parenchymal enhancement.

          (4) Leptomeningeal enhancement.

    5. Complications.

      a. Communicating hydrocephalus.

      b. Subdural effusion and empyema.

      c. Ventriculitis.

      d. Cortical vein and dural sinus thrombosis.

      e. Abscess.

      f. Late: atrophy and encephalomalacia.

  D. Empyema (subdural, epidural): 20% to 30% of intracranial infections.

    1. Most often occurs as complication of sinusitis, otitis, trauma, or surgery.

    2. CT.

      a. Hypodense or isodense, crescentic, lenticular extraaxial fluid collection.

      b. Later: membrane enhancement with or without cerebritis of underlying cortex.

    3. MR.

      a. Hypointense to brain on T1WI (slightly hyperintense compared with CSF); hyperintense on T2WI; membranes enhanced by contrast material.

      b. Hypointense rim medial to collection represents inflamed dura and is seen with epidural (but not subdural) empyema.

      c. Cortical hyperemia, edema, venous thrombosis.

    4. Differential diagnosis: nonpurulent collections (e.g., effusions, hematomas).

III. Specific topics of interest.

  A. CNS complications of HIV.

    1. Pathology: HIV is lymphotropic as well as neurotropic virus.

    2. Incidence: CNS involvement initial complaint in approximately 10%; neurologic complications eventually develop in more than one third of patients (more than 75% in autopsies).

    3. Organisms affecting CNS (most infections are secondary or opportunistic).

      a. *Toxoplasma gondii.*

      b. Cytomegalovirus.

      c. Herpes simplex virus type 1.

      d. *Cryptococcus neoformans.*

      e. *Coccidioides.*

      f. *Aspergillus.*

      g. Others: *Mycobacterium, Mucor, Candida.*

      h. Bacterial infections rare.

4. CT and MR: various findings.
   a. Diffuse cerebral atrophy.
   b. White matter disease.
      (1) HIV encephalopathy in up to 60%; progressive multifocal leu-koencephalopathy (PML) in 2% to 4%. (NOTE: PML is also seen with lymphoma and other malignancies.)
      (2) Diffuse, bilateral, usually symmetric in both HIV encephalopathy and PML. PML often discrete, can involve gray matter, can be more asymmetric.
      (3) CT: low attenuation; MR: high signal on proton density–weighted scans or T2WI.
   c. Neoplasms.
      (1) Kaposi's sarcoma (scalp involvement; brain is rare site).
      (2) CNS lymphoma (6% to 7% of patients): can be primary or secondary; seen as enhancing periventricular solid or ring lesions.
   d. Infections.
      (1) Toxoplasmosis: most common infection. No pathognomonic appearance, but widely distributed, multiple solid or ring enhancing foci with edema are most common. Both primary CNS lymphoma and toxoplasmosis have predilection for basal ganglia.
      (2) Cryptococcosis: bilateral small lesions, hyperintense on T2WI, clustered around basal ganglia (predilection for invading perivascular Virchow-Robin spaces); can cause meningitis.
      (3) Cytomegalovirus: predilection for ependymal and subependymal regions; causes ventriculitis.
B. Cysticercosis: prevalent in developing nations and therefore in immigrants from endemic areas.
   1. Pathology: CNS infection by larval stage of pork tapeworm, *Taenia solium*.
   2. CT.
      a. Approximately 70% have parenchymal calcification.
      b. Approximately 70% have hydrocephalus.
      c. Parenchymal edema common.
   3. MR: Findings vary depending on stage in evolution of infection.
      a. Cysts: parenchymal in 50% to 70% (usually involving gray-white junction), intraventricular in 20% to 50%, subarachnoid in less than 5%.
      b. Most acute cysts produce low signal on T1WI. High-intensity nodule within cyst is scolex of tapeworm (vesicular stage). Contrast enhancement rare at this stage.
      c. Degenerating cysts may be hyperintense on T1WI or T2WI; pe-

ripheral edema; ringlike contrast enhancement in two thirds of cases.

    d. Involuting cysts (granular nodular stage) appear as small nodular or ringlike lesions with or without edema. Fifty percent enhance.

    e. Inactive cysts calcify and either are not seen or are represented by signal voids (nodular calcified stage). Cysts at this stage do not enhance.

C. Tuberculosis (TB): Overall incidence worldwide (and particularly in United States) had been declining but is now rising again because of HIV infection, drug and alcohol abuse, homelessness, and poor sanitation and nutrition. Therefore familiarity with imaging manifestations of intracranial tuberculosis is becoming increasingly important.

  1. Three groups of intracranial TB have been described.

    a. Active meningitis.

    b. Meningitis sequelae.

    c. Tuberculomas (localized parenchymal disease).

  2. Radiology.

    a. Diffuse active: leptomeningitis.

      (1) Most common form of intracranial TB.

      (2) Thick gelatinous exudate with cisternal obliteration (most often suprasellar, followed by ambient cistern and sylvian fissure).

      (3) Cisternal enhancement (predominantly basilar, but convexity meningeal enhancement also occurs).

      (4) Communicating hydrocephalus.

      (5) Infarction (basal ganglia, thalamus, internal capsule, brainstem) secondary to vascular spasm; hemorrhage.

      (6) Parenchymal granulomas common (often suprasellar): isointense to gray matter on both T1WI and T2WI; solid or ring enhancement after administration of contrast material on both CT and MR.

    b. Sequelae of meningitis.

      (1) Calcification (suprasellar, diffuse).

      (2) Variable communicating hydrocephalus.

      (3) Meningeal enhancement, enhancing granulomas.

    c. Tuberculomas (localized granulomatous lesions).

      (1) Solitary or multiple nodular masses, often in cortex or corticomedullary junction, with variable edema.

      (2) Enhancement after administration of contrast media.

D. Lyme disease: tick-borne multisystem inflammatory disease caused by spirochete *Borrelia burgdorferi*.

  1. Recent study shows MR abnormalities in 43% of patients with CNS complaints (CNS manifestations develop in 10% to 15% of patients).

    a. Focal areas of signal abnormality (hypointense on T1WI, hyperintense on T2WI).

    b. Subcortical white matter involvement.

       (1) Frontal lobes most common.

       (2) Parietal lobes also frequently affected.

    c. May represent foci of perivascular inflammation or demyelination.

E. Sarcoidosis: noninfectious systemic disease with characteristic pathologic findings (noncaseating granulomas).

  1. Clinical CNS involvement in 5%.

  2. Pathology.

    a. Granulomatous noncaseating involvement of meninges and brain.

    b. Secondary infarctions.

  3. Radiology.

    a. Nonspecific periventricular high-signal lesions on T2WI.

    b. Diffuse or focal meningeal thickening that is enhanced strongly on T1WI after administration of contrast media.

    c. Thickened infundibulum.

    d. Cranial nerve (especially optic nerve) enhancement.

    e. Focal parenchymal mass lesions usually enhance homogeneously.

    f. Hydrocephalus.

    g. Vasculitis and cerebral infarction.

    h. Spinal cord involvement.

SUGGESTED READINGS

Balakrishnan J, Becker PS, Kuman AJ, et al: Acquired immunodeficiency syndrome: correlation of radiologic and pathologic findings in the brain, *Radiographics* 10:201-215, 1990.

Barkovich AJ: Infections of the nervous system. In *Pediatric neuroimaging,* New York, 1990, Raven Press, pp 293-325.

Boesch CH, Issakainen J, Kewitz G, et al: Magnetic resonance imaging of the brain in congenital cytomegalovirus infection, *Pediatr Radiol* 19:91-93, 1989.

Buckner CB, Leithiser RE, Walker CW, Allison JW: The changing epidemiology of tuberculosis and other mycobacterial infections in the United States: implications for the radiologist, *AJR* 196:255-264, 1991.

Chang KH, Han MH, Roh JK, et al: Gd-DTPA enhanced MR imaging in intracranial tuberculosis, *Neuroradiology* 32:19-25, 1990.

Chang KH, Han MH, Roh JK, et al: Gd-DTPA-enhanced MR imaging of the brain in patients with meningitis: comparison with CT, *AJNR* 11:69-76, 1990.

Chang KH, Lee JH, Han MH, Han MC: The role of contrast-enhanced MR imaging in the diagnosis of neurocysticercosis, *AJNR* 12:509-512, 1991.

Drose JA, Dennis MA, Thickman D: Infection in utero: US findings in 19 cases, *Radiology* 178:369-374, 1991.

Enzmann D, Chang Y, Augustyn G: MR findings in neonatal herpes simplex encephalitis type II, *J Comput Assist Tomogr* 14:453-457, 1990.

Fernandez RE, Rothberg M, Ferencz G, Wujack D: Lyme disease of the CNS, *AJNR* 11:479-481, 1990.

Haimes AB, Zimmerman RD, Morgello S, et al: MR imaging of brain abscesses, *AJNR* 10:279-291, 1989.

Kesselring J, Miller DH, Robb SA, et al: Acute disseminated encephalomyelitis, *Brain* 113:291-302, 1990.

Martinez HR, Rangel-Guerra R, Elizondo G, et al: MR imaging in neurocysticercosis, *AJNR* 10:1011-1019, 1989.

Mathews VP, Kuharik MA, Edwards MK, et al: Gd-DTPA-enhanced MR imaging of experimental bacterial meningitis, *AJNR* 9:1045-1050, 1988.

Miller DH, Kendall BE, Barter S, et al: Magnetic resonance imaging in central nervous system sarcoidosis, *Neurology* 38:378-383, 1988.

Ramsey RG, Geremia GK: CNS complications of AIDS: CT and MR findings, *AJR* 151:449-454, 1988.

Sherman JL, Stern BJ: Sarcoidosis of the CNS, *AJNR* 11:915-923, 1990.

Tassin GB: Cytomegalic inclusion disease, *AJNR* 12:117-122, 1991.

Tien RD, Chu PK, Hesselink JR, et al: Intracranial cryptococcosis in immunocompromised patients, *AJNR* 12:283-289, 1991.

Tsuchiya K, Yamaguchi T, Furui S, et al: MR imaging vs. CT in subacute sclerosing panencephalitis, *AJNR* 9:943-946, 1988.

Weingarten K, Zimmerman RD, Becker RD, et al: Subdural and epidural empyemas: MR imaging, *AJNR* 10:81-87, 1989.

Williams AL: Infectious diseases. In Williams AL, Haughton VM: *Cranial computed tomography: a comprehensive text,* St Louis, 1985, Mosby–Year Book, pp 269-315.

CHAPTER 38

White matter diseases: dysmyelinating disorders

With Wendy R.K. Smoker

KEY CONCEPTS

1. White matter disease is classified into *dys*myelinating disorders (normal myelin not formed or inadequately maintained) and *de*myelinating disorders (normal myelin formed but destroyed).
2. Most white matter changes on computed tomography (CT) and magnetic resonance (MR) are nonspecific, but some are suggestive:
   a. Macrocephaly plus white matter disease in an infant suggests Canavan's or Alexander's disease. The former is diffuse; in the latter, frontal areas are most affected.
   b. Almost complete lack of myelination suggests Pelizaeus-Merzbacher disease.
   c. Hyperdense thalamic, caudate, and white matter foci are seen in Krabbe's disease.
   d. Childhood adrenoleukodystrophy classically has confluent, symmetric bioccipital lesions with ring or edge enhancement.
3. Chromosome and biochemical studies (e.g., blood and urine amino acid determinations, specific enzyme assays) and structural analyses (e.g., of peroxisomes and mitochondria) are needed for definitive diagnosis.

White matter diseases can be classified by many different schemata. A convenient one is to divide them into two basic groups: dysmyelinating diseases (myelin either does not form or is not maintained normally) and demyelinating diseases (myelin forms normally but is then destroyed). This chapter focuses on dysmyelinating disorders. Chapter 39 considers demyelinating diseases. The dysmyelinating diseases can be further divided into leukodystrophies with primary involvement of myelin and miscellaneous storage diseases with secondary involvement of myelin. Some white matter diseases in children (such

251

as Canavan's disease) that are classified as dysmyelinating disorders may form myelin that undergoes very early destruction and are thus technically demyelinating diseases. For convenience, most of the white matter diseases in young children are included in the discussion of dysmyelinating disorders.

I. Leukodystrophies (with primary involvement of myelin).
  A. Alexander's disease (fibrinoid leukodystrophy).
    1. Biochemical or enzymatic defect: unknown.
    2. Clinical findings.
      a. Manifest during first few weeks to 6 months of life.
      b. Macrocephaly and developmental delay.
    3. Course: progressive spastic quadriparesis, intellectual and neurologic deterioration, death in infancy or early childhood (average 2 years of age).
    4. Radiology.
      a. CT.
        (1) Symmetric, well-defined, low-attenuation white matter areas.
        (2) Frontal lobes involved early, then posterior extension.
        (3) External capsule affected; internal capsule relatively spared.
        (4) May have some contrast enhancement around frontal horns.
      b. MR.
        (1) Confluent white matter lesions with prolonged T1 and T2 relaxation times.
        (2) Lesions extend to subcortical arcuate fibers and along external and extreme capsules.
    5. Definitive diagnosis determined by brain biopsy or autopsy.
  B. Canavan's disease (spongiform leukodystrophy).
    1. Biochemical or enzymatic defect.
      a. Recently classified as encephalomyopathy (mitochondrial disorder that affects both central nervous system and skeletal muscle) with deficiency of enzyme asparto-acyclase.
      b. Autosomal recessive (especially in Ashkenazi Jews).
    2. Clinical findings.
      a. Symptom onset before 10 months of age, usually between 3 and 6 months.
      b. Somewhat older children may have megalencephaly with initially normal neurologic status.
      c. Progressive neurologic deterioration with developmental delay, spasticity, optic atrophy, and blindness.
      d. Death usual by 2 or 3 years of age.
    3. Radiology (nonspecific findings).
      a. CT.
        (1) Diffuse low-density changes throughout white matter.
        (2) Later: ventriculomegaly, cerebral atrophy.

      b. MR: symmetric diffusely hyperintense white matter, all locations, no focal predominance.

C. Krabbe's disease (globoid cell leukodystrophy).

  1. Biochemical or enzymatic defect.

      a. Classified as lysosomal disorder.

      b. Deficiency of beta-galactosidase.

      c. Autosomal recessive.

  2. Clinical findings.

      a. Symptom onset between 2 and 6 months (infantile form).

      b. Developmental delay, restlessness, irritability, spasticity.

      c. Dementia, optic atrophy, cortical blindness, immobilizing spastic quadriplegia.

      d. Death within 1 to 3 years (although late-onset form has been described).

  3. Radiology.

      a. CT.

         (1) Early: symmetric hyperdense areas in thalami, caudate nuclei, brainstem, cerebellum, corona radiata.

         (2) Intermediate: patchy periventricular low-attenuation areas.

         (3) Late: diffuse white matter atrophy.

      b. MR.

         (1) Basal ganglia and brainstem are hyperintense on T1-weighted imaging (T1WI); exhibit slightly shortened T2 relaxation.

         (2) White matter shows prolonged T2 relaxation time.

  4. Definitive diagnosis: lymphocyte or skin fibroblast assay for beta-galactosidase.

D. Pelizaeus-Merzbacher disease.

  1. Biochemical or enzymatic deficiency.

      a. Unidentified.

      b. Reduced synthesis of proteolipid protein in white matter.

      c. X-linked recessive.

  2. Clinical findings.

      a. Onset: neonatal or first few months of life.

      b. Nystagmus and abnormal eye movements, optic atrophy.

      c. Slowly progressive pyramidal, dystonic, and cerebellar signs.

  3. Radiology.

      a. CT.

         (1) May be normal early.

         (2) Low-signal white matter; progressive white matter atrophy (nonspecific).

      b. MR.

         (1) Newbornlike pattern with inversion of normal gray-white matter contrast and increased white matter signal on T2WI (myelination may be virtually absent).

(2) Decreased signal intensity in basal ganglia and thalamus.

(3) Atrophy.

E. Metachromatic leukodystrophy.

  1. Biochemical or enzymatic deficiency.

    a. Deficiency of arylsulfatase A leads to abnormal accumulation of sulfatides in metachromatic granules within macrophages and glial cells.

    b. Classified as lysosomal disorder (a sphingolipidosis like Krabbe's and Gaucher's diseases).

  2. Clinical findings.

    a. Subtypes based on age at presentation.

      (1) Congenital.

      (2) Late infantile (less than 3 years of age; death within 3 to 4 years; most common form).

      (3) Juvenile (symptomatic between 5 and 16 years; slow progression).

      (4) Adult (symptomatic after 16 years).

    b. Symptoms of most common form (late infantile) are gait disorder, strabismus, and gradual intellectual deterioration; in adult can be misdiagnosed as Alzheimer's dementia, Pick's disease, schizophrenia, or other disorder.

  3. Radiology (findings nonspecific).

    a. CT.

      (1) Low-attenuation changes in periventricular white matter and centrum semiovale.

      (2) Atrophy.

      (3) Lesions not enhanced by contrast media.

    b. MR.

      (1) Nonspecific; prolonged T1 and T2 relaxation times.

      (2) Some regions of normal myelination can usually be seen.

  4. Definitive diagnosis: lymphocyte or granulocyte enzyme assay.

F. Adrenoleukodystrophy (ALD): childhood variety (most common form).

  1. Biochemical or enzymatic deficiency.

    a. Accumulation of saturated very long chain fatty acids.

    b. X-linked recessive peroxisomal disorder.

    c. Since myelin is formed but destroyed, this is technically a demyelinating disease.

  2. Clinical findings.

    a. Exclusively in males.

    b. Usual presentation at age 4 to 8 years.

    c. Behavioral changes, intellectual deterioration, and visual complaints; may be symptoms of adrenal insufficiency (abnormal skin pigmentation).

    d. Progressive; fatal within a few years.

3. Radiology.
   a. CT: Characteristic classic pattern is:
     (1) Symmetric low-attenuation changes in parietooccipital white matter.
     (2) Peripheral (anterior rim) enhancement.
     (3) Progression from posterior to anterior.
     (4) Progressive atrophy.
   b. MR.
     (1) All patients have bilateral confluent occipital white matter producing increased signal on T2WI and extending into optic radiations and splenium of corpus callosum.
     (2) Auditory tract involvement in 87%.
     (3) Pyramidal tract involvement in 53%.
     (4) Disease advances anteriorly through internal and external capsules and centrum semiovale; relative sparing of subcortical U fibers.
     (5) Occasionally involvement is primarily frontal and progresses posteriorly.

G. Adult ALD (adrenomyeloneuropathy).
  1. Second most common form of ALD.
  2. Sex-linked recessive; affects men 20 to 30 years of age.
  3. Prolonged course with adrenal insufficiency, hypogonadism, cerebellar ataxia, and intellectual deterioration.
  4. Nonspecific imaging findings (normal or mild atrophy; foci of prolonged T1 and T2 relaxation in white matter).

H. Neonatal ALD.
  1. Biochemical, enzymatic, genetic.
    a. Classified as peroxisomal disorder.
    b. Autosomal recessive.
  2. Clinical findings.
    a. Symptomatic between birth and 4 months of age.
    b. Dysmorphic facial features, hypotonia, and retinitis pigmentosa.
    c. Mental retardation and seizures common.
    d. Death by 2 years of age.
  3. Radiology: nonspecific changes of diffuse white matter atrophy and degeneration.

II. Miscellaneous: Host of other enzymatic-metabolic, lysosomal, and mitochondrial encephalopathies may have CNS manifestations. Detailed discussion is beyond scope of this text, but many neurodegenerative disorders (more than 600 in childhood alone) have been described. Some of these, such as lysosomal disorders (e.g., mucopolysaccharidoses, mucolipidoses, Niemann-Pick disease, Gaucher's disease, G_{M2} gangliosidosis), peroxisomal disorders (Zellweger cerebrohepatorenal syndrome, infantile Refsum's disease), and mitochondrial encephalopathies (Menkes', and Kearns-Sayre syndromes) may have secondary involvement of myelin and white matter abnormalities on imaging studies. Imaging findings associated with most of these disorders and others such as aminoacidurias are nonspecific, primarily increased white matter signal on T2WI (see Chapter 40).

SUGGESTED READINGS

Baram TZ, Goldman AM, Percy AK: Krabbe's disease: specific MRI and CT findings, *Neurology* 36:111-115, 1986.

Barkovich AJ: Metabolic and destructive brain disorders. In *Pediatric neuroimaging*, New York, 1990, Raven Press, pp 35-43.

Brismar J, Ageel A, Brismar G, et al: Maple syrup urine disease, *AJNR* 11:1219-1228, 1990.

Brismar J, Ageel A, Gascon G, Ozand P: Malignant hyperphenylalanemia: CT and MR of the brain, *AJNR* 11:135-138, 1990.

Brismar J, Brismar G, Gascon G, Ozand P: Canavan disease: CT and MR imaging of the brain, *AJNR* 11:809-810, 1990.

Dietrich RB, Vining EP, Taira RK, et al: Myelin disorders of childhood: correlation of MR findings and severity of neurological impairment, *J Comput Assist Tomogr* 14:693-698, 1990.

Goebel HH, Warlo I: Biopsy studies in neurodegenerative disease of childhood, *BNI Q* 6:19-27, 1990.

Jensen ME, Sawyer RW, Braun IF, Rizzo WB: MR imaging appearance of childhood adrenoleukodystrophy with auditory, visual, and motor pathway involvement, *Radiographics* 10:53-66, 1990.

Murata R, Nakajima S, Tanaka A, et al: MR imaging of the brain in patients with mucopolysaccharidosis, *AJNR* 10:1165-1170, 1989.

Naidu S, Moser HW: Value of neuroimaging in metabolic disease affecting the CNS, *AJNR* 12:413-416, 1991.

Press GA, Barshop BA, Haas RH, et al: Abnormalities of the brain in nonketotic hyperglycinemia: MR manifestations, *AJNR* 10:315-321, 1989.

Sandhu FS, Dillon WP: MR demonstration of leukoencephalopathy associated with mitochondrial encephalomyopathy: case report, *AJNR* 12:375-379, 1991.

Silverstein AM, Hirsh DK, Trobe JD, Gebarski SS: MR imaging of the brain in five members of a family with Pelizaeus-Merzbacher disease, *AJNR* 11:495-499, 1990.

Uchiyama M, Hata Y, Tada S: MR imaging of adrenoleukodystrophy, *Neuroradiology* 33:25-29, 1991.

Van der Kamp MS, Valk J: The MR spectrum of peroxisomal disorders, *Neuroradiology* 33:30-37, 1991.

Wolpert SM, Anderson ML, Kaye EM: Metabolic disoders. In Wolpert SM, Barnes PD (eds): *MRI in pediatric neuroradiology*, St Louis, Mosby–Year Book, Inc. In press.

CHAPTER 39

White matter disease: demyelinating disorders

With Wendy R.K. Smoker

KEY CONCEPTS

1. Other than vascular age-related white matter changes, multiple sclerosis is the most common demyelinating disease.
2. The broad spectrum of causes for demyelinating disease includes infection, autoimmune disorders, radiation therapy and chemotherapy, a variety of toxic agents, vascular disease, and trauma.
3. Foci of increased white matter signal on T2-weighted images (T2WI) are normal in the healthy elderly.

Demyelinating or myelinoclastic diseases are disorders in which myelin is normally formed and maintained but later destroyed by endogenous or exogenous agents. Demyelinating disease can be subdivided by cause, such as idiopathic (e.g., multiple sclerosis), postinfectious, posttherapy, toxic-degenerative, and vascular. Dozens—if not hundreds—of special etiologic agents could be listed. Only the most common demyelinating diseases are discussed here.

I. Idiopathic.
  A. Multiple sclerosis.
    1. By far most common of all demyelinating diseases except for vascular disease related to aging.
    2. Etiology: unknown; possibly autoimmune or slow virus.
    3. Pathology: demyelination with relative axonal preservation.
    4. Location: periventricular white matter most common site.
    5. Age and sex: 2:1 female to male; between 20 and 50 years of age; childhood and adolescent disease 10:1 female.
    6. Radiology.

257

    a. CT.

       (1) Isointense or hypointense white matter foci.

       (2) Variable contrast enhancement.

       (3) Mass and irregular ring enhancement can mimic neoplasm.

    b. MR: variable findings including:

       (1) Discrete, periventricular, hyperintense white matter foci on T2WI; corpus callosum, pons, medulla, and cerebellar white matter often also involved.

       (2) Lesions may become confluent in severe, long-standing cases.

       (3) Isointense or hypointense on T1WI; may have beveled edge appearance.

       (4) Variable contrast enhancement.

       (5) Atrophy (diffuse); small corpus callosum in severe cases.

       (6) Occasionally, abnormal iron deposition in basal ganglia.

  7. Extensive differential diagnosis of multiple white matter lesions (see box below) because edema, perivascular cellular infiltration, demyelination, and gliosis all show nonspecific prolongation of T1 and T2 relaxation times. Common:

    a. Dilated perivascular spaces (linear in medullary white matter; round lesions tend to be located near base of brain, e.g., in basal ganglia).

    b. Microvascular disease and lacunar infarcts (less common in corpus callosum and posterior fossa); patients usually over 50 years of age.

    c. Multiple sclerosis.

    d. Encephalitis and other infections.

    e. Trauma (diffuse axonal injury).

    f. Metastases.

B. Schilder's disease (myelinoclastic diffuse sclerosis): considered by

---

DIFFERENTIAL DIAGNOSIS OF MULTIFOCAL WHITE MATTER LESIONS

Aging, small vessel vascular disease, lacunar infarcts

Multiple sclerosis

Encephalitis (acute disseminated encephalomyelitis, subacute sclerosing panencephalitis)

Progressive multifocal leukoencephalopathy

Metastases

Trauma (white matter shearing injury)

Normal (in healthy elderly)

some to be more virulent, childhood form of multiple sclerosis. Imaging shows more confluent areas of demyelination; major differential diagnosis is childhood forms of adrenoleukodystrophy.

II. Postinflammatory: Most are postviral or possibly allergic or immune-mediated responses to previous infection.
  A. Acute disseminated encephalomyelitis (see Chapter 37).
  B. Subacute sclerosing panencephalitis (see Chapter 37).
  C. Progressive multifocal leukoencephalopathy (see Chapter 37).
    1. Pathology.
      a. Discrete, multifocal areas of demyelination and intranuclear inclusions found in both deep and superficial white matter and in gray matter.
      b. Associated with papovavirus infection.
    2. Seen in 2% to 4% of patients with acquired immunodeficiency syndrome; increased incidence after organ transplantation and in other immunocompromised states.
    3. Also seen in lymphoproliferative diseases (lymphoma, leukemia) and other malignancies.

III. After therapy.
  A. Disseminated necrotizing leukoencephalopathy.
    1. Occurs primarily in patients undergoing chemotherapy (most often methotrexate); occurs with or without radiation.
    2. Pathology.
      a. Radiation produces fibrinoid white matter necrosis.
      b. Methotrexate produces coagulative necrosis and demyelination.
    3. Radiology: Both CT and MR show white matter lesions in centrum semiovale. Can be focal or diffuse.
      a. Mass effect (focal necrosis) can be present.
      b. Some contrast enhancement, often peripheral, occurs frequently.
      c. Can mimic recurrent or residual neoplasm.
      d. Mineralizing microangiopathy with multiple calcific foci also occurs as sequela of radiation therapy or chemotherapy.
      e. Diffuse radiation injury is seen as widespread confluent areas of increased signal in periventricular white matter on T2WI.

IV. Toxic and degenerative.
  A. Central pontine myelinolysis, also known as osmotic demyelination syndrome.
    1. Associated with:
      a. Malnutrition.
      b. Alcoholism.
      c. Electrolyte abnormalities (especially hyponatremia).
      d. Chronic debilitating disorders.
    2. Radiology.
      a. CT.

(1) Can be normal.
(2) Nonenhancing low-density lesions in pons.
(3) No mass effect.
(4) Other areas (basal ganglia and thalami) may be involved.
  b. MR.
    (1) Hypointense area(s) in pons, usually with sparing of tegmentum on T1WI.
    (2) Hyperintense on T2WI, no mass effect.
    (3) May show other lesions in thalami and basal ganglia.
  3. Differential diagnosis: multiple sclerosis, infarct, and neoplasm.
B. Marchiafava-Bignami disease.
  1. Clinical findings: often (but not always) long history of drinking red wines.
  2. Pathology: toxic demyelination of corpus callosum.
  3. Radiology: low-density lesions in corpus callosum, hemispheric white matter on CT, hyperintense foci on T2WI.
C. Carbon monoxide encephalopathy.
  1. Clinical findings: carboxyhemoglobin in blood.
  2. Radiology: symmetric hypodense foci in globus pallidus, cerebral white matter on CT, hyperintense lesions on T2WI.
D. Hypoxic-ischemic encephalopathy.
  1. Premature infants.
    a. Watershed (most vulnerable to hypoxic-ischemic insults) in premature infant is in deep periventricular white matter (relative paucity of developing penetrating cortical vessels). Germinal matrix hemorrhage also occurs in deep periventricular areas.
    b. Periventricular leukomalacia (PVL) may result in:
      (1) Diminished white matter volume and thinned corpus callosum.
      (2) Ventriculomegaly.
      (3) Increased signal of periventricular white matter on proton density–weighted scans (PD) and T2WI; most common areas are peritrigonal.
      (4) Abnormal areas directly abut ventricular walls; subcortical white matter is relatively spared.
      (5) Differential diagnosis: normal foci of slow myelination in posterior association tracts (these are not directly adjacent to ventricular wall); may persist until third or fourth decade.
    c. NOTE: PVL is *not* specific for, or pathognomonic of, hypoxic-ischemic damage.
      (1) PVL is seen in vast majority of surviving premature infants.
      (2) PVL can be caused by wide spectrum of factors contributing

to adverse intrauterine environment (e.g., infection, metabolic disorders, substance abuse).

    (3) Changes of PVL can occasionally be seen in term infants in absence of asphyxia and probably are due to intrauterine (not perinatal) insult.

2. Term infants and adults.

    a. Watershed is in mature or adult (i.e., parasagittal) distribution.

    b. Imaging findings with perinatal hypoxic-ischemic insults vary with severity of insult and timing of scan.

    (1) Acute: diffuse cerebral edema.

    (2) Basal ganglionic hemorrhage or infarction may occur.

    (3) Later: ischemic changes in cortex, subcortical white matter seen as low density on CT; low signal on T1WI, foci of prolonged T2 on PD or T2WI.

    (4) Other sequelae: multicystic encephalomalacia, white matter atrophy with ventriculomegaly, ulegyria (mushroom-shaped gyri in watershed areas overlying area of white matter tissue loss and gliosis).

E. Trauma (see Chapter 42): white matter shearing injuries.

1. Twisting, shearing injury produces damage in predictable locations.

    a. Subcortical white matter.

    b. Corpus callosum.

    c. Centrum semiovale.

    d. Corticomedullary junction.

2. Radiology.

    a. Hypointense foci on T1WI, hyperintense on T2WI in characteristic locations.

    b. Look for other evidence of trauma (e.g., residual blood products).

3. One of many causes for multifocal white matter disease ("unknown bright objects" [UBOs]).

F. Vascular: Lacunar infarcts, small vessel vascular disease, aging, and migraine headaches have been implicated as causes for small multifocal white matter lesions.

G. Normal: Sixty percent of healthy elderly patients with normal cognitive function have multiple foci of increased white matter signal on T2WI.

SUGGESTED READINGS

Balakrishnan J, Becker PS, Kumar AJ, et al: Acquired immunodeficiency syndrome: correlation of radiologic and pathologic findings in the brain, *Radiographics* 10:201-215, 1990.

Barkovich AJ: Metabolic and destructive brain disorders. In *Pediatric neuroimaging*, New York, 1990, Raven Press, pp 49-75.

Barkovich AJ, Truwit CL: Brain damage from perinatal asphyxia: correlation of MR findings with gestational age, *AJNR* 11:1087-1096, 1990.

Hendrie HC, Farlow MR, Austroni MG, et al: Foci of increased T2 signal intensity on brain MR scans of healthy elderly subjects, *AJNR* 10:703-707, 1989.

Lien HH, Blomlie V, Saeter G, et al: Osteogenic sarcoma: MR signal abnormalities of the brain in asymptomatic patients treated with high-dose methotrexate, *Radiology* 179:547-550, 1991.

Mayer PL, Kier EL: The controversy of the periventricular white matter circulation: a review of the anatomic literature, *AJNR* 12:223-228, 1991.

Nelson MD Jr, Gonzalez-Gomez I, Gilles FH: The search for human telencephalic ventriculofugal arteries, *AJNR* 12:215-222, 1991.

Osborn AG, Harnsberger HR, Smoker WRK, Boyer R: Multiple sclerosis in adolescents: CT and MR findings, *AJNR* 11:489-494, 1990.

Osborn RE, Alder DC, Mitchell CS: MR imaging of the brain in patient with migraine headaches, *AJNR* 12:521-524, 1991.

Smith AS, Meisler DM, Weinstein MA: High-signal periventricular lesions in patients with sarcoidosis: neurosarcoidosis or multiple sclerosis? *AJNR* 10:425-490, 1989.

Valk PE, Dillon WP: Radiation injury of the brain, *AJNR* 12:45-62, 1991.

Yetkin FZ, Haughton VM, Papke RA, et al: Multiple sclerosis: specificity of MR for diagnosis, *Radiology* 178:447-451, 1991.

Zamaroczy D, Schluesener HJ, Jolesz FA, et al: Differentiation of experimental white matter lesions using multiparametric magnetic resonance measurements, *Invest Radiol* 26:317-324, 1991.

CHAPTER 40

Degenerative, toxic, and metabolic diseases

KEY CONCEPTS

1. Cortical atrophy and periventricular and deep white matter lesions are often found in normal elderly people with intact cognition.
2. Considerable clinical overlap in the dementias (e.g., Alzheimer's disease, multiinfarct dementia) is reflected in overlapping computed tomography (CT) and magnetic resonance (MR) appearance and paucity of pathognomonic imaging findings.
3. Extrapyramidal system and movement disorders with frequent imaging abnormalities (not pathognomonic) include:
   a. Huntington's chorea: caudate atrophy
   b. Parkinson's disease: atrophy of substantia nigra
   c. Progressive supranuclear palsy: midbrain atrophy
4. Abnormal signal (diffuse hypointensity from iron deposition, focal hyperintensities from gliosis on T2-weighted image [T2WI]) can be seen in the basal ganglia, as well as other nuclei, the cerebellum, and other locations, in a number of disorders. Some overlap with normal is also present.
5. Pick's disease is characterized by frontotemporal atrophy.
6. In Jakob-Creutzfeldt disease, imaging findings are often normal; occasionally rapidly progressive diffuse cerebral atrophy is seen.
7. In alcohol-induced atrophy, imaging findings are nonspecific but the cerebellum is often disproportionately affected. Alcoholic patients also often have nonspecific white matter hyperintense foci on T2WI.
8. In central pontine myelinolysis, T2WI shows a midpontine area of increased signal.

A comprehensive delineation of all neurodegenerative disease is beyond the scope of this text. Some of the degenerative diseases that primarily affect white matter are discussed in the preceding chapters. This chapter outlines a few of the other more common degenerative brain disorders.

I. Normal brain aging: Just as certain imaging findings reflect changes in brain morphology with fetal and neonatal development, so other CT and MR manifestations mirror normal alterations in the aging brain.
   A. White matter.
      1. Sixty percent of healthy elderly patients with normal cognitive function have multifocal areas of increased white matter signal on T2WI.
      2. Rim of increased signal intensity around lateral ventricles, especially frontal and occipital horns, is normal in elderly (most likely represents gliosis).
      3. Periventricular hypodensities on CT (sometimes called leukoariosis) are also commonly identified in elderly.
   B. Basal ganglia.
      1. Ferric iron not present in brain at birth; increases with age.
      2. Progressive deposition of iron in globus pallidus and substantia nigra; lesser amounts in red nucleus, putamen, and dentate nucleus.
         a. Causes preferential T2 relaxation.
         b. Low signal on T2WI.
         c. Globus pallidus normally shows lower signal than putamen; by eighth decade they may be equal.
   C. Ventricles, sulci, and subarachnoid cisterns.
      1. CSF spaces undergo mild to moderate progressive enlargement with normal aging.
      2. Although some CT- and MR-based criteria for age-related standards of normal ventricular and sulcal size have been published, these often involve complicated computer programs and therefore are difficult to apply in practice, particularly in patients over 70 years of age.
   D. Brain metabolism.
      1. Positron emission tomography has shown that normal aging causes little or no significant change in glucose utilization.
      2. To date, no definitive changes with normal aging have been seen with MR spectroscopy.
      3. Reports of alterations in regional cerebral blood flow (as assessed by stable xenon CT method) and single-photon emission CT in normal elderly are controversial.
II. Dementias: Dementias and memory disorders are not uniformly diffuse and not all alike. Following summarizes current thinking on imaging in cases of dementia.
   A. Alzheimer's disease.
      1. Incidence: most common disorder causing dementia.

2. Pathology (characteristic).
   a. Alzheimer's neurofibrillary degeneration and tangles. (NOTE: These are not specific for Alzheimer's disease, since they can be found in progressive supranuclear palsy, some patients with viral encephalitis, and subacute sclerosing panencephalitis.)
   b. Senile plaques.
   c. Nonspecific neuronal loss, atrophic changes, and reactive astrocytosis.
3. Radiology.
   a. Cerebral atrophy, particularly in anterior temporal lobe and hippocampal formation. (Reported changes include temporal horn greater than 3 mm and dilated hippocampal–choroidal fissure complex.) There is some overlap with normal changes of aging.
   b. Periventricular, and less commonly subcortical, hyperintensities on T2WI. Also has substantial overlap with normal changes of aging.
   c. Progressive ventricular enlargement with time, greater than normal increase with age.
B. Vascular dementia (e.g., multiinfarct dementia, multiinfarct cognitive disorder, Binswanger's encephalopathy, lacunar state).
   1. Incidence: estimated 10% of dementias.
   2. Pathology: wide spectrum of findings, including infarct, myelin pallor, demyelination, hyaline arteriolar sclerosis, gliosis.
   3. Radiology: overlap with Alzheimer's disease, normal changes of aging.
      a. Periventricular and subcortical foci of increased signal on T2WI (prominent subcortical abnormalities thought to be more common in vascular than degenerative dementia).
      b. Cortical (gray matter) infarcts, volume loss.
III. Extrapyramidal system and movement disorders: Number of these disorders are accompanied by cortical loss and enlargement of adjacent subarachnoid spaces. Some (e.g., Huntington's chorea and Parkinson's disease) may also be accompanied by dementia.
A. Huntington's chorea.
   1. Incidence: 5 to 10:100,000.
   2. Inheritance: autosomal dominant with complete penetrance. Locus on chromosome 4 reported.
   3. Age at clinical onset: 20 to 50 years.
   4. Pathology: severe neuronal loss, greatest in caudate nucleus and putamen.
   5. Radiology.
      a. Diffuse cortical atrophy common.

      b. Focal caudate atrophy (frontal horns preferentially enlarged).

      c. Increased iron deposition in striatum.

B. Parkinson's disease.

  1. Incidence: most common movement disorder (1% of people over 50 years of age).

  2. Age at clinical onset: 40 to 70 years.

  3. Pathology: loss of pigment-bearing neurons in substantia nigra (particularly zona compacta), locus ceruleus, and dorsal vagal nucleus; associated changes of reactive gliosis.

  4. Radiology.

      a. Atrophy of substantia nigra (pars compacta) is characteristic.

      b. Most patients do not have significantly decreased putaminal signal on T2WI.

      c. Generalized cortical atrophy; overlaps with normal changes of aging.

C. Progressive supranuclear palsy.

  1. Clinical findings: parkinsonian clinical features plus abnormalities in central control of extraocular muscles; ataxia; sometimes dementia.

  2. Pathology: neuronal loss with Alzheimer's neurofibrillary tangles in basal ganglia (particularly pallidum), brainstem, and cerebellum.

  3. Radiology: no consistent abnormalities.

      a. Midbrain atrophy (50% of cases).

      b. Some earlier reports of decreased putaminal signal but is highly variable.

      c. Some patients have decreased signal in colliculi on T2WI.

D. Multisystem atrophy.

  1. Clinical findings: parkinsonian features plus involvement of additional systems (e.g., sympathetic nervous system).

  2. Incidence: about one fifth as common as Parkinson's disease.

  3. Pathology: Spectrum includes:

      a. Shy-Drager syndrome.

      b. Olivopontocerebellar atrophy.

      c. Striatonigral degeneration.

  4. Radiology.

      a. Atrophy.

        (1) Olivopontocerebellar degeneration involving cerebellum, pons, brachium pontis.

        (2) Shy-Drager syndrome: numerous nuclei (especially putamen) affected.

      b. Hypointensity on T2WI.

        (1) Olivopontocerebellar degeneration: transverse pontine fibers, cerebellum, brachium pontis.

    (2) Shy-Drager syndrome: all nuclei, particularly putamen, substantia nigra, red nucleus.
  E. Hallervorden-Spatz disease.
    1. Incidence: rare.
    2. Inheritance: autosomal recessive.
    3. Onset of symptoms: second decade.
    4. Pathology: abnormal iron accumulation in basal ganglia with variable degrees of neuronal loss.
    5. Radiology: diffusely hypointense globus pallidus, thalami, red nuclei, and substantia nigra on T2WI (iron deposition) with focal hyperintensities (gliosis).
IV. Miscellaneous degenerative and toxic disorders.
  A. Pick's disease ("lobar atrophy").
    1. Incidence: rare.
    2. Pathology.
      a. Severe neuronal loss with cortical and subcortical astrocytosis in frontal and temporal lobes, sometimes in basal ganglia and substantia nigra.
      b. Argentophilic inclusions and Pick's cells.
    3. Radiology: selective frontotemporal atrophy.
  B. Jakob-Creutzfeldt disease.
    1. Incidence: one per million per year.
    2. Clinical findings: Rapid progressive dementia, myoclonus; invariably fatal.
    3. Pathology.
      a. Transmissible; probably slow or atypical viral infection; no specific agent yet identified.
      b. Widespread spongiform changes in cerebral cortex.
    4. Radiology.
      a. Often normal or only mild atrophy.
      b. Rapidly progressive severe atrophy rare.
  C. Wilson's disease (hepatolenticular degeneration).
    1. Inheritance: autosomal recessive.
    2. Pathology: increased absorption of copper from intestine; failure of conversion to ceruloplasmin with deposition of copper-aluminum complex (especially in brain and liver).
      a. Copper deposition, spongy degeneration of basal ganglia.
      b. Gliosis of affected areas.
    3. Radiology.
      a. Copper has minimal magnetic susceptibility effects and therefore is not hypointense on T2WI.
      b. Gliotic changes (high-signal foci) in basal ganglia, as well as brainstem and white matter.

    D. Alcoholic atrophy: Changes are nonspecific, but often cerebellum is disproportionately affected. Presence of multiple round hyperintense white matter foci in asymptomatic alcoholics was recently reported.

    E. Marchiafava-Bignami disease.
      1. Occurs mainly in alcoholic, malnourished persons.
      2. Pathology: selective myelinolysis in corpus callosum, less often in deep white matter.
      3. Radiology.
        a. CT: hypodense corpus callosum.
        b. MR: foci of prolonged T1 and T2 relaxation in corpus callosum and deep white matter.

    F. Central pontine myelinolysis.
      1. Reported in alcoholic, malnourished patients and those with electrolyte or acid-base abnormalities (especially hyponatremia with rapid correction).
      2. Pathology: Myelinoclastic changes are most striking in pons but have been reported in other areas.
      3. Radiology: prolonged T1 and T2 in central region of basis pontis.
      4. Differential diagnosis: multiple sclerosis, infarct, encephalitis, neoplasm.

    G. Degenerative brain diseases secondary to proven or putative inborn errors of metabolism: Reported imaging findings are sparse; nonspecific subtle signal abnormalities can sometimes be found in white matter.
      1. Disorders of lipid metabolism.
        a. Tay-Sachs disease (infantile G_{M3} gangliosidosis).
        b. Niemann-Pick disease (sphingomyelinosis).
        c. Gaucher's disease (glucocerebroside lipidosis).
        d. Metachromatic leukodystrophy (cerebroside sulfatidosis).
        e. Krabbe's disease (galactocerebrosidosis).
        f. Batten's disease (neuronal ceroid lipofuscinosis).
      2. Disorders of mucopolysaccharide metabolism.
        a. Type I (Hurler's syndrome).
        b. Type II (Hunter's syndrome).
        c. Type III (Sanfilippo's syndrome).
      3. Disorders of carbohydrate metabolism.
        a. Glycogen storage disease.
        b. Galactosemia.
        c. Subacute necrotizing encephalopathy (Leigh's disease).
      4. Disorders of amino acid metabolism.
        a. Phenylketonuria.
        b. Tyrosinosis.
        c. Leucinosis (maple syrup urine disease).
        d. Homocystinuria.
        e. Hartnup disease.

5. Disorders of metal metabolism.
    a. Wilson's disease (see preceding).
    b. Hypoparathyroidism, pseudohypoparathyroidism. (NOTE: Widespread calcification in basal ganglia, other nuclei, and white matter was once thought to be characteristic but is more often seen in *absence* of demonstrable metabolic disorders.)
H. Wallerian degeneration.
    1. Pathology: anterograde degeneration of axons and their myelin sheaths secondary to either axon injury or death of axon's cell body. In brain, seen most commonly with cerebral infarction, less often with trauma.
    2. Radiology: linear foci of prolonged T1 and T2 relaxation times along white matter fiber tracts (e.g., internal capsule, brainstem); ipsilateral atrophy of affected structure (e.g., peduncle, pons).

SUGGESTED READINGS

Bowen BC, Barker WW, Loewenstein DA: MR signal abnormalities in memory disorder and dementia, *AJNR* 11:283-290, 1990.

Braffman BH, Grossman RI, Goldberg HI, et al: MR imaging of Parkinson disease with spin-echo and gradient-echo sequences, *AJNR* 9:1093-1099, 1988.

Brown JJ, Hesselink JR, Rothrock JF: MR and CT of lacunar infarcts, *AJNR* 9:477-482, 1988.

de Leon MJ, George AE, Reisberg B, et al: Alzheimer's disease: longitudinal CT studies of ventricular change, *AJNR* 10:371-376, 1989.

Drayer BP: Imaging of demyelinating and degenerative diseases of the brain, RSNA Categorical Course Syllabus in Neuroradiology, Chicago, 1987, Radiological Society of North America, pp 113-124.

Fazekas F, Chewluk JB, Alvai A, et al: MR signal abnormalities at 1.5T in Alzheimer's dementia and normal aging, *AJNR* 8:421-426, 1987.

Gallucci M, Amicarelli I, Rossi A, et al: MR imaging of white matter lesions in uncomplicated chronic alcoholism, *J Comput Assist Tomogr* 13:395-398, 1989.

George AE, de Leon MJ, Stylopoulos CA, et al: CT diagnostic features of Alzheimer disease, *AJNR* 11:101-107, 1990.

Jack CR Jr, Bentley MD, Twomey CK, Zinsmeister AR: MR imaging-based volume measurements of the hippocampal formation and anterior temporal lobe: validation studies, *Radiology* 176:205-209, 1990.

Johnson DW, Stringer WA, Marks MP, et al: Stable xenon CT cerebral blood flow imaging: rationale for and role in clinical decision making, *AJNR* 12:201-213, 1991.

Kido DK, Caine ED, LeMay M, et al: Temporal lobe atrophy in patients with Alzheimer disease, *AJNR* 10:551-555, 1989.

Kuhn MJ, Johnson KA, Davis DR: Wallerian degeneration: evaluation with MR imaging, *Radiology* 168:199-202, 1989.

Miller GM, Baker HL Jr, Okazaki H, Whisnant JP: Central pontine myelinolysis and its imitators: MR findings, *Radiology* 168:795-902, 1988.

Mirowitz SA, Sartor K, Prensky AJ, et al: Neurodegenerative diseases of childhood: MR and CT evaluation, *J Comput Assist Tomogr* 15:210-222, 1991.

Mutoh K, Okuno T, Ito M, et al: MR imaging of a group I case of Hallervorden-Spatz disease, *J Comput Assist Tomogr* 12:851-853, 1988.

Naidu S, Moser HW: Value of neuroimaging in metabolic diseases affecting the CNS, *AJNR* 12:413-416, 1991.

Okazaki H: Degenerative disease. In *Fundamentals of neuropathology,* New York, 1989, Igaku-Shoin, pp 163-182.

Okazaki H: Metabolic and toxic diseases. In *Fundamentals of neuropathology,* New York, 1989, Igaku-Shoin, pp 183-282.

Onishi T, Hoshi H, Nagamuchi S, et al: Regional cerebral blood flow study with ^{123}I-IMP in patients with degenerative dementia, *AJNR* 12:513-520, 1991.

Prayer L, Wimberger D, Kramer J, et al: Cranial MRI in Wilson's disease, *Neuroradiology* 32:211-214, 1990.

Rusinek H, de Leon MJ, George AE, et al: Alzheimer disease: measuring loss of cerebral gray matter with MR imaging, *Radiology* 178:109-114, 1991.

Savoiardo M, Strada L, Geiotti F, et al: MR imaging in progressive supranuclear palsy and Shy-Drager syndrome, *J Comput Assist Tomogr* 13:555-560, 1989.

Savoiardo M, Strada L, Girotti F, et al: Olivopontocerebellar atrophy: MR diagnosis and relationship to multisystem atrophy, *Radiology* 174:693-698, 1990.

Schlenska GK, Walter GF: Serial computed tomography in Creutzfeldt-Jakob disease, *Neuroradiology* 31:303-306, 1989.

Shaw DMW, Maravilla KR, Weinberger E, et al: MR imaging of phenylketonuria, *AJNR* 12:403-406, 1991.

Simmons JT, Pastakia B, Chase TN, Shults CW: Magnetic resonance imaging in Huntington disease, *AJNR* 7:25-28, 1986.

CHAPTER 41

Intracranial hemorrhage

KEY CONCEPTS

1. Magnetic resonance (MR) signal of hematoma depends on:
   a. Age of clot
   b. Oxygenation
      (1) Peripheral versus central
      (2) Parenchymal versus cisternal
   c. Hemoglobin status (electron configuration of iron) and potential for dipole-dipole interactions
   d. Red blood cell status (intact versus lysed) and physical state of clot (e.g., liquid versus semisolid)
   e. Dilution effects
   f. Magnetic field strengths
   g. Pulse sequences and flip angles
2. **MR of blood**

	T1WI	T2WI
a. Oxyhemoglobin	Isointense	Isointense
b. Deoxyhemoglobin	Dark	Darker
c. Methemoglobin		
(1) Intracellular	Bright	Dark
(2) Extracellular	Bright	Bright
d. Hemosiderin, ferritin	Dark	Dark (even darker on gradient echo scans)

3. CAVEAT: MR signal of blood clots is highly variable and multifactorial. Other factors *besides* hemoglobin state include field strength, pulse sequences elected, status of red blood cells, age, and even size of the clot, and presence of water or fibrin.

I. Pathology.
   A. Pathochemistry. (NOTE: Temporal evolution of hemorrhage is variable.)

  1. Intracerebral hemorrhage most often has arterial origin.
  2. Hyperacute.
     a. Occurs in minutes to a few hours.
     b. Active bleeding; both clotted and nonclotted blood present.
     c. Oxygen-saturated hemoglobin. (High water content of hyper-acute clots may produce high signal intensity of clot on T2WI.)
  3. Acute.
     a. Within hours.
     b. Progressive clotting, clot retraction, hemoconcentration.
     c. Deoxyhemoglobin protein clot with intact red blood cells.
     d. Adjacent edema.
  4. Subacute.
     a. Twenty-four hours to several days.
     b. Deoxyhemoglobin converted to methemoglobin.
     c. Lysis of red blood cells with time; lysis and methemoglobin formation occur from peripheral to central.
     d. Edema decreases.
  5. Chronic.
     a. Days to weeks.
     b. Hemosiderin and ferritin in macrophages at periphery.
     c. Fibrosis and marginal gliosis.
     d. Edema absent.
 B. Etiology (Table 41-1).
  1. Trauma, hypertension, and stroke most common causes.
  2. Vascular (vascular malformation, aneurysm).
  3. Neoplastic: *Any tumor can hemorrhage.*
     a. Primary: Highly vascular neoplasms such as glioblastoma often bleed; meningiomas rarely do.
     b. Metastatic: lung, breast, and melanoma common sources of brain metastases; choriocarcinoma, melanoma, and metastases from lung and kidney most common lesions to hemorrhage.
  4. Spontaneous.
  5. Infection (rare).
  6. Miscellaneous: coagulopathy, angiopathy (e.g., amyloid), dural sinus and cortical vein occlusion.
 C. Location: Intracranial hemorrhage may be:
  1. Epidural.
  2. Subdural.
  3. Subarachnoid.
  4. Parenchymal.
  5. Intraventricular.
II. MR imaging of brain hemorrhage (see box, p. 274). Some controversy exists on this subject, but following probably represents dominant viewpoints:
 A. Pathophysiology.

Table 41-1 Causes of intracranial hemorrhage

Pathology	Typical location(s)	Comments
Congenital-developmental: prematurity (germinal plate)	Periventricular: intraventricular	
Trauma	Epidural; subdural; subarachnoid; white matter (shearing); cortical contusions	
Hypertension	External capsule; basal ganglia; pons; cerebellum	
Stroke	Vascular distribution; gyrus	
Vascular malformation		
Anteriovenous malformation	Anywhere	Typical age 20-40 yr
Venous angioma	White matter near ventricular angle	Look for transcortical draining vein
Cavernous angioma	White matter; gray-white junction	Often multiple, familial
Aneurysm	Subarachnoid; basal clots	Acute subarachnoid hemorrhage hard to see on magnetic resonance image
Neoplasm		
Primary	White matter	Any tumor anywhere can bleed
Metastatic	Gray-white junction	Frequently multiple; lung; kidney; melanoma; choriocarcinoma
Miscellaneous		
Amyloid	Lobar: gray-white junction	In elderly; multiple recurring lobar bleeds common
Coagulopathy	Anywhere	Circulating anticoagulants (e.g., in lupus), platelet disorders, etc.
Dural sinus or cortical vein occlusion	Petechial clots; edema	Sinus thrombosis (usually high signal on T1-weighted image); "empty delta" sign on computed tomography classic but not always present

BLOOD PRODUCT EVOLUTION IN BRAIN HEMORRHAGE

OXYHEMOGLOBIN

1. Onset to 12 hours
2. Fe^{2+}
3. Diamagnetic
4. No T1 or T2 shortening (isointense)

DEOXYHEMOGLOBIN

1. 1 to 7 days
2. Fe^{2+} (but has four unpaired electrons in high-spin state)
3. Paramagnetic
4. Relaxivity
   a. T1 shortening: none (isointense)
   b. T2 shortening: yes (hypointense)

METHEMOGLOBIN

1. 5 days to months or years
2. Fe^{3+}
3. Paramagnetic
4. Relaxivity
   a. T1 shortening: yes (hyperintense)
   b. T2 shortening: yes if intracellular
   c. T2 prolongation: yes if extracellular (hyperintense; undiluted may be isointense)

HEMOSIDERIN

1. Weeks to years
2. Fe^{3+}
3. Paramagnetic
4. Relaxivity
   a. T1 shortening: none (isointense); may be slightly hypointense if large lesion)
   b. T2 shortening: yes (hypointense)
   c. Magnetic susceptibility effects (profoundly hypointense on gradient echo scans)

1. Oxyhemoglobin has ferrous iron, is diamagnetic, and does not affect relaxation times.
2. Deoxyhemoglobin has ferrous iron but also has four unpaired electrons, is paramagnetic, causes local field magnetic susceptibility effects (preferential T2 shortening), and is isointense on T1, darker on T2.

3. Methemoglobin is ferrous, has five unpaired electrons, and has proton-electron dipole-dipole relaxation.
   a. Intact red blood cells: both T1 and T2 shortening; bright on T1WI, hypointense on proton density–weighted scan (PD), even more hypointense on T2WI.
   b. Free methemoglobin: T1 shortening; no T2 shortening with extracellular; bright on both T1WI and T2WI.
4. Hemosiderin: ferric; paramagnetic with high magnetic susceptibility.
   a. Water-insoluble, therefore does not shorten T1 because proton-electron dipole-dipole interactions cannot occur. Isointense to hypointense on T1WI.
   b. Enhances T2 relaxation, therefore dark on T2WI.
   c. Strong magnetic susceptibility effects make hemosiderin profoundly hypointense on gradient echo scans.
   d. Recent studies indicate that ferritin also contributes to MR appearance of chronic hemorrhage.
5. Proton density changes affect appearance on MR. Dilution causes increased proton density. Effects:
   a. Concentrated intracellular methemoglobin is hyperintense on T1WI, hypointense on T2WI.
   b. Concentrated (undiluted) free methemoglobin is hyperintense on T1WI, isointense on T2WI.
   c. Dilute free methemoglobin is hyperintense on both T1WI and T2WI.
   d. Recent studies indicate ferritin also contributes to MR appearance of late hemorrhage.
B. MR pulse sequence for hemorrhage evaluation.
   1. Spin echo.
      a. T1WI: TR 500-800 msec/TE 20 msec.
      b. Proton density: TR 2500 msec/TE 20-40 msec.
      c. T2WI: TR 2500-3000 msec/TE 70-90 msec.
   2. Gradient echo. (NOTE: Even T1-weighted partial flip angle scans are very sensitive to magnetic susceptibility effects of iron and show decreased signal.)
      a. T1WI: TR 500 msec/TE 8 msec/60° flip angle.
      b. Proton density: TR 500 msec/TE 20 msec/20° flip angle.
      c. T2WI: TR 500 msec/TE 40 msec/20° flip angle.
C. Hematoma signal on MR depends on multiple factors.
   1. Age of clot.
   2. Oxygenation (peripheral versus central, parenchymal versus cisternal).
   3. Hemoglobin status.

4. Red blood cells: intact or lysed.
5. Dilution effects.
6. Magnetic field strength.
7. Pulse sequences and flip angles (determine T1 and T2 weighting and magnetic susceptibility effects).
  D. Location and MR appearance of extraaxial blood.
    1. Subarachnoid hemorrhage.
      a. Acute: may be difficult to detect on MR because of:
        (1) Absence of clot formation.
        (2) Low deoxyhemoglobin concentration (cerebrospinal fluid has relatively high oxygen saturation).
      b. Subacute: hyperintense on T1WI.
      c. Chronic hemorrhage can produce superficial siderosis seen as marked hypointensity on T2WI.
    2. Subdural hematoma.
      a. Acute: isointense on T1WI, hypointense on T2WI.
      b. Subacute: varies, usually hyperintense.
      c. Chronic.
        (1) Most are isointense to slightly hypointense (relative to gray matter) on T1WI.
        (2) Most hyperintense on T2WI.
        (3) Some are hyperintense on both T1WI and T2WI (probably because of repeated hemorrhage).
III. CT imaging of brain hemorrhage.
  A. Density of clot depends on:
    1. Hematocrit.
    2. Hemoglobin concentration (protein, not iron, is major determinant of density).
    3. Clot retraction.
    4. Lysis and degradation.
  B. Age and CT appearance.
    1. Acute: hyperdense; exceptions:
      a. May be isodense in extremely anemic patients.
      b. Very rapid hemorrhage can appear hypodense within hyperdense clot.
      c. May be isodense in patients with coagulopathies and normal hematocrit.
    2. Subacute (several days to weeks): isodense.
    3. Chronic: hypodense.
  C. Location and CT appearance.
    1. Epidural hematoma: usually lentiform.
    2. Subdural hematoma.
      a. Acute usually crescentic; chronic can be either crescentic or lentiform.

   b. Effaces underlying sulci.
   c. Displaces interface of gray and white matter; displaces cortical veins.
   d. Subacute subdural hematomas may have enhanced underlying vascular membrane.
  3. Subarachnoid.

SUGGESTED READINGS

Fobben ES, Grossman RI, Atlas SW, et al: MR characteristics of subdural hematoma and hygromas at 1.5T, *AJNR* 10:687-693, 1989.

Gomori JM, Grossman RI, Goldberg HI, et al: Intracranial hematomas: imaging by high-field MR, *Radiology* 157:87-93, 1985.

Grossman RI, Gomori JM, Goldberg HI, et al: MR imaging of hemorrhagic conditions of the head and neck, *Radiographics* 8:441-454, 1988.

Hayman LA, Taber KH, Ford JJ, et al: Effect of clot formation and retraction on spin-echo MR images of blood, *AJNR* 10:1155-1158, 1989.

Taber KH, Migliore PJ, Pagani JJ, et al: Temporal changes in the oxidation state in in vitro blood, *Invest Radiol* 25:240-244, 1990.

Thulborn KR, Sorenson AG, Kowall NW, et al: The role of ferrition and hemosiderin in the MR appearance of cerebral hemorrhage, *AJNR* 11:291-297, 1990.

Zyed A, Hayman LA, Bryan RN: MR imaging of intracerebral blood: diversity in the temporal pattern at 0.5 and 1.0 T, *AJNR* 12:469-474, 1991.

CHAPTER 42

Trauma

KEY CONCEPTS

1. Skull roentgenograms have no role in management of an acute head injury.
2. Computed tomography (CT) is the procedure of choice for evaluating head injuries.
3. Magnetic resonance (MR) is the procedure of choice for evaluating subacute or chronic head injuries and suspected cases of nonaccidental trauma.

Head trauma can affect the calvarium and skull base, leptomeninges, brain parenchyma, and cerebral vasculature in various ways and combinations. A significant number of patients with head trauma also have cervical spine injuries. Numerous studies have shown that plain skull roentgenograms have little if any useful role in the evaluation of acutely injured patients with craniocerebral trauma. If plain films of the head and neck are obtained, the most useful studies are of the cervical spine. This chapter focuses on imaging skull and brain trauma, primarily with CT and to a lesser extent with MR.

   I. Calvarium and base of skull fractures.
      A. Linear skull fractures.
         1. Most common type.
         2. Linear nondisplaced lucency.
         3. Bone windowing of CT scans required for detection.
         4. Absence of fracture: no prognostic significance regarding presence or absence of underlying brain damage. Small linear fractures parallel to scan plane can be missed but are not usually significant.
         5. Complications.

---

    a. Of fractures of posterior wall of frontal sinus or at base of skull.
      (1) Infection.
      (2) Cerebrospinal fluid leak.
      (3) Posttraumatic cephalocele.
      (4) Hearing loss or facial nerve damage with temporal bone fractures.
      (5) Pneumocephalus.
    b. Of dural tear: leptomeningeal cyst or "growing fracture."
    c. Of vessel tear: epidural hematoma.
  B. Depressed skull fracture.
  C. Sutural diastasis.
II. Epidural and subdural hematomas.
  A. Epidural hematoma (EDH).
    1. Outer layer of dura normally is tightly attached to inner table of skull.
      a. Blood collecting in this confined potential space typically assumes biconvex or lentiform shape.
      b. Although occasionally very large, most EDHs are relatively small.
    2. Etiology.
      a. Laceration of meningeal arteries.
      b. Disruption of dural sinuses and veins (venous EDHs particularly common in children).
    3. Location: nearly two thirds temporoparietal; frontal and occipital poles are less common sites.
    4. Radiology.
      a. Biconvex high-density extraaxial mass on CT.
        (1) Displacement of adjacent interface between gray and white matter.
        (2) Subfalcine and descending transtentorial herniation and signs of increased intracranial pressure are common associated findings.
        (3) Look for contrecoup and other injuries.
      b. Mixed isodense to hypodense areas within hyperdense hematoma indicate rapid bleeding and accumulation of unclotted blood.
  B. Subdural hematoma (SDH).
    1. Etiology: rupture of bridging cortical veins.
    2. Location.
      a. Typically convexity (frontoparietal).
      b. Interhemispheric SDH in child without SDH elsewhere should raise suspicion of nonaccidental trauma.

      c. Small subtemporal, subfrontal, and tentorial SDHs best seen on coronal scans.

      d. Usually unilateral in adults; bilateral in 80% to 85% of infants.

   3. Radiology: Findings depend on age of SDH.

      a. CT of acute SDH.

        (1) Crescentic high-density extraaxial fluid collection.

        (2) May extend into interhemispheric fissure and along falx.

        (3) Displacement of interface between gray and white matter.

        (4) Often associated with underlying brain injury (e.g., contusion, focal hematoma).

      b. CT of subacute SDH (SDH typically few days to 3 weeks old).

        (1) Depending on age of clot, may be isodense compared with adjacent brain and difficult to see.

        (2) Look for mass effect (e.g., displacement of interface between gray and white matter, medial displacement of surface veins after administration of contrast material).

        (3) Underlying membrane may be enhanced by contrast media.

        (4) "Balanced" or bilaterally symmetric subacute SDHs can be isodense with underlying cortex and difficult to detect. (Look for indirect signal of mass effect; consider MR or contrast-enhanced CT.)

      c. CT of chronic SDH (SDH greater than 3 weeks old).

        (1) Low-density crescentic extraaxial fluid collection on CT.

        (2) Repeat hemorrhage into preexisting chronic SDH can give mixed density collection, fluid-fluid levels.

        (3) Underlying membrane is enhanced by contrast material.

      d. MR of SDH (see Chapter 40).

        (1) Evolution of acute and subacute hematomas similar to that of intraparenchymal hemorrhage.

        (2) Chronic SDH: isointense or slightly hypointense on T1WI; hyperintense on T2WI; hemosiderin rarely seen.

        (3) Layering phenomena and hemosiderin deposition occur with repeat hemorrhage.

III. Subarachnoid hemorrhage (SAH): often concomitant to other cerebral injury (e.g., intraventricular hemorrhage, contusion; also with rupture of parenchymal hematoma into subarachnoid space or ventricles). Appearance is similar to SAH from aneurysmal rupture. Subtle signs of SAH include high-density collection in foramen cecum of interpeduncular fossa, slight thickening or hyperdensity of falx or tentorium with "feathered" appearance caused by blood extending into adjacent sulci.

IV. Intraventricular hemorrhage (IVH).

  A. Common causes.

   1. Hypertensive hemorrhage in adult (rupture of caudate or basal ganglionic hematoma into ventricle).

2. Germinal matrix hemorrhage in premature infant.
3. Choroid plexus injury with trauma; also rupture of adjacent parenchymal hematoma into ventricle.
4. Aneurysm rupture (from anterior communicating artery into frontal horn of lateral ventricle; from posterior inferior cerebellar artery into fourth ventricle).
   B. Radiology: high-density intraventricular collection on CT; fluid-fluid level common, especially in occipital horns.
V. Parenchymal hemorrhage.
   A. Contusion.
   1. Caused by forcible contact between parenchyma and skull or by depressed skull fracture.
   2. Most common parenchymal injury.
   3. Pathology: petechial hemorrhage, capillary rupture followed by edema, liquefaction.
   4. Location: frontal and anterior temporal most common.
   5. Direct blow causes "coup" injury; "contrecoup" injury occurs at remote site (usually opposite direct injury).
   6. Radiology: CT spectrum varies from normal or minimal focal edema to small, scattered, high-density foci to large lobar collections. Recent studies of ultra-early hemorrhage indicate that bleeding and hematoma enlargement often continue after first hour of hemorrhage. MR of parenchymal hematoma is outlined in Chapter 40.
   B. Shearing injury (diffuse axonal injury).
   1. Etiology: rotational forces with stretching and tearing of axons in white matter fiber tracts.
   2. Location.
      a. Subcortical white matter.
      b. Corpus callosum and deep centrum semiovale.
      c. Internal capsule and basal ganglia.
      d. Brainstem.
   3. High mortality (greater than 50%), often significant morbidity.
   4. Radiology: CT findings may be relatively normal. In subacute or chronic phase, MR can show foci of old hemorrhage, gliosis, and scarring. Shearing injury is one cause of multiple hyperintense white matter foci on T2WI (see Chapter 39).
VI. Increased intracranial pressure: Early changes include sulcal and cisternal effacement, loss of gray-white matter interface on CT, and by diffuse low density of cerebral hemispheres.
VII. Nonaccidental trauma.
   A. Etiology.
   1. Direct blow.
   2. Shaking (shearing injuries).

   B. Incidence: intracranial abnormalities in 10% to 44% of abused children; leading cause of morbidity and mortality in abused children.

   C. CT: Suggestive findings include:

      1. SDH: most common injury; especially suggestive are hematomas of different ages and interhemispheric hematomas.

      2. SAH.

      3. Contusions.

      4. Presence of healing skull fracture, evidence of acute injury.

   D. MR: imaging modality of choice in suspected nonaccidental trauma.

      1. Can more precisely delineate small SDH or cortical contusion.

      2. Can detect shearing injuries and nonhemorrhagic contusions.

      3. Can delineate coexisting hematomas of different ages.

SUGGESTED READINGS

Barkovich AJ: Metabolic and destructive brain disorders. In *Pediatric neuroimaging,* New York, 1990, Raven Press, pp 68-75.

Boyko O, Cooper DF, Grossman CB: Contrast-enhanced CT of acute isodense subdural hematoma, *AJNR* 12:341-343, 1991.

Broderick JP, Brott TG, Tomsick T, et al: Ultra-early evaluation of intracerebral hemorrhage, *J Neurosurg* 72:195-199, 1990.

Fobben ES, Grossman RI, Atlas SW, et al: MR characteristics of subdural hematomas and hygromas at 1.5T, *AJNR* 10:687-693, 1989.

Kleinman PK: Diagnostic imaging in infant abuse, *AJR* 155:703-712, 1990.

Sato Y, Yuh WTC, Smith WL, et al: Head imaging in child abuse: evaluation with MR imaging, *Radiology* 173:653-657, 1989.

Zimmerman RA: Evaluation of head injury: supratentorial. In Taveras JM, Ferrucci JT (eds): *Radiology: diagnosis-imaging-intervention.* Vol 3. *Neuroradiology and radiology of the head and neck,* Philadelphia, 1986, Lippincott, Chapter 37.

CHAPTER 43

Intracranial neoplasms: introduction

KEY CONCEPTS

1. Primary central nervous system (CNS) neoplasms are classified according to the putative cell of origin.
2. The general classification is into glial and nonglial neoplasms.
3. Glial neoplasms include those arising from astrocytes, oligodendrocytes, ependymal cells, and choroid plexus cells. They account for 40% to 50% of primary intracranial tumors.

The basic human urge to classify or group things has with brain tumors—as with many other lesions—produced more controversy than consensus. Although any scheme for categorizing CNS neoplasms has its share of detractors, the system proposed by Bailey and Cushing in the 1920s has, with some modifications, remained the most widely used. The Bailey-Cushing system is based on supposed histogenesis or "cell of origin." Although the shortcomings of this approach are numerous and both immunologic and ultrastructural techniques have greatly expanded the identification of specific cell types composing CNS tumors, the imaging features of brain tumors and their radiologic-pathologic correlations are presented using the modified Bailey-Cushing approach delineated in Okazaki's recent text *Fundamentals of Neuropathology*.

I. Origin of intracranial tumors by cell type: With possible exception of neuron itself, any of following cell types (or precursors thereof) can give rise to primary CNS tumors.
   A. Neurons: Mature neurons do not divide and therefore do not have derivative CNS neoplasms. The only actively dividing neural tissue that could be considered to belong to CNS is olfactory mucosa, which gives rise to olfactory neuroblastomas (esthesioneuroblastoma).

    B. Glial cells: These outnumber the trillion neurons by 5 to 10 times and constitute over half of CNS by volume. Numerous types of glial (sometimes termed "neuroglial") cells exist; some of more important are:

      1. Protoplasmic astrocyte.

      2. Fibrous astrocyte.

      3. Oligodendrocyte.

      4. Ependymal cells.

      5. Choroid plexus (modified ependyma).

    C. Nerve sheath.

      1. Schwann cells.

      2. Fibroblasts (exiting spinal roots and cutaneous nerves only).

    D. Mesenchymal tissue.

      1. Meninges.

      2. Blood vessels.

      3. Bone.

    E. Lymphocytes and leukocytes.

    F. Germ cells.

    G. Pituitary and pineal glands.

  II. CNS neoplasms: general classification and incidence.

    A. Primary neoplasms (70% to 75% of intracranial neoplasms).

      1. Glial tumors (40% to 50% of primary brain tumors).

      2. Nonglial neoplasms.

        a. Tumors of primitive bipotential precursors and nerve cells.

        b. Nerve sheath tumors.

        c. Mesenchymal tumors.

        d. Lymphoreticular tumors and leukemia.

        e. Tumors of maldevelopmental origin.

        f. Phakomatoses.

    B. Metastatic neoplasms (25% to 30% of intracranial tumors).

 III. CNS neoplasms: age and location.

    A. Less than 15 years of age (15% to 20% of intracranial tumors).

      1. CNS tumors second most common pediatric neoplasm (leukemia is most common).

      2. Between 50% and 70% of pediatric brain tumors are infratentorial (in children under 2 years of age, two thirds are supratentorial).

      3. Metastases rare.

    B. More than 15 years of age (adult).

      1. Supratentorial in 70%.

      2. Metastases common.

 IV. Spine tumors: constitute 5% to 10% of CNS neoplasms.

  V. Clinical presentation of primary CNS tumors: primary symptoms generally related to size of neoplasms, location, presence of edema or hemorrhage, and other factors; secondary symptoms related to increased intracranial pressure.

A. Focal neurologic deficit (most common symptom).

B. Seizure (second most common symptom; incidence varies with tumor type, location).

C. Headaches symptom in 30%.

SUGGESTED READING

Okazaki H: Neoplastic and related lesions. In *Fundamentals of neuropathology*, New York, 1989, Igaku-Shoin, pp 203-273.

CHAPTER 44

Intracranial neoplasms: glial tumors

KEY CONCEPTS

1. Glial neoplasms include astrocytomas, oligodendrogliomas, ependymomas, and choroid plexus tumors.
2. Between 40% and 50% of primary central nervous system (CNS) neoplasms are gliomas; 70% of gliomas are astrocytomas; and 75% of astrocytomas are anaplastic astrocytomas or glioblastoma multiforme.
3. The magnetic resonance (MR) signal of neoplasms is nonspecific and tells little about histologic characteristics, benignity, or malignancy.

I. General.
 A. Some general comments about neuroglial cells.
  1. Astrocytes: location.
   a. Fibrous type in white matter and at junction between gray and white matter.
   b. Protoplasmic astrocytes in gray matter.
   c. Microglial cells ubiquitous.
   d. Oligodendrocytes in white matter and some gray matter.
   e. Ependymal cells lining ventricle and central canal of cord.
   f. Modified ependymal cells in choroid plexus.
  2. Functions of glial cells.
   a. Developmental lattice.
   b. Mechanical support.
   c. Do not generate or propagate impulses but do react passively and probably have significant role in augmenting neuronal functions.

    d. Oligodendrocytes make myelin.
    e. Microglial cells phagocytose debris.
    f. Astrocytes make scar and reactive tissue.
    g. Ependymal cells move cerebrospinal fluid (CSF) and are responsible for secretion and transport of CSF.
  3. Glial cells have enormous potential for abnormal growth and are chief source of primary CNS neoplasms.
B. Corresponding to three major types of glial cell are three major types of glioma.
  1. Astrocyte—astrocytoma.
  2. Oligodendrocyte—oligodendroglioma.
  3. Ependymal cell—ependymoma.
  4. NOTE: "Mixed" gliomas (tumors with more than one cell type present) also occur. A fourth category of glial neoplasms, choroid plexus tumors, is less common than the three major types.
C. Incidence.
  1. Between 40% and 50% of primary CNS tumors are gliomas.
  2. Seventy percent of gliomas are astrocytomas.
  3. Fifty percent of astrocytomas are glioblastoma multiforme (most malignant variety of astrocytoma).
D. Types of astrocytoma.
  1. Fibrillary.
  2. Pilocytic.
  3. Subependymal giant cell (most common in tuberous sclerosis).
  4. Gemistocytic.
  5. Pleomorphic xanthoastrocytoma.
  6. Anaplastic.
E. Grading of astrocytomas.
  1. Traditional (Kernohan).
    a. Grade 1: normal to slightly increased cellularity, anaplasia minimal to absent.
    b. Grade 2: slightly increased cellularity, early anaplastic changes in roughly half of cells.
    c. Grade 3 or anaplastic astrocytoma: cellularity increased by 50% or more, moderate anaplasia, average of one mitotic figure per high power field.
    d. Grade 4 or glioblastoma multiforme: marked cellularity, anaplasia, numerous mitoses, necrosis, neovascularity.
  2. National Brain Tumor Study Group modification of World Health Organization classification groups astrocytomas into three categories.
    a. Low-grade ("benign" or well-differentiated) astrocytoma: proliferation of well-differentiated fibrillary astrocytes, mild nu-

clear pleomorphism, mild cellularity, mitoses rarely encountered, no endothelial proliferation.
  b. Anaplastic astrocytoma: greater hypercellularity and pleomorphism, mitoses and endothelial proliferation common, necrosis absent.
  c. Glioblastoma multiforme: highly cellular, marked pleomorphism, prominent endothelial proliferation; necrosis present.
II. Low-grade astrocytoma ("benign" astrocytoma).
  A. Incidence: 25% to 30% of astrocytomas.
  B. Age: generally occur in younger patients.
    1. Childhood.
    2. Adults from 20 to 40 years.
  C. Location: proportional to amount of white matter present.
  D. Pathology: See preceding.
    1. No necrosis.
    2. No neovascularity; hemorrhage rare; edema uncommon.
    3. May be either focal or diffusely infiltrating.
    4. Calcification in 15% to 20% of patients.
  E. Radiology.
    1. Computed tomography (CT): typically well-delineated, low-density mass with little or no enhancement.
    2. MR: well-defined, isointense or hypointense on T1-weighted image (T1WI), hyperintense on T2WI; hemorrhage and signal heterogeneity uncommon; little mass effect or edema. May also be diffusely infiltrating, causing slight enlargement of affected hemisphere.
  F. Survival: 3 to 10 years; death from tumor dedifferentiating into more malignant astrocytoma more common than death from progressive low-grade disease.
  G. Juvenile pilocytic astrocytoma is distinctive subtype of astrocytoma.
    1. Tumor of children and young adults; often (but not always) associated with neurofibromatosis.
    2. Pilocytic ("hairlike") astrocytes and loosely aggregated protoplasmic astrocytes; often cystic.
    3. Location: tend to occur around third and fourth ventricles.
      a. Optic chiasm and hypothalamus most common.
      b. Cerebellar vermis next most common.
      c. Cerebellar hemispheres.
      d. Less common: cerebral hemispheres.
    4. Radiology.
      a. Sharply marginated, well delineated.
      b. Edema rare.
      c. Cyst formation common (with mural nodule).
      d. Calcification occasionally.

     e. CT: isodense or hypodense, marked enhancement of nodule.

     f. MR: isointense or hypointense on T1WI, hyperintense on T2WI; enhancement by contrast media in nodule but not cyst wall.

III. Anaplastic ("malignant") astrocytoma.
  A. Incidence: 25% to 30% of astrocytomas.
  B. Age: greater than 40 years.
  C. Location: proportional to amount of white matter.
  D. Pathology: See preceding (often histologic overlap at either end with low-grade astrocytoma or glioblastoma).
  E. Radiology: compared with benign astrocytoma:
    1. Less well defined.
    2. More mass effect.
    3. More contrast enhancement.
    4. More heterogeneity on both CT and MR.
    5. Less commonly calcified.
  F. Survival: 2 to 3 years.

IV. Glioblastoma multiforme.
  A. Incidence: 50% of astrocytomas.
  B. Age: fifth to seventh decades. Age at diagnosis is single most powerful predictor of histologic findings and survival. In general, the older the patient, the more malignant the astrocytoma and the worse the prognosis.
  C. Location: supratentorial cerebral hemispheres (posterior fossa glioblastoma multiforme rare).
  D. Pathology: characterized by necrosis and hemorrhage.
  E. Radiology: compared with benign astrocytoma, greater mass effect, vasogenic edema, heterogeneity, and enhancement. NOTE: In glioblastome multiforme, viable tumor cells can almost always be found in edematous areas *outside* region of contrast enhancement.

V. Oligodendroglioma.
  A. Incidence: 5% of primary brain tumors.
  B. Adults/children, 8:1; peak age 35 to 40 years.
  C. Location: 85% supratentorial, mostly hemispheric.
    1. Often cortical or subcortical.
    2. Intraventricular rare.
    3. Frontal lobe most common.
  D. Pathology.
    1. Well-defined, circumscribed, globular.
    2. Hemorrhage and cyst formation rare.
    3. Calcification in more than 70%.
    4. Nearly 50% considered "mixed" (i.e., some astrocytic elements).
  E. Radiology.
    1. CT: heterogeneous mass, usually partially calcified, with variable enhancement.

2. Edema in less than one third.
3. MR: mixed isointense and hypointense on T1WI, hyperintense on T2WI; variable enhancement.
4. Tumors often extend to or involve cortex.

VI. Ependymoma.
- A. Incidence: 5% of intracranial tumors (but third most common intracranial neoplasm in children).
- B. Age.
  1. Children and adolescents (50% younger than 5 years); second, much smaller peak in adults 30 to 40 years of age.
  2. Middle-aged and elderly: subependymoma (only about one third of these are symptomatic; majority are incidental findings at autopsy).
- C. Location.
  1. Between 60% to 70% infratentorial (mostly in children); 70% from fourth ventricle; often extend into cerebellopontine angle or vallecula.
  2. Between 30% and 40% supratentorial (often extraventricular); distributed evenly throughout all age groups.
- D. Pathology.
  1. Several types: cellular (most common; forms perivascular pseudorosettes), epithelial (rosettes), papillary (uncommon), myxopapillary (found exclusively in conus medullaris or filum terminale). Most are slow growing with low mitotic index. Malignancy is rare. A variant, subependymoma, is often found at autopsy in older adults and most frequently occurs in caudal fourth ventricle.
  2. Calcification in 50%.
  3. Cysts common; hemorrhage relatively uncommon (less than 14%).
- E. Radiology.
  1. CT: Most common appearance is a mostly isodense (on nonenhanced CT), calcified (in 50%), partially cystic midline posterior fossa mass with variable enhancement. Tumor often extends laterally into cerebellopontine angles and posteriorly into vallecula. Supratentorial ependymoma is often periventricular or parenchymal, not intraventricular, less often calcified, and may be indistinguishable radiographically from astrocytoma.
  2. MR: typically, solid fourth ventricular mass; nonspecific heterogeneous signal; propensity to spread via foramina of Magendie and Luschka ("plastic" configuration).
- F. Survival: Despite low mitotic index, most ependymomas recur and have relatively poor outcomes (25% to 50% 5-year survival).

VII. Choroid plexus tumors.
- A. Incidence: 0.5% of all intracranial neoplasms; 2% to 3% of gliomas.
- B. Age.

1. Childhood (50% to 80% less than 5 years; 40% less than 1 year).
2. Adults (uncommon).
C. Location.
   1. Childhood: at least 70% in atria of lateral ventricles; 10% in third ventricle.
   2. Adults: fourth ventricle.
D. Pathology.
   1. Histologically benign; approximately 10% malignant.
   2. Reddish cauliflower-like mass.
   3. Cystic degeneration.
   4. Hydrocephalus (cause controversial; "overproduction" of cerebrospinal fluid or communicating hydrocephalus secondary to hemorrhage has been suggested).
   5. Implantation and cerebrospinal fluid seeding can occur with both benign and malignant choroid plexus neoplasms.
E. Radiology.
   1. CT: well-marginated, smooth or lobulated, isodense intraventricular mass with strong, relatively uniform enhancement; calcification in 25% to 80%.
   2. MR: often intermediate intensity on both T1WI and T2WI; areas of signal void. Calcification and old hemorrhage are common. Extension outside ventricle should suggest possibility of malignancy.

SUGGESTED READINGS

Atlas SW: Adult supratentorial tumors, *Semin Roentgenol* 25:130-154, 1990.

Coates TL, Hinshaw DB Jr, Peckman N, et al: Pediatric choroid plexus neoplasms: MR, CT and pathologic correlation, *Radiology* 173:81-88, 1989.

Dean BL, Drayer BP, Bird CR, et al: Gliomas: classification with MR imaging, *Radiology* 174:411-415, 1990.

Domingues RC, Taveras JM, Reimer P, Rosen BR: Foramen magnum choroid plexus papilloma with drop metastases to the lumbar spine, *AJNR* 12:564-565, 1991.

Ellenbogen RG, Winston KR, Kupsky WJ: Tumors of the choroid plexus in children, *Neurosurgery* 28:327-335, 1989.

Gusnard DA: Cerebellar neoplasms in children, *Semin Roentgenol* 25:263-278, 1990.

Jelinek J, Smirniotopoulos JJ, Paresi JE, Kanger M: Lateral ventricular neoplasms of the brain, *AJNR* 11:567-574, 1990.

Lee YY, Van Tassel P: Intracranial oligodendrogliomas: imaging findings in 35 untreated cases, *AJNR* 10:119-127, 1989.

Lee YY, Van Tassel P, Bruner JM, et al: Juvenile pilocytic astrocytomas: CT and MR characteristics, *AJR* 152:1263-1270, 1989.

Spoto GP, Press GA, Hesselink JR, Solomon M: Intracranial ependymoma and subependymoma: MR manifestations, *AJNR* 11:83-91, 1990.

Vertosick FT Jr, Selker RG, Arena VC: Survival of patients with well-differentiated astrocytomas diagnosed in the era of computed tomography, *Neurosurgery* 28:496-501, 1991.

CHAPTER 45

Intracranial neoplasms (nonglial neoplasms): tumors of primitive bipotential precursors and nerve cells

KEY CONCEPTS

1. Primitive neuroectodermal tumors (PNETs) are histologically similar to other undifferentiated small cell central nervous system (CNS) tumors such as medulloblastomas, neuroblastomas, and pineoblastomas.
2. Medulloblastomas are the second most common pediatric brain tumor (astrocytomas are the first). Some pathologists consider medulloblastomas to be posterior fossa PNETs.
3. Imaging studies alone cannot reliably predict the histologic features of pineal tumors or show whether they are malignant. Knowledge of the patient's age and findings of a tumor marker assay and biopsy are necessary.

The first major subgroup of nonglial neoplasms is tumors of primitive bipotential precursors and nerve cells. This category includes medulloblastomas, PNETs, ganglioneuromas and gangliogliomas, primary cerebral neuroblastomas, and pineal parenchymal tumors.

I. Medulloblastoma.
   A. Incidence.
      1. Six percent of all primary intracranial tumors.
      2. Second most common childhood brain tumor.
         a. Between 15% and 20% of childhood intracranial neoplasms (second only to astrocytoma).
         b. Between 30% and 40% of childhood posterior fossa tumors.
   B. Age.
      1. Seventy-five percent less than 15 years of age; 50% less than 10 years.

      2. Second peak at 20 to 30 years of age.

      3. Occurs rarely up to late forties.

  C. Location: exclusively cerebellar.

      1. Midline cerebellar in 75% to 90% (mostly children).

        a. Usually completely fill fourth ventricle.

        b. May extend through vallecula into cisterna magna; lateral extension into cerebellopontine angles less common.

      2. Lateral location in 10% to 15% (mostly adults).

  D. Pathology: Some pathologists consider medulloblastoma to be infratentorial PNET.

      1. Thought to arise from residual germinative cells in external granular layer of posterior medullary velum.

      2. Densely cellular neoplasms with hyperchromatic nuclei, high nuclear/cytoplasmic ratios.

      3. May form pseudorosettes (highly characteristic of medulloblastoma, found in less than one third of patients).

      4. Neoplasm is poorly differentiated in 50%, is desmoplastic in 25%, and shows glial or neuroglial differentiation in 25%.

      5. Early spread into brainstem; dissemination throughout cerebrospinal fluid (CSF) pathways in up to half of patients at time of initial diagnosis.

  E. Radiology.

      1. Computed tomography (CT).

        a. Approximately 90% are well-defined, hyperdense, midline posterior fossa mass on nonenhanced CT.

        b. Enhancement strong and relatively uniform in more than 90%.

        c. Hemorrhage rare; calcification in 10% to 15%; small cysts or areas of inhomogeneous enhancement in up to 40%; hydrocephalus in 95%.

      2. Magnetic resonance (MR): variable.

        a. Isointense to hypointense with brain on T1-weighted image (T1WI); mostly variable (isointense or hyperintense), often mixed signal on T2WI.

        b. Enhancement usually strong but may occasionally be patchy or absent.

        c. Enhancement discloses CSF pathway metastases in 25% to 50% at time of diagnosis. Spinal cord, cauda equina, and thecal sac "drop metastases" are common.

        d. Recent studies show that not all recurrent medulloblastomas are enhanced and therefore absence of enhancement does not necessarily indicate absence of recurrent tumor.

II. Gangliocytoma and ganglioglioma.

  A. Incidence: uncommon (less than 1% of intracranial tumors).

    B. Age: children and young adults (80% less than 30 years).
    C. Location.
        1. Mainly cerebral hemispheres (frontal, temporal occipital lobes).
        2. Ventricles: mainly third, occasionally fourth ventricle.
        3. Cerebellum.
    D. Pathology: spectrum; ganglion neoplasms are classified according to stage of differentiation and to relative proportion of neuronal to glial elements; from most to least well differentiated: gangliocytoma, ganglioglioma, ganglioneuroblastoma, anaplastic ganglioglioma, neuroblastoma.
        1. Ganglioneuroma: pure ganglionic neuronal tumor.
        2. Ganglioglioma: abnormal ganglion cells with glial stroma.
        3. Dysplastic gangliocytoma of cerebellum (Lhermitte-Duclos disease) is rare variant. It is typically found in adults and consists of markedly thickened and enlarged cerebellar folia. Not a true neoplasm.
        4. CAUTION: Some cases of congenitally dysplastic cerebral hemispheres have been called gangliocytomas or gangliogliomas. These dysplastic hemispheres are congenital malformations or hamartomas, not true neoplasms.
    E. Radiology.
        1. CT.
           a. Well-circumscribed low- or mixed-density lesion with little mass effect.
           b. Cysts common (40% to 50%), calcification in one third.
           c. Variable enhancement.
           d. Can erode inner table of skull.
        2. MR: nonspecific.
           a. Well delineated.
           b. Variable signal but usually hypointense on T1WI; generally hyperintense on T2WI.
III. Primitive neuroectodermal tumor (PNET or "peanut" tumor).
    A. Incidence: less than 5% of supratentorial tumors.
    B. Age: Most under 5 years; rarely seen into late teens.
    C. Location: typically deep cerebral white matter; can be intraventricular.
    D. Pathology: controversial; some pathologists consider medulloblastomas, pineoblastomas, and other undifferentiated small cell tumors of the CNS to be PNETs.
        1. Large, bulky masses.
        2. Cysts, necrosis, and hemorrhage common.
        3. Grossly well circumscribed, microscopically invasive.
        4. Densely cellular with greater than 90% undifferentiated cells resembling germinal matrix cells of embryonic neural tube.

    E. Radiology.
       1. CT.
          a. Hyperdense on nonenhanced CT.
          b. Cysts and calcification in 50%.
          c. Hemorrhage in 10%.
          d. Some contrast enhancement nearly always present but variable pattern (solid or patchy; rim; often inhomogeneous).
       2. MR.
          a. Large hemispheric mass that appears well marginated.
          b. No significant edema.
          c. Signal very heterogeneous (cysts and hemorrhage common).
          d. Enhancement patterns similar to those of CT.
    F. Survival: highly malignant; extensive CSF dissemination frequently found at autopsy.
IV. Primary cerebral neuroblastoma.
    A. Incidence: rare (less than 1% of intracranial neoplasms).
    B. Age: generally regarded as tumor of infants and children (80% less than 10 years; 25% less than 2 years; recent series has found cases up to 50 years of age.
    C. Location.
       1. Intraparenchymal mass.
       2. Often juxtaventricular.
       3. Can be intraventricular.
       4. Olfactory neuroblastoma (esthesioneuroblastoma).
    D. Pathology: often considered subset of PNETs.
       1. Densely cellular.
       2. Poorly differentiated (like peripheral neuroblastoma but with rarer evidence of maturation toward mature ganglion cells); pseudorosettes sometimes seen.
       3. Calcification, cysts, and hemorrhage common.
       4. Recurrence and leptomeningeal seeding common.
    E. Radiology: highly variable and nonspecific; resembles other PNETs and gliomas.
       1. CT.
          a. Periventricular or intraventricular mass.
          b. Calcification, cysts, and hemorrhage frequent.
          c. Little edema.
          d. Inhomogeneous enhancement.
       2. MR: inhomogeneous on both T1WI and T2WI; low-signal foci from calcification, flow void, and old hemorrhage common.
    F. Survival: 30% at 5 years.
V. Pineal parenchymal tumors (pineoblastoma, pineocytoma).

A. Incidence: rare (less than 1% of intracranial tumors).
B. Age.
  1. Pineoblastoma: usually in young children but has been reported up to 60 years of age.
  2. Pineocytoma: any age; often older adults.
C. Location: pineal, posterior third ventricle.
D. Pathology.
  1. Pineal parenchymal tumors are thought to arise from pineal parenchymal cells called "pineocytes" (modified nerve cells, fibers of which may arise in superior cervical ganglion).
  2. Pineocytoma: relatively mature cells.
  3. Pineoblastoma: primitive cells histologically similar to those in medulloblastoma (some consider pineoblastoma to be variety of PNET).
E. Radiology.
  1. Pineocytoma.
    a. Isodense or hyperdense on nonenhanced CT; usually strong enhancement.
    b. Calcification common; tumor tends to engulf calcified pineal gland.
    c. MR: variable and nonspecific; can be very similar to benign pineal cysts (hypointense on T1WI, hyperintense on T2WI), although spin density scans are sometimes helpful in this distinction (tumors more intense than CSF on proton density–weighted scans).
    d. NOTE: Many authors warn that histologic features and malignancy cannot be determined with imaging studies alone. Correlation with patient's age, assay for tumor markers, and biopsy are necessary for differential diagnosis and optimal treatment.
  2. Pineoblastoma.
    a. Isodense or hyperdense on nonenhanced CT.
    b. Variable MR signal: usually isointense or hypointense to brain on T1WI; isointense or hyperintense on T2WI: often mixed.
    c. Enhanced by contrast media on both CT and MR.
    d. May invade tectum and thalami.
    e. Tend to be larger and more lobulated than pineocytomas.

SUGGESTED READINGS

Benitez WI, Glasier CM, Husain M, et al: MR findings in childhood gangliomas, *J Comput Assist Tomogr* 14:712-716, 1990.

Castello M, Davis PC, Takei Y, Hoffman JC Jr: Intracranial ganglioglioma, *AJNR* 11:109-115, 1990.

Davis PC, Wickman RD, Takei Y, Hoffman JK Jr: Primary cerebral neuroblastoma, *AJNR* 11:115-120, 1990.

Figueroa RE, El Gammal T, Brorks BS, et al: MR findings in primitive neuroectodermal tumors, *J Comput Assist Tomogr* 13:773-778, 1989.

Gusnard DA: Cerebellar neoplasms in children, *Semin Roentgenol* 25:263-278, 1990.

Klein P, Rubinstein W: Benign symptomatic glial cysts of the pineal gland: a report of seven cases and reviews of the literature, *J Neurol Neurosurg Psychiatry* 52:991-995, 1989.

Nakagawa H, Iwasaki S, Kichikawa K, et al: MR imaging of pineocytoma: report of two cases, *AJNR* 11:195-198, 1990.

Robbins N, Mendelsohn D, Mulne A, et al: Recurrent medulloblastoma, *AJNR* 11:583-587, 1990.

Russell DS, Rubinstein LJ: Medulloblastomas (including cerebellar neuroblastoma). In *Pathology of tumors of the nervous system,* ed 5, Baltimore, 1989, Williams & Wilkins, pp 251-279.

Tien RD, Barkovich AJ, Edwards MSB: MR imaging of pineal tumors, *AJNR* 11:109-115, 1990.

Zimmerman RA: Pediatric supratentorial tumors, *Semin Roentgenol* 25:225-248, 1990.

CHAPTER 46

Intracranial neoplasms (nonglial neoplasms): nerve sheath tumors

KEY CONCEPTS

1. Nerve sheath tumors include schwannomas, neurofibromas, and malignant nerve sheath tumors.
2. Cranial nerve tumors are schwannomas.
3. Cutaneous and most peripheral nerve sheath tumors are neurofibromas. Neurofibromas are tumors of Schwann cells and fibroblasts.
4. Spinal nerve root tumors can be either schwannomas or neurofibromas.
5. Schwannomas almost never degenerate; malignant degeneration of neurofibromas occurs in 3% to 13% of cases.
6. Schwannomas are primarily associated with neurofibromatosis type 2 (NF-2); neurofibromas with NF-1.

Three clinicopathologic subtypes of nerve sheath tumors are recognized: schwannomas (term preferred to "neurinoma" or "neurilemoma"), neurofibromas, and malignant nerve sheath tumors. Schwannomas and neurofibromas are compared in Table 46-1.

I. Schwannoma.
  A. Incidence: 5% to 10% of central nervous system (CNS) tumors (only 2% of posterior fossa tumors in children; very uncommon in absence of NF).
  B. Age and sex: Spontaneous cases typically occur in thirties to sixties; younger age in patients with NF-2. Female/male ratio 2:1.
  C. Pathology.
    1. Schwann cells are neoplastic element.

Table 46-1 Comparison between schwannoma and neurofibroma

Schwannoma	Neurofibroma
Schwann cells	Schwann cells plus fibroblasts
Focal, rounded	Fusiform, plexiform
Often cystic, necrotic, hemorrhagic	Rarely cystic, necrotic, or hemorrhagic
Cranial and spinal nerves; isolated schwannomas of peripheral nervous system trunks occur	Exiting spinal nerves, peripheral or cutaneous nerves
Do not become malignant	3%-13% have malignant degeneration
Association with NF-2	Association with NF-1

NF, Neurofibromatosis.

2. Two histologic types: Antoni type A (compact tissue); Antoni type B (loose).
3. Fatty degeneration, cysts, and vascular changes common.
4. Encapsulated with hyalinization, sinusoidal dilatation, and thrombosis common.
5. Almost never become malignant.
6. Most spontaneous lesions single; multiple lesions in NF-2.
D. Location.
   1. Cranial nerves (CNs) III to XII (especially vestibular division of CN VIII, followed by CNs V, VII, and X).
   2. Spinal nerves (sensory roots): Schwannomas involve dorsal, not ventral, roots.
   3. Peripheral nerve trunks: Schwannomas can occur spontaneously; very rare in NF.
   4. Cutaneous nerves: Schwannomas almost never occur there.
E. Radiology.
   1. Rounded, well-delineated mass; occasionally calcification present.
   2. Isodense or mixed isodense and hypodense to brain parenchyma on nonenhanced computed tomography (CT); strong enhancement.
   3. Magnetic resonance (MR): isointense or hypointense on T1-weighted image (T1WI); typically hyperintense on T2WI; often cystic and necrotic; hemorrhage occasionally.
   4. Enlarged bony canals (internal auditory canals enlarged in 75% to 90% of patients with vestibular schwannoma or "acoustic neuroma").
II. Neurofibroma.
A. Incidence: uncommon as isolated lesions; seen in patients with NF-1.
B. Age: Plexiform cutaneous neurofibromas are seen in children with NF-1. Spontaneously occurring, solitary, circumscribed neurofibromas in general population are uncommon; usually appear in fourth decade.

C. Pathology.
1. Mixture of Schwann cells, fibroblasts, neurons, and mucopolysaccharide matrix.
2. Little tendency toward fatty degeneration, vascular change, or hemorrhage.
3. Usually unencapsulated.
4. Occasionally undergo malignant degeneration.
5. Often multiple.
6. Associated with NF-1.
D. Location.
1. Intracranial cranial nerves: never (can occur in region of posterior ganglia as central extension of peripheral tumors). Plexiform neurofibromas in children with NF-1 involve orbital cranial nerve branches (usually CN V).
2. Spinal roots: rare as site of spontaneous neurofibroma. Neurofibromas found in spinal root, even if solitary, are usually part of von Recklinghausen's disease (NF-1).
3. Peripheral nerve trunks: exiting spinal nerve plexuses and trunks in multiple neurofibromatosis (NF-1).
4. Cutaneous nerves: may be site of isolated neurofibromas; 30% to 50% are associated with von Recklinghausen's disease. Plexiform neurofibromas occur in NF-1 (see preceding discussion).
E. Radiology.
1. Fusiform enlargement of spinal nerve root that appears as intradural extramedullary or dumbbell-shaped mass.
2. CT: hypodense to isodense with muscle; usually is not enhanced.
3. MR: tumors slightly hyperintense on T1WI; mixed hyperintense and hypointense on T2WI; variable enhancement.
III. Malignant nerve sheath tumors.
A. Malignant transformation of preexisting schwannomas very rare.
B. Frequency of malignant transformation into neurofibrosarcoma estimated to be 3% to 13% in von Recklinghausen's disease.
C. Can arise spontaneously; common site is from supraorbital or maxillary branch of cranial nerve V. Primary malignant schwannomas have been reported.
D. Imaging cannot reliably distinguish malignant nerve sheath tumor from benign neurofibroma or schwannoma.

SUGGESTED READINGS

Aoki S, Barkovich AJ, Nishimura K, et al: Neurofibromatosis types 1 and 2: cranial MR findings, *Radiology* 172:527-534, 1989.
Braffman BH, Bilaniuk LT, Zimmerman RA: MR of central nervous system neoplasia of the phakomatosis, *Semin Roentgenol* 25:198-217, 1990.

Carney JA: Psammomatous melanotic schwannoma, *Am J Surg Pathol* 14:206-222, 1990.

Halliday AL, Sobel RA, Martuza RL: Benign spinal nerve sheath tumors: their occurrence sporadically and in neurofibromatosis types 1 and 2, *J Neurosurg* 74:248-253, 1991.

Okazaki H: Nerve sheath tumors. In *Fundamentals of neuropathology,* New York, 1989, Igaku-Shoin, pp 231-239.

CHAPTER 47

Intracranial neoplasms (nonglial neoplasms): tumors of mesenchymal tissue

KEY CONCEPTS

1. The three basic types of meningioma are meningothelial, fibroblastic, and transitional.
2. So-called angioblastic meningiomas are probably meningeal hemangiopericytomas.
3. Imaging criteria are not reliable for predicting histologic type or whether neoplasm is benign or malignant.
4. Most hemangioblastomas arise spontaneously; 10% to 20% occur with von Hippel–Lindau disease.
5. Cranial fibrosarcomas and osteogenic sarcomas are rare and most often arise from irradiated or pagetoid bone.

The three major categories of intracranial tumors with mesenchymal tissue origin are meningioma, hemangioblastoma, and sarcoma. A fourth category, xanthomatous tumors, is sometimes included but is not discussed here.

I. Meningioma.
  A. Incidence.
    1. Between 15% and 20% of primary intracranial tumors.
    2. Most common nonglial neoplasm.
    3. Rare in children and adolescents (1% to 2% of pediatric intracranial tumors).
  B. Age and sex.
    1. Peak incidence 40 to 60 years; rare under 2 years of age unless patient has neurofibromatosis.
    2. Female/male ratio 2:1 in brain, 4:1 in spine.
  C. Location: Because meningiomas are thought to arise from meningothe-

lial cells of arachnoid villi, they are found adjacent to dural venous sinuses, in areas of sutural confluence, and in other sites where arachnoid granulations and arachnoidal rests occur (e.g., choroid plexus). Tumors can be globular, en plaque, or intraosseous.

1. Parasagittal or convexity (30% to 40%).
2. Sphenoid wing (15% to 20%).
3. Olfactory groove or planum sphenoidale (10%).
4. Suprasellar (10%).
5. Falx (5%).
6. Other miscellaneous (10% to 15%).
   a. Posterior fossa (5% to 10%).
      (1) Cerebellopontine angle.
      (2) Clivus and foramen magnum.
   b. Cavernous sinus (2%).
   c. Ventricles (typically trigone) (2%).
   d. Orbit (less than 1%).
   e. Pineal (less than 1%).
   f. Intradiploic (less than 1%).
   g. Ectopic (nose, paranasal sinuses, parotid gland).
7. Spine (2% to 3% of meningiomas).
8. Multiple in 5% to 10%; 75% localized to one hemicranium.

D. Pathology: A variety of different forms have been described, but no prognostic significance can be attached to any type. Two basic types and transitional forms between them are:
1. Meningothelial (syncytial): whorls.
2. Fibroblastic: sheets.
3. Transitional.

Malignant meningiomas are rare, tend to invade brain, and can metastasize extracranially (but so can "benign" meningiomas). Term "angioblastic meningioma" is misleading; most of these are more appropriately called "vascular" meningiomas. Some so-called angioblastic meningiomas are probably hemangiopericytomas and are unrelated to meningeal cells, although they may behave much like meningiomas.

E. Radiology.
1. Skull films.
   a. Sclerosis.
   b. Increased vascular channels.
   c. Calcification.
   d. Bone destruction.
   e. Pneumosinus dilatans.
2. Computed tomography (CT).
   a. Sharply delineated; 75% homogeneously hyperdense on nonenhanced CT; 25% isodense; 1% hypodense.

    b. Abut dural surface (often broad based, forming obtuse angle with dura).

    c. Calcification in 15% to 20%.

    d. Hemorrhage rare; central necrosis in 3% to 14%.

    e. Adjacent osseous changes in 15% to 20%.

       (1) Hyperostosis (diffuse or focal).

       (2) Bone destruction and erosion.

       (3) Lucent line can sometimes be seen between hyperostosis and calcified meningioma-en-plaque.

    f. Edema of underlying brain in 60%; follows white matter tracts with relative sparing of internal capsule.

    g. Enhancement strong and uniform in 90% following contrast administration; mild in 10%. Densely calcified meningiomas may show no appreciable increase in attenuation with contrast media.

    h. Thin low-density halo may be present around mass and indicates its extraaxial location.

    i. Displacement of interface between gray and white matter.

  3. Magnetic resonance (MR): variable appearance.

    a. Most typical appearance is isointense with gray matter on all sequences.

    b. Some very hyperintense on T2-weighted image (T2WI); densely fibrous or heavily calcified tumors can be hypointense on T2WI.

    c. Low-signal rim around tumor common (cerebrospinal fluid cleft, vascular rim, or dura).

    d. High-velocity signal loss in enlarged feeding and draining vessels.

    e. Eighty-five percent enhance strongly.

    f. Adjacent dural "tail" or "collar" of thickened meninges in continuity with mass seen in 60% (can be tumor). Presence of dural tail sign is highly suggestive of—but not specific for—meningioma. Dural tail can represent either actual tumor extension or nonneoplastic dural reaction. Also reported with sarcoid, lymphoma, chloroma, and histiocytic granulomatosis.

    g. Dural sinus involvement or occlusion can often be assessed with flow-sensitive scans.

  4. MR spectroscopy studies show typical spectral pattern in meningiomas (strongly increased Cho peak).

B. Miscellaneous meningioma items.

  1. Difficult to determine histologic type of meningioma from imaging studies.

  2. Histologic criteria for malignancy are difficult to define; classically

benign meningiomas with typical histology can have neural axis metastasis or even extraneural metastases (e.g., to lung). In general, clinical and radiologic criteria do not distinguish malignant meningiomas from their benign counterparts.

3. Mimics of meningiomas on imaging studies.
   a. Dural metastases (breast, lymphoma, lung).
   b. Extramedullary hematopoieses.
   c. Other benign causes of meningeal thickening (e.g., sarcoid).

II. Hemangioblastoma.
   A. Incidence.
      1. Between 1% and 2% of primary intracranial tumors; 8% to 12% of posterior fossa tumors.
      2. Most arise sporadically; 10% to 20% occur as part of von Hippel–Lindau disease (tumors often multiple).
   B. Age.
      1. Young and middle-aged adults (between 20 and 40 years).
      2. Not a tumor of childhood.
      3. Age at presentation in patients with von Hippel–Lindau disease.
         a. With retinal angioma, early twenties.
         b. With cerebellar hangioblastoma, early thirties (but may become symptomatic as early as middle to late teens).
         c. With renal cell carcinoma, early to middle forties.
   C. Location.
      1. More than 90% in cerebellar hemispheres.
      2. Medulla occasional site.
      3. Spinal cord.
      4. Location above tentorium comparatively rare (less than 100 reported cases) but can occur anywhere.
   D. Pathology: benign tumors with thin-walled vessels, islands of mesenchyma.
   E. Radiology.
      1. Solid in 40%, cystic in 60% (cyst wall not neoplastic).
      2. Nearly always in contact with leptomeninges at some point.
      3. Calcification rare.
      4. CT and MR: cystic or solid mass with strong enhancement (rarely, cyst may be present without nodule). Cystic part of lesion typically hypointense compared with brain on T1WI, hyperintense on T2WI. Signal may be complex if hemorrhage has occurred.
      5. High-velocity signal loss (flow voids) in feeding and draining vessels on MR.
   F. Survival: tumors benign but up to 25% recur (tumors most likely to recur in younger patients with multicentric neoplasms or von Hippel–Lindau disease).

III. Sarcomas.
  A. Incidence: 1% to 2% of primary intracranial tumors.
  B. Fibrosarcoma and meningeal sarcomatosis.
    1. Occur at any age.
    2. Largest group of central nervous system (CNS) sarcomas.
    3. Usually arise from or are attached to dura.
    4. The most malignant, highly undifferentiated fibrosarcomas occur in children.
    5. Some follow irradiation (5 to 10 years later) or occur in pagetoid bone; rarely arise from malignant degeneration of meningioma.
  C. Chondrosarcoma (usually arise from skull base).
  D. Osteogenic sarcoma (skull is a rare site of primary tumor).
    1. Occurs in children and young adults; rare in older patients in absence of Paget's disease.
    2. Can occur if brain has been irradiated (up to 20 years later).
  E. Gliosarcoma.
    1. Rare malignant primary brain tumor (less than 5% of astrocytomas).
    2. Pathology: both gliomatous and sarcomatous elements present (either neoplastic gliomatosis and sarcomatous elements appear spontaneously, or sarcoma arises in malignant astrocytoma or glioblastoma multiforme, possibly from neoplastic degeneration of hypertrophied, hyperplastic vascular endothelium).
    3. Radiology: often hyperdense on CT (because of high vascularity or cellularity), strongly enhancing. Some patients have large necrotic areas and inhomogeneous enhancement. Tumor may resemble meningioma (if cortical location) or glioblastoma.
  F. Hemangiopericytoma.
    1. Many so-called angioblastic meningiomas are probably hemangiopericytomas. These tumors are sometimes therefore called meningeal hemangiopericytoma or angioblastic meningioma (hemangiopericytic type).
    2. Incidence: less than 1% of CNS tumors.
    3. Cell of origin is pericyte (modified smooth muscle cell), not meningothelial cell.
    4. Radiology: CT like vascular meningioma; MR isointense with brain on both T1WI and T2WI.
    5. Propensity for both local recurrence and extraneural metastasis (25%).
    6. Survival at 5 years 67%, 10 years 40%, 15 years 23%.

SUGGESTED READINGS

Aoki S, Sasaki Y, Machida T, Tanioka H: Contrast-enhanced MR images in patients with meningioma: importance of enhancement of the dura adjacent to the tumor, *AJNR* 11:933-938, 1990.

de la Monte S, Horowitz SA: Hemangioblastomas: clinical and histopathological factors correlated with recurrence, *Neurosurgery* 25:695-698, 1989.

Demaerel P, Johannik D, Van Hecke P, et al: Localized ^{1}H NMR spectroscopy in fifty cases of newly diagnosed intracranial tumors, *J Comput Assist Tomogr* 15:67-76, 1991.

Demaerel P, Wilms G, Lammens M, et al: Intracranial meningiomas: correlation between MR imaging and histology in fifty patients, *J Comput Assist Tomogr* 15:45-51, 1991.

Elster AD, Challa VR, Gilbert TA: Meningiomas: MR and histopathologic features, *Radiology* 170:857-862, 1989.

Goldsher D, Litt AW, Pinto RS: Dural "tail" associated with meningiomas on Gd-DTPA-enhanced MR images: characteristics, differential diagnostic value, and possible implications for treatment, *Radiology* 176:447-450, 1990.

Guthrie BL, Ebersold MJ, Scheithauer BW, Shaw EG: Meningeal hemangiopericytoma: histopathological features, treatment, and long-term follow-up of 44 cases, *Neurosurgery* 25:514-522, 1989.

Kipes JJ: *Meningiomas: biology, pathology, differential diagnosis,* Masson monographs in diagnostic pathology, vol 4, New York, 1982, Masson.

Maiuri F, Stella L, Benvenuti D, et al: Cerebral gliosarcomas, *Neurosurgery* 26:261-267, 1990.

Naidich TP: Imaging evaluation of meningiomas. In *Categorical course: neoplasms of the central nervous system,* Chicago, 1990, American Society of Neuroradiology, pp 39-51.

Rohringer M, Sutherland GR, Lou DF, Sima AAF: Incidence and clinicopathological features of meningioma, *J Neurosurg* 71:665-672, 1989.

Tien RD, Yang PJ, Chu PK: "Dural tail sign": a specific MR sign for mengioma? *J Comput Assist Tomogr* 15:64-66, 1991.

Wilms G, Lammens M, Marchal G, et al: Thickening of dura surrounding meningiomas: MR features, *J Comput Assist Tomogr* 13:763-768, 1989.

CHAPTER 48

Intracranial neoplasms (nonglial neoplasms): tumors of the lymphoreticular system and leukemia

KEY CONCEPTS

1. Primary lymphoreticular disorders affecting the central nervous system (CNS) include non-Hodgkin lymphoma (NHL) and histiocytosis X.
2. Leukemia and myeloma of the CNS are rarely primary.
3. The incidence of primary CNS NHL is rising sharply.
4. Three groups are at risk for CNS NHL:
   a. Children with inherited immunosuppressive disorders
   b. Immunosuppressed transplant patients
   c. Patients with acquired immunodeficiency syndrome (AIDS)

Primary CNS lymphomas are non-Hodgkin lymphomas, mostly of B cell origin. Although primary intracranial lymphomas were formerly considered rare (approximately 1% of primary brain tumors), their incidence is rising sharply. The frequency has at least trebled over the last decade with the increase in AIDS and other immunocompromised patients (e.g., transplant recipients), and some authors are predicting that lymphoma will become one of the most common CNS tumors in the 1990s.

I. Lymphoma (NHL).
   A. Incidence.
      1. Historically about 1% of primary intracranial neoplasms.
      2. Incidence increasing rapidly with increase in AIDS and in immunocompromised and immunosuppressed patients.
      3. May become most common CNS tumor in the 1990s.
   B. Age.
      1. Historically tumor of older patients (median age 55 years).

2. Children with inherited immunosuppressive disorders (median age 10 years).
3. Transplant recipients with NHL (median age 37 years).
4. AIDS patients with NHL (median age 39 years).

C. Location.
1. Solitary or multiple (50%) focal intracranial mass(es), often in thalamus, basal ganglia, or corpus callosum; 75% have ventricular or meningeal border; 75% to 85% supratentorial.
2. Diffuse meningeal or periventricular lesions.
3. Uveal or vitreous deposits.
4. Localized spinal intradural masses.

D. Pathology.
1. Origin controversial, since CNS does not have endogenous lymphoid tissue or lymphatic circulation.
2. Almost all primary CNS lymphomas are non-Hodgkin type.
3. Ill-defined mass with irregular borders or diffusely infiltrative.
4. Tends to spread along blood vessels and Virchow-Robin perivascular spaces.
5. Relatively homogeneous, uniformly cellular tumor with aggressive histologic characteristics; immunosuppressed patients may have heterogeneous mass with necrosis.

E. Radiology.
1. CT.
   a. Isodense or hyperdense mass on nonenhanced CT most often involving deep gray matter or corpus callosum.
   b. Most are enhanced strongly and relatively uniformly.
   c. Calcification and hemorrhage rare.
   d. Necrosis rare; exception is AIDS, in which lesions may appear ringlike and can be indistinguishable from infection (e.g., toxoplasmosis).
2. MR.
   a. Variable but often hypointense to brain on T1WI, isointense to hyperintense on T2WI.
   b. Usually enhanced strongly and uniformly with contrast material.
   c. Multiple lesions common.
   d. Leptomeningeal seeding sometimes detected with contrast-enhanced MR.
   e. Combination of paranasal sinus masses and hypothalamic-infundibular mass suggestive of lymphoma, leukemia, or rarely histiocytosis (non-X type).

F. Survival: if untreated, 1½ months after diagnosis.

II. Myeloma and leukemia: Primary CNS tumors rare; most cases of CNS leukemia or myeloma reflect secondary involvement.

III. Langerhans' cell histiocytosis (previously known as histiocytosis X): Localized primary masses can occur, especially in hypothalamic-infundibular region; diffuse involvement of leptomeninges and cranial nerves has also been reported. Focal masses of histiocytosis usually isodense to hyperdense on nonenhanced CT; enhanced strongly and uniformly. Histiocytosis typically is isointense to brain on both T1WI and T2WI; strong enhancement following contrast material administration.

SUGGESTED READINGS

Atlas SW: Adult supratentorial tumors, *Semin Roentgenol* 25:130-154, 1990.

Castellino RA: The non-Hodgkin lymphomas: practical concept for the diagnostic radiologist, *Radiology* 178:315-321, 1991.

Goldstein ID, Zeifer B, Chao C, et al: CT appearance of primary CNS lymphoma in patients with acquired immunodeficiency syndrome, *J Comput Assist Tomogr* 15:39-44, 1991.

Hochberg FH, Miller DC: Primary central nervous system lymphoma, *J Neurosurg* 68:835-853, 1988.

Jack CR Jr, O'Neill BP, Banks PM, Reese DF: Central nervous system lymphoma: histologic types and CT appearance, *Radiology* 167:211-215, 1988.

O'Sullivan RM, Sheehan M, Poskitt KJ, et al: Langerhans cell histiocytosis of hypothalamus and optic chiasm: CT and MR studies, *J Comput Assist Tomogr* 15:52-55, 1991.

Schwaighofer BW, Hesselink JR, Press GA, et al: Primary intracranial CNS lymphoma: MR manifestations, *AJNR* 10:725-729, 1989.

Shibata S: Sites of origin of primary intracerebral malignant lymphoma, *Neurosurgery* 25:14-19, 1989.

Sze G, Soletsky S, Bronen R, Krol G: MR imaging of the cranial meninges with emphasis on contrast enhancement and meningeal carcinomatosis, *AJNR* 10:965-975, 1989.

CHAPTER 49

Intracranial neoplasms (nonglial neoplasms): tumors of maldevelopmental origin and phakomatoses

---

KEY CONCEPTS

1. Imaging findings in pineal region tumors are nonspecific; in general, histologic features cannot be distinguished nor can malignancy be determined.
2. In general, on magnetic resonance (MR) epidermoid tumors behave more like cerebrospinal fluid (CSF) whereas dermoid tumors appear more like fat.
3. A hypothalamic hamartoma looks like a collar button of gray matter stuck in the suprasellar cistern between the infundibulum and mammillary bodies. It is most often seen in boys with isosexual precocious puberty.

Included in the group of tumors of maldevelopmental origin are primary germ cell tumors (germinomas and teratomas), epidermoid and dermoid tumors, lipoma (although some recent investigators believe that lipoma is actually a malformation and not a true neoplasm), neuroepithelial tumors (craniopharyngioma and Rathke's cleft cyst), and hamartomas.

I. Germ cell tumors.
   A. Incidence.
      1. Between 1% and 2% of all primary intracranial tumors.
      2. In childhood 2% to 4% of primary brain neoplasms.
   B. Age and sex.
      1. Striking male preponderance (as high as 10:1).
      2. Peak incidence in second decade.
   C. Location.
      1. Pineal gland in 60% to 80%.

2. Others (so-called ectopic germinomas).
   a. Suprasellar in 20% to 30%.
   b. Basal ganglia or thalamus in less than 5%.
   c. Multiple (usually pineal plus suprasellar) 10%.
D. Pathology: two major types of primary intracranial germ cell tumors.
   1. Germinoma.
      a. Sixty percent of germ cell neoplasms.
      b. Histologically identical to testicular seminoma and ovarian dysgerminoma.
      c. Pineal gland most common site; germinomas represent more than half of neoplasms in this area.
   2. Teratomatous group.
      a. Twenty percent of germ cell neoplasms.
      b. Three subtypes.
         (1) Embryonal carcinomas and endodermal sinus (yolk sac) tumors.
         (2) Teratomas: variable differentiation along more than one of the three germ layers; can be composed of primitive neuroectoderm, mesoderm, or ectodermal derivatives; may be intermediate stage with maturation to tissue such as cartilage, bone, fat, or hair; may be mature differentiated or "organoid" tumor such as neural, respiratory, or gastrointestinal; or may be mixture. "Malignant teratoma" has various meanings but usually refers to more primitive or undifferentiated teratomas, whereas "benign" refers to mature differentiated type. Immunochemical tests often positive for alpha-fetoprotein and human chorionic gonadotropin (beta subunit).
         (3) Choriocarcinoma: rare; composed of trophoblastic cells; immunochemical tests demonstrate human chorionic gonadotropin.
      c. Locations of intracranial teratomas.
         (1) Most common site is pineal gland.
         (2) Others: suprasellar or third ventricle, occasionally fourth ventricle.
   3. Mixed forms (both germinoma and teratoma): 20% of germ cell tumors.
E. Radiology.
   1. Germinoma.
      a. Computed tomography (CT).
         (1) Well-delineated pineal or suprasellar mass that often involves infundibulum (rarely basal ganglia).
         (2) Hyperdense on nonenhanced CT in 80%.

(3) Calcification in 80%.

(4) Strong homogeneous enhancement in majority of cases.

  b. MR.

    (1) Isointense on T1-weighted image (T1WI); isointense to slightly hyperintense (relative to gray matter) on T2WI; may have small cysts and necrotic foci.

    (2) Intense but often heterogeneous enhancement.

    (3) Metastases shown well with contrast-enhanced MR (direct local extension or diffuse CSF seeding).

 2. Teratoma.

  a. CT.

    (1) Heterogeneous, often with calcification, fat, and cystic and solid areas.

    (2) Enhancement usually minimal or absent.

  b. MR.

    (1) Inhomogeneous; hypointense on T1WI (hyperintense foci if fat present); usually heterogeneously hyperintense on T2WI.

    (2) Malignant teratomas invade locally (e.g., tectum, thalamus) and often have CSF metastases.

 3. Endodermal sinus tumors, choriocarcinoma, and mixed germ cell tumors all have variable, nonspecific CT and MR characteristics.

 4. NOTE: Many authors have concluded that imaging findings for pineal region neoplasms are nonspecific; neither histologic features nor malignancy can be determined by CT or MR alone. At least 17 histologically different tumor types, as well as other nonneoplastic masses, occur in pineal region (see box, p. 314).

II. Epidermoid, dermoid tumors (Table 49-1).

  A. Epidermoid tumors.

    1. Incidence: Epidermoid tumors account for approximately 1% of primary intracranial tumors but 7% to 9% of cerebellopontine angle tumors.

    2. Age: peak incidence fourth to sixth decades.

    3. Location (typically off midline).

      a. Cerebellopontine angle (most common).

      b. Parapituitary.

      c. Middle fossa.

      d. Cranial diploë.

      e. Spine (all levels, with or without skin defect or dermal sinus).

    4. Pathology.

      a. Irregular, cauliflower-like outer surface with desquamated epithelial debris filling cyst lined by squamous epithelium and keratinized connective tissue.

      b. Tends to insinuate into CSF spaces and invaginate vessels.

DIFFERENTIAL DIAGNOSIS OF PINEAL REGION MASSES*

1. Parenchymal origin tumor
   a. Pineocytoma
   b. Pineoblastoma
2. Germ cell origin tumor
   a. Germinoma
   b. Teratoma
   c. Embryonal carcinoma, endodermal sinus (yolk sac) tumor
   d. Choriocarcinoma
3. Cysts
   a. Arachnoid and glial cysts
   b. Epidermoid and dermoid cysts
4. Gliomas (e.g., tectal plate glioma)
5. Nonglial neoplasms (e.g., meningioma, schwannoma)
6. Miscellaneous
   a. Vertibrobasilar dolichoectasia
   b. Basilar tip aneurysm
   c. Aneurysmal dilatation of the vein of Galen
   d. Lipoma (quadrigeminal cistern)

---

*At least 17 different neoplasms of the pineal region have been described; this list includes the more common lesions.

5. Radiology.
   a. CT.
      (1) Low-density (near CSF attenuation) lobulated mass.
      (2) Calcification may be present but is relatively uncommon.
      (3) Contrast enhancement rare.
   b. MR.
      (1) Classically resembles CSF in signal: hypointense to brain on T1WI, hyperintense on T2WI.
      (2) Occasionally have short T1 (these tumors also frequently have negative Hounsfield numbers on CT).

Table 49-1 Comparison between epidermoid and dermoid tumors

Epidermoid tumors	Dermoid tumors
More common	Less common
Squamous epithelium	Epithelium plus dermal appendages
Keratin	Keratin, fat, calcification
Tend to be off midline (cerebellopontine angle, middle fossa)	Midline location (vermis, fourth ventricle)
Look more like CSF on imaging studies	Look more like fat
Local insinuation into CSF space	Can rupture, diffusely seed subarachnoid space and ventricles

CSF, Cerebrospinal fluid.

B. Dermoid tumors.
1. Incidence: intracranial dermoid tumors less common than epidermoid; reverse is true in spine.
2. Age at presentation: first two decades for intraspinal dermoid tumors, third to fifth decades for intracranial lesions.
3. Location: tend to be midline.
   a. Parasellar region.
   b. Posterior fossa (vermis, fourth ventricle).
   c. Lumbosacral.
4. Pathology.
   a. Smooth, lobulated mass with squamous epithelial lining plus dermal appendages.
   b. Fat and calcification common.
   c. Dermal sinus may be present in spinal and occipital regions.
5. Radiology.
   a. CT.
      (1) Well-delineated midline mass.
      (2) Fat density.
      (3) No enhancement.
      (4) Look for subarachnoid fat and intraventricular fat (from rupture), presence of dermal sinus.
   b. MR.
      (1) Signal like fat (short T1 and T2).
      (2) Dermoid tumors do not insinuate themselves as do epidermoid tumors.
      (3) Look for evidence of rupture into subarachnoid space; look for skull base defects that indicate possible dermal sinus tract.
      (4) No enhancement unless infected.
III. Lipoma.
A. Incidence: less than 1% of primary intracranial tumors.
B. Age: all ages.
C. Pathology.
1. Probably not true neoplasm but represents malformation of primitive meningeal tissue (meninx primitiva).
2. Composed of adipose tissue, variable amounts of vascular elements, collagen and muscle fibers, glial cells.
3. Calcification and ossification common.
4. Over half are associated with other brain malformations.
D. Location: Intracranial lipomas occur primarily in midline.
1. Interhemispheric 45% (often with partial or complete agenesis of the corpus callosum).
2. Quadrigeminal plate and superior cerebellar 25%.

3. Suprasellar and interpeduncular 14%.
4. Cerebellopontine angle 9%; sylvian cistern 5%.
5. Spinal (most thoracic; one third of spinal lipomas are associated with other congenital anomalies such as spina bifida, tethered cord, or meningomyelocele).

E. Radiology.
   1. CT.
      a. Fat density mass.
      b. Callosal lipomas often associated with corpus callosum agenesis (complete or partial).
      c. Curvilinear or nodular calcification.
      d. No enhancement.
   2. MR.
      a. Fat signal (hyperintense on T1WI, hypointense on T2WI).
      b. Chemical shift artifact.
      c. Intracranial vessels and nerves course through more than one third of lesions.

IV. Neuroepithelial tumors.
A. Craniopharyngioma.
   1. Incidence.
      a. Three percent of primary intracranial tumors.
      b. In children: 9% of primary brain neoplasms (15% of supratentorial and 50% of suprasellar tumors).
   2. Age.
      a. Half occur before 20 years of age (peak between 10 and 14 years).
      b. Second peak in middle age (fourth to sixth decades).
   3. Location.
      a. Both intrasellar and suprasellar in 70%.
      b. Suprasellar in 20%.
      c. Intrasellar in 10%.
      d. Third ventricle in less than 1%.
   4. Pathology.
      a. Precise origin unknown but may be remnants of Rathke's pouch.
      b. Epithelium-lined cyst with variable contents (e.g., keratin, cholesterol, blood products).
      c. Often calcified.
      d. May form epithelial fronds that insinuate widely into and around brain; 25% extend into anterior, middle, or posterior fossa.
   5. Radiology.
      a. CT.
         (1) Multilobulated sellar or suprasellar mass with both cystic and solid components.

        (2) Calcification in 90%.

        (3) Cystic in 90%.

        (4) Enhancement in 90% (pattern varies from nodular to rim).

    b. MR: signal extremely variable depending on cyst contents (most are hyperintense on T2WI, variable on T1WI but often also hyperintense).

  B. Rathke's cleft cyst.

    1. Incidence: 13% to 33% of autopsies (most are found incidentally).

    2. Age: any age.

    3. Location: Two thirds intrasellar, one third suprasellar or both.

    4. Pathology: probably arise from Rathke's pouch (stomodeal epithelial remnant between pars distalis and pars intermedialis). Cyst has variable contents and is lined with cuboidal epithelium.

    5. Radiology.

      a. CT: cystic or solid intrasellar or suprasellar mass with no enhancement.

      b. MR: variable but often isointense or hypointense on T1WI, hyperintense on T2WI.

V. Hamartomas: Hamartomas are abnormal but nonneoplastic collections of hamartomatous tissue. Occasionally they represent collections of neuronal tissue in ectopic location (e.g., "nasal glioma," which is not gliomatous neoplasm at all but hamartomatous mixture of fibrillary glial tissue and vascular connective tissue). Most important intracranial hamartoma, aside from hamartomas associated with tuberous sclerosis and neurofibromatosis, is hypothalamic (tuber cinereum hamartoma). Features of this lesion are:

  A. Incidence: rare.

  B. Age and sex: usually young boy (less than 2 years) with isosexual precocious puberty or, less commonly, seizures.

  C. Location: tuber cinereum (between optic chiasm and infundibulum anteriorly, mammillary bodies posteriorly).

  D. Pathology: hamartomatous overgrowth of neuronal tissue.

  E. Radiology.

    1. CT.

      a. Rounded suprasellar mass.

      b. Isodense with brain.

      c. No enhancement with contrast media.

      d. Rare: cystic areas.

    2. MR.

      a. Sessile or pedunculated ("collar button") mass between infundibulum and mammillary bodies.

      b. Usually isointense with gray matter on all sequences (may be minimally hyperintense on protein density scans or T2WI).

c. No enhancement.

d. Usually less than 2 cm in diameter but occasionally larger.

VI. Phakomatoses (see Chapter 29).

SUGGESTED READINGS

Barkovich AJ: Brain tumors of childhood. In *Pediatric neuroimaging,* New York, 1990, Raven Press, pp 149-203.

Boyko OB, Curnes JT, Okes WJ, Burger PC: Hamartomas of the tuber cinereum: CT, MR, and pathologic findings, *AJNR* 12:309-314, 1991.

Burton EM, Ball WS, Crone K, Dolan LM: Hamartoma of the tuber cinereum: a comparison of MR and CT findings in four cases, *AJNR* 10:497-501, 1989.

Chang T, Teng MMH, Guo W-Y, Shentg W-C: CT of pineal tumors and intracranial germ-cell tumors, *AJNR* 10:1039-1044, 1989.

Horowitz BL, Chari MV, Reese J, Bryan RN: MR of intracranial epidermoid tumors, *AJNR* 11:299-302, 1990.

Hubbard AM, Egelhoff JC: MR imaging of large hypothalamic hamartomas in two infants, *AJNR* 10:1277, 1989.

Okazaki H: In *Fundamentals of neuropathology,* New York, 1989, Igaku-Shoin, pp 252-258.

Smith AS, Benson JE, Blaser SI, et al: Diagnosis of ruptured intracranial dermoid cyst: value of MR over CT, *AJNR* 12:175-180, 1991.

Tien RD, Barkovich AJ, Edwards MSB: MR imaging of pineal tumors, *AJNR* 11:557-565, 1990.

Truwit CL, Barkovich AJ: Pathogenesis of intracranial lipoma, *AJNR* 11:665-674, 1990.

Zee C-S, Segall H, Apuzzo M, et al: MR imaging of pineal region neoplasms, *J Comput Assist Tomogr* 15:56-63, 1991.

CHAPTER 50

Intracranial neoplasms: metastatic neoplasms

KEY CONCEPTS

1. Most cerebral metastases are multiple and supratentorial, often at junction between gray and white matter.
2. Histologic identification of the primary site is not possible from appearance on computed tomography (CT) and magnetic resonance (MR) alone.
3. Lung, breast, melanoma, colon, and prostate gland are the most common sites of origin; the primary site is unknown in l0% to 15%.

Involvement of the central nervous system (CNS) and its meninges by neoplasms arising in extracranial tissues may result either from direct extension of a primary tumor or from blood-borne metastases. Primary intracranial neoplasms can also spread to other parts of the CNS. Finally, primary brain tumors occasionally metastasize outside the CNS. Identifying CNS metastases is important because therapy is often altered when these lesions are detected.

I. Pathology.
   A. Incidence (varies according to type of data used, e.g., clinical, autopsy, or radiographic).
      1. Twenty percent of patients with systemic cancer have intracranial metastases at postmortem examinations.
      2. Approximately 15% to 30% of intracranial tumors identified on CT scans are metastases.
   B. Location.
      1. Parenchyma most common, typically at corticomedullary junction (interface between gray and white matter).
      2. Supratentorial in 80%.

3. Multiple in 70% to 80%.
4. Other sites: calvarium, leptomeninges (epidural, subdural spaces), subarachnoid space, and cerebrospinal fluid (CSF). Uncommon but reported sites include choroid plexus, pineal body, and pituitary gland.
C. Clinical findings.
1. Peak incidence in sixth to seventh decades. Only 6% of pediatric CNS tumors are metastases from extracranial primary neoplasms. Leptomeningeal metastases in children are more likely from primary CNS neoplasm such as medulloblastoma, ependymoma, or pineal tumors.
2. Most patients with CNS metastases have neurologic abnormalities, although occurrence of asymptomatic lesions may be as high as 5% to 12%.
3. Brain metastasis can be initial clinical presentation of many tumors (e.g., lung carcinoma first detected in brain in up to 30%).
D. Source.
1. Most common: lung, breast (these two account for 50% to 60% of metastatic tumors), melanoma (up to 15% in some series), kidney, and colon. Prostate common metastatic source to bone (e.g., calvarium, spine).
2. Primary site unknown in 10% to 15%.
3. Incidence of sarcoma, lymphoma, and leukemia with CNS involvement rising because of increase in immunocompromised patients.
E. Spread of tumors involving CNS occurs:
1. Along natural passages (e.g., head and neck tumors spread to skull base along anatomic compartments, then extend intracranially through foramina, and fissures).
2. Along surfaces.
   a. Pia (over cortex).
   b. Ependyma (along ventricles).
3. Along tracts (white matter).
4. Along leptomeninges (with or without calvarial involvement).
5. Via CSF.
6. Via bloodstream.
II. Radiology: In general, CT and MR scans lack distinctive features that allow histologic identification of primary tumor.
A. CT: Some authors have advocated double-dose (up to 80 g organically bound iodine), contrast-enhanced, delayed (up to 45 minutes) scans to detect metastases. However, contrast-enhanced MR is superior to contrast-enhanced CT (even with double-dose, delayed studies) in lesion detection, localization, and differentiation between solitary and multiple lesions.
1. Parenchymal metastases.
   a. Nonenhanced CT: Intensity can be less than, equal to, or greater

than that of normal brain. Hyperdense metastases are sometimes seen with densely cellular neoplasms (e.g., medulloblastoma and lymphoma), as well as other tumors such as melanoma, choriocarcinoma, and osteosarcoma. Hemorrhage is relatively uncommon but does occur with melanoma, hypernephroma, and other highly vascular primary neoplasms. Calcification in untreated metastases is rare.

  b. Typically metastases are enhanced by contrast material. Necrosis and cavitation are common. Metastases are usually thick walled and irregular, but occasionally thin-walled metastases occur and can mimic abscess. Because metastases lack blood-brain barrier, moderate to marked vasogenic edema is common, even with small lesions.

  c. Contrast enhancement in postoperative site after removal of gliomas and metastatic tumors is diagnostic dilemma. Enhancement up to 2 or 3 days after surgery is usually due to residual neoplasm. After 5 to 7 days, enhancement often reflects neovascularization in postoperative brain; distinguishing residual neoplasm from postsurgical changes is difficult. Delayed radiation necrosis can also mimic tumor recurrence many months later.

2. Other CNS metastases.

  a. Calvarium is site of approximately 5% of brain metastases. Bone destruction with either well-defined or diffuse epidural or subdural involvement occurs in 15% of patients with calvarial metastasis. Bone window settings are vital; surprisingly large lesions can otherwise be overlooked.

  b. Leptomeningeal metastases can appear as sulcal and basilar cisternal obliteration, with enhancement following administration of contrast material. Detection of disseminated meningeal metastases can be difficult (enhancing tissue lying just under dense calvarium). This is especially true with lymphoma and leukemia in which scans often show no abnormality even though cytologic examination of CSF is positive for tumor.

  c. Subarachnoid or ependymal spread of neoplasm is common with ependymoma, medulloblastoma, primitive neuroectodermal tumor, lymphoproliferative malignancy, and high-grade astrocytoma (e.g., approximately 25% of patients with glioblastoma have CSF metastases at autopsy).

  d. Choroid plexus is occasional site for metastases and usually appears as strongly enhanced focal enlargement of choroid plexus. Pituitary metastases are common at autopsy but are usually microscopic and asymptomatic unless they also involve infundibulum or hypothalamus and cause diabetes insipidus. Pineal gland is uncommon site for metastasis.

B. MR.
1. Recent studies show contrast-enhanced T1-weighted images (T1WI) to be superior to other studies in detecting metastases. Non-contrast- and contrast-enhanced T1WI plus T2WI are recommended for evaluation of these patients.
2. Parenchymal metastases.
   a. Isointense or hypointense on T1WI, isointense or hyperintense on T2WI.
   b. Hemorrhage may produce complex appearance with mixed signal.
   c. Edema common, seen on T2WI as peritumoral high signal that spreads along white matter tracts.
   d. Most metastases are enhanced strongly with contrast material. Subtle metastases in depths of sulci and at interface of gray and white matter can be missed entirely on nonenhanced MR.
3. Leptomeningeal metastases.
   a. Contrast enhancement increases ability of MR to detect lepto-meningeal metastases (especially in spine).
      (1) Overall sensitivity without contrast material is low (about 20%).
      (2) Sensitivity with contrast enhancement is higher (between one third and two thirds of cases).
   b. Findings.
      (1) Nodular subarachnoid masses (less common than diffuse thickening of leptomeninges).
      (2) Thickened meninges (usually isointense on T1WI).
      (3) Extension of intraaxial lesions into subarachnoid space.
      (4) Spinal cord or nerve root thickening or nodules.
      (5) Diffusely enhanced meninges.
4. Ventricular and ependymal metastases.
5. Calvarial metastases.
   a. Replacement of fatty diploic space (patchy, diffuse loss of high signal on T1WI).
   b. Recognizable destruction of inner and outer tables is variable.
   c. Enhancement of metastases by contrast material is common (except for enhancement of diploic veins and meninges near pacchionian granulations, normal diploic space is not enhanced).
   d. Adjacent meningeal and subgaleal soft tissue masses sometimes present.

SUGGESTED READINGS

Davis PC, Hudgins PA, Peterman SB, Hoffman JC Jr: Diagnosis of cerebral metastases: double-dose delayed CT vs. contrast-enhanced MR imaging, *AJNR* 12:293-300, 1991.

Hayman LA, Evans CA, Hinck VC: Delayed high iodine dose contrast computed tomography: cranial neoplasm, *Radiology* 136:677-684, 1980.

Lee Y-Y, Tien RD, Bruner JM, et al: Loculated intracranial leptomeningeal metastases: CT and MR characteristics, *AJNR* 10:1171-1179, 1990.

Mathews VP, Broome DR, Smith RR, et al: Neuroimaging of disseminated germ cell neoplasms, *AJNR* 11:319-324, 1990.

Orda K, Tanaka R, Takahashi H, et al: Cerebral glioblastoma with cerebrospinal fluid dissemination: a clinicopathological study of 14 cases examined by complete autopsy, *Neurosurgery* 25:533-540, 1989.

Potts DG, Abbot GF, von Sneidern JV: NCI study: evaluation of CT on the diagnosis of intracranial neoplasms. III. Metastatic tumors, *Radiology* 136:664-675, 1980.

Rippe DJ, Boyko OB, Friedman HS, et al: Gd-DTPA-enhanced MR imaging of leptomeningeal spread of primary intracranial CNS tumor in children, *AJNR* 11:329-332, 1990.

Rodesch G, Van Bogaert P, Maviodakis N, et al: Neuroradiologic findings in leptomeningeal carcinomatosis: the value interest of gadolinium-enhanced MRI, *Neuroradiology* 32:26-32, 1990.

Russell EJ, Geremia GK, Johnson CE, et al: Multiple cerebral metastases: detectability with Gd-DTPA-enhanced MR imaging, *Radiology* 165:609-617, 1987.

Smirniotopoulos J: Intracranial neoplasms. In *Radiologic-pathologic correlations,* course syllabus, Washington, DC, 1991, Armed Forces Institute of Pathology.

Sze G, Milano E, Johnson C, Heier L: Detection of brain metastases: comparison of contrast-enhanced MR with unenhanced MR and enhanced CT, *AJNR* 11:785-791, 1990.

Sze G, Soletsky S, Bronen R, Krol G: MR imaging of the cranial meninges with emphasis on contrast enhancement and meningeal carcinomatosis, *AJNR* 10:965-975, 1989.

Taphoorn MJB, Heimans JJ, Kaiser MCRLE, et al: Imaging of brain metastases, *Neuroradiology* 31:391-395, 1989.

Trattnig S, Schindler E, Ungersbock K, et al: Extra-CNS metastases of glioblastoma: CT and MR studies, *J Comput Assist Tomogr* 14:294-296, 1990.

Wakai S, Audoh Y, Ochiai C, et al: Postoperative contrast enhancement in brain tumors and intracerebral hematomas: CT study, *J Comput Assist Tomogr* 14:267-271, 1990.

West MS, Russell EL, Breit R, et al: Calvarial and skull base metastases: comparison of nonenhanced and Gd-DTPA-enhanced MR images, *Radiology* 174:85-91, 1990.

Yousem DM, Patione PM, Grossman RI: Leptomeningeal metastases: MR evaluation, *J Comput Assist Tomogr* 14:255-261, 1990.

CHAPTER 51

Intracranial neoplasms: pediatric brain tumors

KEY CONCEPTS

1. Overall, primary brain tumors in children are divided almost evenly between supratentorial (more common in neonates and infants) and infratentorial (more common in young children).
2. The three main posterior fossa tumors in children are astrocytomas (cerebellar/brainstem ratio approximately 2:1), medulloblastomas, and ependymomas.
3. The following intracranial tumors common in adults are rare in children: metastases, glioblastomas, pituitary adenomas, hemangioblastomas, meningiomas (in the absence of neurofibromatosis), and colloid cysts.

Both the histologic spectrum and anatomic location of primary brain tumors in children differ significantly from those in adults. In addition, tumors occurring in neonates and infants are different from those in older children. The pathologic and radiologic characteristics of specific neoplasms are delineated in previous chapters. This chapter summarizes the special features of pediatric brain tumors and how they differ from tumors in adults.

   I. Incidence.
      A. From 15% to 20% of intracranial tumors occur in childhood.
      B. Central nervous system (CNS) tumors are second most common cancer in children (leukemia is first).
  II. Location.
      A. Overall, nearly equal incidence of tumors above and below tentorial incisura.

      1. Supratentorial in 52%.

      2. Infratentorial in 48%.

  B. Neonate to 2 years of age: supratentorial/infratentorial ratio 2:1.

  C. Ages 2 to 10 years: infratentorial more common than supratentorial.

  D. Ages 10 to 15 years: supratentorial and infratentorial have equal incidence.

III. Pathology.

  A. Astrocytomas account for slightly more than half of all primary CNS neoplasms in children. In order of frequency these are located in:

      1. Cerebral hemispheres.

      2. Cerebellum (hemispheres and vermis).

      3. Brainstem.

      4. Optic tract.

      5. Hypothalamus.

  B. Approximate statistics for *supra*tentorial neoplasms.

      1. Astrocytoma 30%.

      2. Craniopharyngioma 15%.

      3. Opticochiasmatic hypothalamic glioma 12% to 15%.

      4. Giant cell astrocytoma 5% to 15%.

      5. Ganglioglioma and ganglioneuroma 6%.

      6. Primitive neuroectodermal tumor (PNET) 5%.

      7. Choroid plexus tumor 5%.

      8. Germ cell tumor 2%.

      9. Oligodendroglioma 1%.

     10. Epidermoid and dermoid tumors less than 1%.

     11. Meningioma less than 1%.

     12. Pituitary adenoma rare.

     13. Metastases rare (except: Wilms' tumor and osteogenic sarcoma).

     14. Hemangioblastoma rare.

     15. Colloid cyst rare.

  C. Approximate statistics for *infra*tentorial neoplasms:

      1. Cerebellar astrocytoma 30% to 35%.

      2. Brainstem glioma 20% to 25%.

      3. Medulloblastoma 20% to 25%.

      4. Ependymoma 10% to 15%.

      5. Other (e.g., dermoid and epidermoid tumors) 5%.

      6. Metastases rare.

  D. Astrocytomas in children.

      1. Most are low grade.

      2. Most common histologic pattern is pilocytic astrocytoma (especially in younger children).

      3. Anaplastic astrocytomas less common (when they occur, are usually seen in older children).

4. Glioblastoma multiforme is rare.
5. Oligodendroglioma is uncommon.
E. Neonatal tumors (less than 60 days of age).
1. Two thirds supratentorial.
2. Pathology: approximately 50% of neonatal tumors are composed of primitive or poorly differentiated tissues.
a. Teratoma 27%.
b. PNET 27%.
c. Astrocytoma 20%; glioblastoma 9%.
d. Choroid plexus papilloma 7%.
F. Intracranial tumors in infants less than 1 year.
1. Can be considered congenital.
2. Supratentorial/infratentorial ratio 2:1.
3. Clinical findings: hydrocephalus, focal neurologic deficit.
4. Pathology.
a. Astrocytoma (often nonmalignant) 32%.
b. PNET 27%.
c. Choroid plexus tumors 14%.
d. Dermoid tumors 9%.
e. Malignant teratoma 9%.
IV. Radiology.
A. Calcification in pediatric brain tumors (overall approximately 20%).
1. Craniopharyngioma 80% to 90%.
2. Choroid plexus tumor 75%.
3. Oligodendroglioma 75%.
4. Ependymoma 50%.
5. Ganglioglioma 35%.
6. PNET 30%.
7. Astrocytoma 10% to 20%.
8. Medulloblastoma 10% to 15%.
9. Brainstem glioma less than 5%.
B. Hyperdense (high-attenuation) tumors on non-contrast-enhanced CT scans are calcified or hemorrhagic or have high cellularity with high nuclear/cytoplasmic ratio. Excluding calcification, most common hyperdense tumors on nonenhanced CT in children are:
1. Medulloblastoma, PNET, and pineoblastoma.
2. Choroid plexus neoplasms.
3. Lymphoma.
4. Germ cell tumors.
C. MR signal of CNS neoplasms in both children and adults is usually nonspecific; most tumors tend to be isointense or hypointense to brain on T1-weighted image (T1WI) and hyperintense on T2WI. More important factors in establishing appropriate differential diagnosis are age, location, and extension.

D. Contrast enhancement in pediatric CNS neoplasms (at least partial enhancement).
   1. Choroid plexus neoplasms approximately 100%.
   2. Giant cell astrocytoma 100%.
   3. Medulloblastoma 90%.
   4. Cerebellar astrocytoma 90%.
   5. Craniopharyngioma 90%.
   6. Ependymoma 70%.
   7. Brainstem glioma 50%.
E. Prominent cysts are common in craniopharyngiomas and astrocytomas; PNETs, ependymomas, and gangliogliomas also often have cystic areas.
F. Brain tumors in children under 1 year of age tend to be large, supratentorial, and bulky. Often attenuation or signal is mixed because large proportion are teratomas, PNETs, and the more malignant astrocytomas.
G. Cerebrospinal fluid and meningeal dissemination is common with medulloblastomas, ependymomas, PNETs, germ cell neoplasms, and lymphoreticular neoplasms; less common with astrocytomas and choroid plexus neoplasms. Histiocytosis X can mimic diffuse meningeal neoplasm.

ACKNOWLEDGMENT

Helpful in preparing this outline have been lectures delivered over the past several years by Drs. Derek Harwood-Nash, Robert A. Zimmerman, and Thomas P. Naidich (in a variety of categorical courses and postgraduate seminars). Their contributions to the field of pediatric neuroradiology are gratefully acknowledged.

SUGGESTED READINGS

Barkovich AJ: Brain tumors of childhood. In *Pediatric neuroimaging*, New York, 1990, Raven Press, pp 149-203.

Buetow PC, Smirniotopoulos JG, Done S: Congenital brain tumors: a review of 45 cases, *AJNR* 11:793-799, 1990.

Gusnard DA: Cerebellar neoplasms in children, *Semin Roentgenol* 25:263-278, 1990.

Harwood-Nash DC: Brain tumors in children, *Riv Neuroradiol* 3(suppl 2):83-88, 1990.

Lapras C, Guilburd JN, Guyotat J, Patet JD: Brain tumors in infants: a study of 76 patients operated upon, *Childs Nerv Syst* 4:100-103, 1988.

Radkowski MA, Naidich TP, Tomita T, et al: Neonatal brain tumors: CT and MR findings, *J Comput Assist Tomogr* 12:10-20, 1988.

Smith RR: Brain stem tumors, *Semin Roentgenol* 25:219-262, 1990.

Zimmerman RA: Pediatric supratentorial tumors, *Semin Roentgenol* 25:225-248, 1990.

DISEASE PROCESSES BY ANATOMIC LOCATION

CHAPTER 52

Intracranial lesions (differential diagnosis by anatomic location): sellar and juxtasellar masses

With Carol M. Andrews

KEY CONCEPTS

1. An upward bulge of the pituitary gland less than 10 mm in young women (or up to 7 mm in male adolescents) is normal.
2. Origin of posterior pituitary gland "bright spot" on T1-weighted magnetic resonance (MR) scans is controversial but probably due to vasopressin-neurophysin complexes, is present in 50% to 90% of studies, varies physiologically, and can be absent normally. (Lack of "bright spot" does not indicate diabetes insipidus.)
3. Up to 15% of asymptomatic patients have intrapituitary focal low-signal areas on contrast-enhanced scans. These can represent asymptomatic microadenomas, pars intermedia cysts, or colloid cysts. Clinical and endocrinologic correlation with imaging findings is therefore crucial.
4. The most common sellar or juxtasellar mass in adults is adenoma, followed by aneurysm, meningioma, and glioma. In children glioma (hypothalamic or chiasmatic) and craniopharyngioma are the most common lesions in this location.
5. The differential diagnosis of an enlarged infundibulum in a child includes glioma, germinoma, lymphoma, and Langerhans' cell histiocytosis. In an adult the differential diagnosis includes all of the former plus sarcoid and hypophysitis. Patients with central diabetes insipidus often have thickened infundibulum and absence of posterior pituitary "bright spot."
6. An appearance suggesting pituitary adenoma in a child is almost always *not* adenoma; pituitary hyperplasia is much more likely.

I. Sella and juxtasellar region: normal gross and radiographic anatomy (Fig. 52-1).

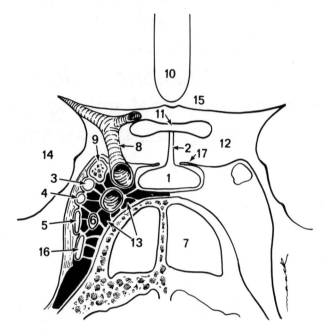

Fig. 52-1 Coronal anatomic drawing of sella turcica, cavernous sinus, and adjacent structures.

1. Pituitary gland
2. Infundibulum
3. Cranial nerve III
4. Cranial nerve IV
5. Cranial nerve V_1
6. Cranial nerve VI
7. Sphenoid sinus
8. Internal carotid artery
9. Anterior clinoid process
10. Third ventricle
11. Optic chiasm
12. Suprasellar cistern
13. Venous spaces of cavernous sinus
14. Temporal lobe
15. Hypothalamus
16. Cranial nerve V_2
17. Diaphragma sellae

A. Sella turcica: part of basisphenoid.
B. Pituitary gland.
    1. Anterior and posterior lobes; pars intermedia.
    2. Infundibulum.
C. Pituitary gland is bordered by following.

1. Superiorly.
   a. Diaphragma sellae.
   b. Suprasellar subarachnoid space.
   c. Optic chiasm.
   d. Anterior recesses of third ventricle.
   e. Hypothalamus.
2. Laterally: cavernous sinus and its contents (cavernous internal carotid artery [ICA], cranial nerves III, IV, VI, and V_1 and V_2, and meninges).
3. Inferiorly: sphenoid bone (nasopharynx below).
4. Circle of Willis lies above, surrounds suprasellar cistern.
D. Radiology.
   1. Computed tomography (CT): typically isodense with brain; uniform strong enhancement.
   2. MR: typically isointense with gray matter; strong uniform enhancement. Up to 15% of asymptomatic patients have low-signal foci suggestive of adenoma on contrast-enhanced MR. (Similar incidence of asymptomatic microadenomas is found at autopsy. These foci can also represent pars intermedia cysts, colloid-type inclusions, and other benign cysts).
   3. MR: posterior pituitary "bright signal."
      a. Present in 50% to 90%.
      b. Results from vasopressin-neurophysin complexes.
      c. Considerable physiologic variation normal.
      d. Absence can be normal and does not necessarily indicate diabetes insipidus.
   4. Height of normal pituitary gland.
      a. Less than 10 mm in females.
      b. Less than 8 mm in males.
      c. Maximum mean height in both sexes occurs from 10 to 19 years.
      d. Pituitary height gradually decreases after 20 years of age.
   5. Convex upper margin normal in teenage girls.
II. Pathology: Nearly 30 different pathologic entities have been described as affecting sella and juxtasellar region (see box, p. 336). Incidences of most of these masses are listed in box on p. 337. Table 52-1 summarizes CT and MR appearances of five most common lesions. Precise radiographic differential diagnosis of sellar and juxtasellar masses varies significantly depending on whether mass is predominantly intrasellar, suprasellar, juxtasellar, or combination. We therefore divide consideration of these lesions into three categories depending on principal anatomic location of abnormality.
A. Intrasellar.
   1. Congenital and developmental.
      a. Empty sella.

Table 52-1   Typical magnetic resonance (MR) and computed tomographic (CT) appearance of the five common suprasellar lesions

Lesions	CT scan		MR scan		Comments
	Unenhanced	Enhanced	T1WI	T2WI	
Pituitary macroadenoma	Isodense	Modest uniform enhancement	Isointense	Isointense or slightly hyperintense	Calcification rare; displacement rather than invasion of adjacent structures; often lobulated
Pituitary macroadenoma (hemorrhagic)	Hyperdense	Hyperdense	Often complex mixed signal: isointense and hyperintense	Complex mixed signal	
Meningioma	Slightly hyperdense	Strong uniform enhancement	Isointense (may be inconspicuous); enhances strongly	Variable: hypointense, isointense, or slightly hyperintense	Smooth well-delineated lesion; calcification common; look for dural "tail"
Craniopharyngioma	Heterogeneous: solid—isodense or slightly hyperdense; cystic—hypodense	Variable: solid may show enhancement; cystic—rim enhances	Variable: solid—isointense; cystic—variable, often hyperintense; enhancement in rim or tumor nodule	Variable: solid—hyperintense; cystic—hyperintense	Focal calcification common; location: 70% both intrasellar and suprasellar, 20% suprasellar only, 10% intrasellar only

Lesion	CT	Enhancement	T1WI	T2WI	Comments
Glioma (opticochiasmatic or hypothalamic)	Isodense or slightly hypodense	May show enhancement	Isointense	Slightly hyperintense (may remain isointense)	May be chiasmal enlargement; calcification uncommon; retrochiasmatic extension virtually pathognomonic[*]
Aneurysm (patent)	Slightly hyperdense	Strong uniform enhancement	Flow void	Flow void	Turbulent flow may give inhomogeneous signal; internal carotid or anterior communicating artery most common location; may be rim calcification
Aneurysm (partially thrombosed)	Slightly hyperdense (thrombus is hypodense compared with gray matter)	Nonenhancing in areas of thrombus	Thrombus variable	Variable	Thrombus may appear heterogeneous secondary to various stages of clot formation with resulting lamination of methemoglobin and hemosiderin

T1WI and *T2WI*, T1- and T2-weighted images.
[*]Exception: long-standing compressive lesion such as craniopharyngioma or meningioma may have high signal in chiasm and optic tracts, caused by edema or gliosis.

PATHOLOGIC ENTITIES AFFECTING THE SELLA AND JUXTASELLAR REGION

Abscess	Histiocytosis
Aneurysm	Hyperplasia
Arachnoid cyst	Hypophysitis
Cephalocele	Lipoma
Chloroma	Lymphoma
Chordoma (granulocytic sarcoma)	Meningioma
Colloid cyst	Meningitis
Craniopharyngioma	Metastasis
Dermoid tumor	Mucocele
Ectopic neurohypophysis	Neuroma
Empty sella	Pituitary macroadenoma
Epidermoid tumor	Pituitary microadenoma
Germinoma	Rathke's cleft cyst
Glioma	Sarcoid
Hamartoma	Tuberculosis

---

      (1) Sella partially or completely filled with cerebrospinal fluid (CSF).

      (2) CT: low attenuation.

      (3) MR: follows CSF signal on all sequences.

  b. Epithelial (Rathke's cleft) cyst.

      (1) Distended stomodeal remnant situated in pars intermedia.

      (2) Usually asymptomatic (found in 13% to 33% of autopsies; rarely symptomatic).

      (3) May cause visual disturbances, pituitary dysfunction, and aseptic meningitis.

      (4) CT: usually homogeneous low-density cystic mass without calcification. Cyst wall may be enhanced by contrast media.

      (5) MR: variable according to contents (may follow CSF; may be hyperintense on T1-weighted image [T1WI], hypointense on T2WI if fatty or mucoid).

      (6) Differential diagnosis: cystic pituitary adenoma, craniopharyngioma, epidermoid tumor, arachnoid cyst, empty sella.

      (7) NOTE: In one third of cases suprasellar extension is present; purely suprasellar Rathke's cleft cyst is rare.

  c. Intrasellar arachnoid and colloid cysts.

      (1) Usually found incidentally at autopsy.

      (2) Can mimic microadenoma.

 2. Vascular.

  a. Medially positioned ICA (so-called kissing carotids). *Paramed-*

MOST FREQUENT SELLAR AND JUXTASELLAR LESIONS
(450 CASES)

Adenoma	36%
Glioma	11%
Meningioma	10%
Craniopharyngioma	9%
Aneurysm	7%
Empty sella	3%
Metastasis	2%
Arachnoid cyst	2%
Rathke's cleft cyst	2%
Hamartoma	2%
Hyperplasia	1%
Hypophysitis	1%
Lymphoma	1%
Chordoma	1%
Germinoma	1%
Neuroma	1%
Ectopic neurohypophysis	1%

 ian carotid arteries are important surgical consideration.
 b. Intrasellar aneurysm.
  (1) CT: well delineated and hyperdense on nonenhanced CT; strong enhancement.
  (2) MR: flow void or inhomogeneous signal because of turbulent flow, thrombosis, blood degradation products.
3. Inflammatory.
 a. Pituitary abscess: rare.
 b. Adenohypophysitis.
  (1) Granulomatous or lymphocytic infiltration.
  (2) Sometimes seen in thyrotoxicosis and in postpartum women.
  (3) Also occurs in tuberculosis, sarcoid, histiocytosis, syphilis, giant cell granulomatous hypophysitis.
  (4) Pituitary gland may be normal or enlarged.
  (5) CT: isodense (can be indistinguishable from adenoma); enhanced with contrast media.
  (6) MR: enlarged gland similar in signal to normal; enhanced with contrast media.
4. Neoplastic.
 a. Pituitary microadenoma (less than 10 mm in diameter).
  (1) CT: seen as low-density mass within strongly enhancing normal gland. Infundibulum and vascular tuft may be displaced.

Upward bulging is not reliable sign because it occurs normally in young menstruating females. Bone erosion is unreliable sign.

(2) MR: variable and depends on timing of scan following contrast administration. Usually isointense or hypointense on routine T1WI, variable signal on T2WI. Lesion seen as low-signal area following administration of contrast material if very rapid scans obtained during and immediately following contrast administration; may become isointense with normal gland on delayed scans.

b. Intrasellar craniopharyngioma.
(1) Ten percent of craniopharyngiomas are purely intrasellar.
(2) CT: low density; calcification frequent; may have cystic or solid enhanced areas.
(3) MR: variable calcification gives signal loss; may be hyperintense on T1WI, usually hyperintense on T2WI.

c. Meningioma: purely intrasellar meningioma rare; isointense mass that enhances strongly; difficult to distinguish from adenoma.

d. Metastases.
(1) Skull base: direct invasion from sinus or nasopharyngeal tumor (displaced pituitary gland can often be distinguished on MR).
(2) Pituitary gland: hematogenous spread fairly common; usually from breast, bronchus, kidney, or colon primary site.

5. Miscellaneous.
a. Hyperplasia.
(1) Normal in young menstruating females.
(2) Normal in puberty, pregnancy.
(3) End-organ failure (child with enlarged pituitary gland is much more likely to have hyperplasia than pituitary adenoma).

b. Surgical: Fat, muscle, and dura (after resection and packing) may appear bizarre. Clinical history is obviously important here.

B. Suprasellar mass: Suprasellar space is anatomically complex region containing CSF (in subarachnoid cisterns and anterior recesses of third ventricle), infundibulum, chiasm, hypothalamus, and circle of Willis. Masses arising in this region can originate from any of these or adjacent pituitary gland, meninges, bone, or brain parenchyma (Fig. 52-1).

1. Congenital and developmental.
a. Suprasellar arachnoid cyst.
(1) CSF is contained within layers of arachnoid and enlarges basal cisterns.
(2) CT: low density, without enhancement or calcification.

      (3) MR: follows CSF on all sequences.

      (4) Mass effect and obstructive hydrocephalus common.

      (5) Differential diagnosis: dilated third ventricle (e.g., in aqueductal stenosis), ependymal or parasitic cyst, cystic neoplasm.

  b. Epithelial (Rathke's cleft) cyst.

      (1) See discussion earlier in chapter.

      (2) MR: variable depending on histologic features. If simple serous cyst, approximates CSF on all sequences; if cyst produces mucus or contains cholesterol, bright on T1WI, variable (often bright) on T2WI.

  c. Colloid cyst.

      (1) Not true suprasellar mass, since epicenter is at foramen of Monro.

      (2) CT: typically hyperdense and nonenhancing but occasionally is isodense or even hypodense with ring enhancement.

      (3) MR: highly variable; often bright on T1WI, hyperintense or isointense on T2WI.

  d. Ependymal (third ventricular) cyst.

      (1) Nonenhancing mass; signal like that of CSF.

      (2) Obstructive hydrocephalus common.

  e. Dilated third ventricle.

      (1) Obstructive hydrocephalus (e.g., aqueductal stenosis).

      (2) Neoplasm (e.g., pineal midbrain tumor).

  f. Tuber cinereum hamartoma.

      (1) Sessile or pedunculated mass that lies in interpeduncular cistern; attached to posterior hypothalamus between infundibular stalk and mammillary bodies.

      (2) Stable in size over time; noninvasive.

      (3) CT: well-defined; nonenhancing; noncalcified; isodense to gray matter.

      (4) MR: isointense to gray matter on T1WI; isointense or mildly hyperintense to gray matter on protein density scan or T2WI; nonenhancing; occasionally, cystic foci present.

      (5) Differential diagnosis: craniopharyngioma, chiasmatic-hypothalamic glioma, germinoma.

2. Vascular.

  a. Aneurysm (see Chapter 13).

  b. Arteriovenous malformation (see Chapter 14).

  c. Dolichoectasia of ICA or basilar artery.

      (1) CT: elongated and tubular; strongly enhancing; often mural calcification present.

      (2) MR: looks like vessel.

3. Inflammatory and infectious (see Chapter 37).
    a. Parasitic cysts (echinococcosis, cysticercosis).
        (1) CT: calcification; low-density, often rim-enhancing mass; adjacent edema common.
        (2) MR: cyst content usually slightly hyperintense compared with CSF; may see hyperintense rim and nodule; can sometimes identify scolex; edema common.
    b. Abscess: pituitary abscesses very rare.
    c. Granulomatous disease.
        (1) Tuberculosis: diffuse basal cistern enhancement.
        (2) Sarcoid: enlarged enhancing infundibulum; may cause diffuse or focal meningeal thickening and enhancement.
        (3) Langerhans' histiocytosis.
            (a) Clinical findings: visual disturbance, endocrine dysfunction.
            (b) Enlarged infundibulum; posterior pituitary "bright spot" often absent.
            (c) Isodense and isointense without contrast material; enhances strongly.
            (d) Differential diagnosis: germinoma or glioma in child, sarcoid or lymphoma in adult.
            (e) Important to consider this as possible cause of infundibular mass in child or young adult, since low-dose radiation therapy, not surgery, is treatment of choice.
        (4) Meningitis.
            (a) Exudative bacterial meningitis can cause diffuse basal cistern enhancement.
            (b) Vascular spasm and stroke may result.
4. Neoplastic.
    a. Pituitary adenoma (macroadenoma).
        (1) Rare in children.
        (2) Normal pituitary gland usually cannot be identified, and mass is not distinct from pituitary gland.
        (3) Well-delineated, lobulated suprasellar mass that extends to sellar floor.
        (4) CT: isodense enhancing mass, sometimes cystic or necrotic with enhancing rim; calcification rare (1% to 8%).
        (5) MR: variable; typically isointense or hypointense to gray matter on T1WI, slightly hyperintense on T2WI; mass may contain hemorrhage in various stages of evolution and necrotic or proteinaceous fluid.
    b. Craniopharyngioma.
        (1) Arises from squamous epithelial remnants of Rathke's pouch; benign, slow growing.

      (2) Combined suprasellar and intrasellar in 70%; suprasellar in 20%; purely intrasellar in 10%; rarely may arise within third ventricle.

      (3) Primarily tumor of children and young adults but second peak in middle age.

      (4) Histologic features and therefore radiographic appearance highly variable; can be cystic or solid, calcified or not, variable density and signal; variable enhancement.

      (5) CT (typical): cystic, enhancing rim with partially calcified, enhancing mural nodule.

      (6) MR (typical): slightly or markedly hyperintense on T1WI (correlates with high cholesterol content or presence of methemoglobin). Most craniopharyngiomas are hyperintense on T2WI.

c. Meningioma.

      (1) Fourth or fifth most common intracranial location.

      (2) Smooth well-delineated mass with broad dural base (look for "tail" of tumor along tentorium or into cavernous sinus).

      (3) CT: isodense or hyperdense; often calcification; strongly enhancing; may have adjacent hyperostosis or "blistering" of skull.

      (4) MR: hypointense or isointense to gray matter on T1WI; isointense or hypointense on T2WI; strong enhancement. Look for clear separation from and different signal than pituitary gland.

d. Glioma.

      (1) Hypothalamic-opticochiasmatic glioma in children associated with neurofibromatosis behaves more like hamartoma, whereas more aggressive behavior is characteristic of solitary (spontaneous) lesion.

      (2) Ill-defined borders.

      (3) Optic nerve tract involvement is characteristic of glioma. (Differential diagnosis: edema or reactive gliosis secondary to extraaxial compressive lesion such as craniopharyngioma or meningioma.)

      (4) CT: variable density and enhancement; calcification uncommon but does occur.

      (5) MR: isointense on T1WI, hyperintense on T2WI.

e. Dermoid tumor.

      (1) Typically midline.

      (2) Often contains fat and calcification.

      (3) CT: nonenhancing isodense or hypodense suprasellar mass.

      (4) MR: variable, often hyperintense on T1WI. Subarachnoid or intraventricular high-signal foci indicates rupture of cyst.

f. Epidermoid tumor.
   (1) Congenital tumor of ectodermal origin.
   (2) Common in cerebellopontine angle and cerebellopontine angle cisterns, middle fossa; suprasellar area less common location.
   (3) CT: low density; irregular, cauliflower-like margin; can be difficult to distinguish from suprasellar arachnoid cyst (latter do not calcify, are not enhanced, and have smooth margin).
   (4) MR: variable on T2WI, intensity intermediate between CSF and brain; most are hyperintense on T2WI; MR helpful in distinguishing epidermoid tumor from suprasellar arachnoid cyst.

g. Teratoma.
   (1) Fat and calcification common.
   (2) CT: hypodense or hyperdense; heterogeneous enhancement.
   (3) MR: hyperintense on T1WI, hypointense on T2WI.

h. Germinoma.
   (1) Look for associated mass in posterior third ventricle.
   (2) Lobulated enlargement of infundibulum and recesses of anterior third ventricle.
   (3) CT: isodense, strongly enhancing.
   (4) MR: isodense on T1WI, slightly hyperdense on T2WI; strong enhancement.

i. Lymphoma.
   (1) CT: isodense; moderate enhancement.
   (2) MR: isodense on T1WI; variable density on T2WI; strong enhancement; often multiple lesions. Coexisting paranasal sinus masses may be present.

j. Lipoma of infundibulum: characteristic appearance of fat on CT and MR.

k. Granular cell tumor (choristoma) of neurohypophysis.
   (1) Primary tumors of the neurohypophysis and infundibulum are rare.
   (2) Two types.
      (a) Glioma (also termed pilocytic astrocytoma or pituicytoma).
      (b) Granular cell tumor (also known as choristoma, myoblastoma, or granular cell myoblastoma).
   (3) Radiology: suprasellar mass that is isointense to brain on protein density–weighted scan, T1WI, and T2WI; may be enhanced by contrast material on both CT and MR.

l. Metastases.
   (1) Hematogenous to pituitary gland and infundibulum.

(2) Leptomeningeal to basal cisterns.

(3) Direct extension (e.g., nasopharyngeal carcinoma, chordoma, retinoblastoma, optic nerve glioma).

5. Miscellaneous.

   a. Often occurs in setting of trauma or idiopathic growth hormone deficiency.

   b. MR: small or absent infundibular stalk; ectopic neurohypophysis seen on T1WI as small, well-delineated "bright spot" in median eminence of hypothalamus.

C. Juxtasellar masses. (See Chapter 21 discussion of lesions affecting skull base from below.)

SUGGESTED READINGS

Abrahams JJ, Trefelner E, Boulware SD: Idiopathic growth hormone deficiency: MR findings in 35 patients, *AJNR* 12:155-160, 1991.

Asari S, Ito T, Tsuchida S, Tsutsui T: MR appearance and cyst content of Rathke cleft cysts, *J Comput Assist Tomogr* 14:532-535, 1990.

Boyko OB, Curnes JT, Oakes WJ, Burger PC: Hamartomas of the tuber cinereum: CT, MR, and pathologic findings, *AJNR* 12:309-314, 1991.

Bradko BS, El Gammal T, Allison JD, Hoffman WH: Frequency and variation of the posterior pituitary bright signal on MR imaging, *AJNR* 10:943-948, 1989.

Cone L, Srinivasan M, Romanul FCA: Granular cell tumor (choristoma) of the neurohypophysis: two cases and a review of the literature, *AJNR* 11:403-406, 1990.

Elster AD, Chen MYM, Williams DW III, Key LL: Pituitary gland: MR imaging of physiologic hypertrophy in adolescence, *Radiology* 174:681-685, 1990.

Freeman MP, Kessler RM, Allen JH, Price AC: Craniopharyngioma: CT and MR imaging in nine cases, *J Comput Assist Tomogr* 11:810-814, 1987.

Hall WA, Luciano MG, Doppman JL, et al: A prospective double-blind study of high resolution pituitary MRI in normal human subjects: occult pituitary adenomas in the general population [Abstract], *J Neurosurg* 72:342A, 1990.

Loes DJ, Barloon TJ, Yuh WTC, et al: MR anatomy and pathology of the hypothalamus, *AJR* 156:579-585, 1991.

Mark LP, Haughton VM, Hendrix LE, et al: High-intensity signals within the posterior pituitary fossa, *AJNR* 12:529-532, 1991.

Newton DR, Dillon WP, Norman D, et al: Gd-DTPA-enhanced MR imaging of pituitary adenomas, *AJNR* 10:949-954, 1989.

Rasmussen C, Larsson SG, Bergh T: The occurrence of macroscopical pituitary calcifications in prolactinomas, *Neuroradiology* 31:507-511, 1990.

Sakamoto Y, Takahashi M, Korogi Y, et al: Normal and abnormal pituitary glands: gadopentelate diglumine–enhanced MR imaging, *Radiology* 178:441-445, 1991.

Suzuki M, Takashima T, Kadaya M, et al: Height of normal pituitary gland on MR imaging: age and sex differentiation, *J Comput Assist Tomogr* 14:36-39, 1990.

Tien RD, Kucharczyk J, Kucharczyk W: MR imaging in patients with diabetes insipidus, *AJNR* 12:533-542, 1991.

Wilms G, Marchal G, Van Hecke P, et al: Colloid cysts of the third ventricle: MR findings, *J Comput Assist Tomogr* 14:527-531, 1990.

Zimmerman RA: Imaging of intrasellar, suprasellar, and parasellar tumors, *Semin Roentgenol* 25:174-197, 1990.

CHAPTER 53

Intracranial lesions (differential diagnosis by anatomic location): cerebellopontine angle and internal auditory canal

---

KEY CONCEPTS

1. Normal structures that can be mistaken for a cerebellopontine angle (CPA) mass include the cerebellar flocculus, choroid plexus, and prominent jugular tubercles.
2. By far the most common CPA mass is acoustic schwannoma, followed by meningioma, epidermoid tumor, paraganglioma, and schwannomas of other cranial nerves.
3. Important internal auditory canal (IAC) lesions include schwannomas of cranial nerves (CNs) VII and VIII, metastases, sarcoidosis, arachnoiditis (including postsurgical meningeal fibrosis), and neuritis (nerve enhancement with acute Bell's palsy, viral infection, demyelinating disease).
4. Most acoustic schwannomas arise from the vestibular division of CN VIII.

An excellent detailed description of the normal and diseased CPA cistern with clinical and imaging findings can be found in Chapter 18 of H. Ric Harnsberger's book *Head and Neck Imaging* in the Mosby–Year Book series "Handbooks in Radiology." The following outline summarizes some key features of lesions in the CPA cistern and IAC.

I. CPA lesions (see box, p. 345).
  A. Normal structures that can mimic a CPA mass (CPA "pseudotumors").
    1. Flocculus of cerebellum.
    2. Choroid plexus (tuft protrudes through foramen of Luschka into CPA cistern).
    3. Jugular tubercles.

CEREBELLOPONTINE ANGLE LESIONS AND INCIDENCE

Acoustic schwannoma	60% to 75%
Meningioma	10%
Epidermoid	5%
Schwannomas of other cranial nerves	5%
Paraganglioma	2% to 10%
Vertebrobasilar dolichoectasia	3% to 5%
Aneurysm, arteriovenous malformation	1% each
Brainstem or cerebellar astrocytoma	1% to 2%
Metastases	1% to 2%
Hemangioma, lipoma, chordoma	< 1% each
Arachnoid cyst	< 1%

4. High jugular bulb.
5. Prominent anterior inferior cerebral artery (AICA).
B. Congenital.
    1. Arachnoid cyst.
        a. Incidence: less than 1%.
        b. Pathology: split or duplicated arachnoid membranes containing cerebrospinal fluid (CSF).
        c. Age: any.
        d. Radiology.
            (1) CT: well-delineated, smoothly marginated mass isodense with CSF (margins may appear angulated); 50% erode adjacent bone.
            (2) MR: CSF-signal mass on all sequences.
    2. Dandy-Walker cyst (see Chapter 28).
C. Vascular.
    1. Vertebrobasilar dolichoectasia.
        a. Incidence: 3% to 5% of CPA masses.
        b. Pathology: atherosclerotic and degenerative.
        c. Age: typically over 50 years.
        d. Radiology.
            (1) CT: tubular, hyperdense on nonenhanced CT; often calcification; strong enhancement.
            (2) MR: signal varies depending on rate and direction of flow (from high-velocity signal loss to high signal).
    2. Aneurysm.
        a. Incidence: 1% to 2% of CPA masses.
        b. Pathology: berry aneurysm (see Chapter 13) from vertebral ar-

tery (VA), superior cerebellar artery (SCA), posterior inferior cerebral artery (PICA).

   c. Age: 20 to 50 years.

   d. Radiology: See Chapter 13; varies according to whether aneurysm is patent or thrombosed.

  3. Arteriovenous malformation.

   a. Incidence: 1% of CPA masses.

   b. Pathology: See Chapter 14.

   c. Age: 20 to 40 years.

   d. Radiology: CPA mass may be dilated feeding artery, venous varix, etc.

  4. Vessel loops: AICA, PICA, SCA, and VA can have vessel loop that impinges on CN VII, producing hemifacial spasm.

D. Infectious and inflammatory (see Chapter 37): Bacterial meningitis, tuberculosis, syphilis, and other infections can produce diffuse enhancement of leptomeninges, including those in CPA. *Focal* masses are uncommon but can be seen with sarcoid, histiocytosis, and cysticercosis.

E. Trauma.

  1. Subdural hematoma.

  2. Postsurgical (e.g., hematoma, thickened leptomeninges).

F. Primary neoplasms.

  1. Acoustic schwannoma.

   a. Incidence: most common CPA mass (60% to 75%).

   b. Pathology: schwannoma arising from CN VIII at glial–Schwann cell interface, usually from vestibular nerve (schwannomas arising from cochlear division in absence of vestibular involvement or neurofibromatosis are rare). If schwannoma is bilateral, patient has neurofibromatosis.

   c. Age: 20 to 50 years most common.

   d. Radiology.

    (1) CT: isodense mass forming acute angle with temporal bone (looks like ice cream on cone), homogeneous enhancement. Necrosis, inhomogeneous density, and enhancement occur less commonly. Calcification is rare. Associated arachnoid cyst in 5%. IAC often widened.

    (2) MR: isointense on T1WI; isointense to slightly hyperintense on T2WI; strong enhancement, extending into IAC.

    (3) Can be purely intracanalicular and apparent only after administration of contrast material.

  2. Meningioma.

   a. Incidence: second most common CPA mass (10%).

   b. Pathology: See Chapter 47.

    c. Age: 30 to 60 years.

    d. Radiology.

        (1) CT: isodense or hyperdense mass adjacent to— but usually not centered on— internal auditory canal. Broad dural base (obtuse angle with temporal bone, in contrast to acute angle seen in typical acoustic schwannoma). Calcification may be present; hyperostosis of adjacent temporal bone is sometimes seen. Strong, uniform contrast enhancement. IAC not widened.

        (2) MR: variable signal (see Chapter 47). Strongly enhancing. Extension into IAC occurs but is relatively rare. (CAUTION: Meningioma overlying IAC may cause vascular congestion and irritation of nerves within IAC, resulting in secondary, nonneoplastic enhancement.)

  3. Epidermoid tumor (congenital cholesteatoma).

    a. Incidence: third most common CPA mass (4% to 5%).

    b. Pathology: arises from intracranial or intraosseous ectodermal inclusions; found in CPA as well as petrous temporal bone. Contains variable combination of keratin debris from desquamated epithelium and solid cholesterin.

    c. Age: 20 to 50 years.

    d. Radiology: insinuates around structures.

        (1) CT: hypodense irregular or lobulated nonenhancing CPA mass.

        (2) MR: irregular cauliflower-like surface. Most common signal pattern parallels CSF, but may occasionally be hyperintense on T1WI if solid cholesterin component is dominant.

  4. Paraganglioma.

    a. Incidence: fourth or fifth most common CPA mass (2% to 10%).

    b. Location: typically from jugular foramen extending into CPA.

    c. Pathology: chemodectoma.

    d. Age: 40 to 60 years.

    e. Radiology.

        (1) CT: isodense, strongly enhancing mass with enlargement of jugular foramen and erosion of jugular spine.

        (2) MR: mixed ("spongy") appearance with hypointense or isointense signal on T1WI; may be hyperintense if hemorrhage has occurred. Foci of high-velocity signal loss from enlarged feeding vessels. Strong enhancement.

  5. Schwannomas of other cranial nerves (see Chapter 46): much less common than schwannomas of vestibulocochlear nerve; from CNs

VI, VII, IX, X, and XI (CNs V and VII probably most common sites of nonacoustic schwannomas; CN XII rare). Incidence: 5% of CPA masses.

6. Hemangioma.
   a. Incidence: 0.5% to 1% of CPA masses.
   b. Pathology, age, and appearance like hemangiomas elsewhere.
7. Lipoma.
   a. Incidence: less than 1% of CPA masses.
   b. Pathology, age, and appearance like lipomas elsewhere.
8. Exophytic brainstem or cerebellar astrocytoma: incidence: 1% to 2% of CPA masses.
9. Chordoma.
   a. Incidence: 1% of CPA masses.
   b. Age: older adults (mean in fifth decade); can occur rarely in children.
   c. Pathology: arises from notochordal remnants in clivus.
   d. Radiology.
      (1) CT: large destructive clival and skull base mass, typically midline; may contain calcification and bony spicules; minimal enhancement.
      (2) MR: lobulated mass, sometimes septated; variable mixed, inhomogeneous signal, but most are isointense or hypointense on T2WI; most are moderately to extremely hyperintense on protein density–enhanced scan or T2WI.
10. Choroid plexus tumor (see Chapter 44): Fourth ventricular choroid plexus papillomas can extend laterally through foramen of Luschka into cerebellopontine angle. Rarely they arise primarily within cistern itself.

II. IAC lesions (see box, p. 349).
   A. Neoplasm.
      1. Acoustic schwannoma.
      2. Facial schwannoma.
      3. Hemangioma.
      4. Lipoma.
      5. Melanoma, lymphoma.
      6. Metastases.
   B. Nonneoplastic IAC lesions.
      1. Vascular loop or aneurysm (from AICA).
      2. Sarcoidosis.
      3. Histiocytosis.
      4. Arachnoiditis (including postoperative or chemical meningitis; can mimic recurrent acoustic schwannoma).

INTERNAL AUDITORY CANAL LESIONS

Acoustic schwannoma	Metastasis
Facial schwannoma	Sarcoid
Hemangioma	Histiocytosis
Lipoma	Arachnoiditis, postoperative
Melanoma	changes
Lymphoma	Neuritis

---

5. Neuritis.
   a. Incidence: unknown.
   b. Age: any.
   c. Pathology: Bell's palsy, herpes (Ramsey Hunt syndrome), probably viral neuritis, vestibulitis.
   d. MR: isointense nerve with or without mass on T1WI, with strong linear contrast enhancement following course of nerve; may be hyperintense on T2WI.

SUGGESTED READINGS

Armington WG, Harnsberger HR, Smoker WRK, et al: Normal and diseased acoustic pathway: evaluation with MR imaging, *Radiology* 167:509-515, 1988.

Brogan M, Chakeres DW: Gd-DTPA enhanced MR imaging of cochlear schwannoma, *AJNR* 11:407-408, 1990.

Hasso AN, Smith DS: The cerebellopontine angle, *Semin US CT MR* 10:280-301, 1989.

King TT, Morrison AW: Primary facial nerve tumors within the skull, *J Neurosurg* 72:1-8, 1990.

Lo WWM: Cerebellopontine angle tumors. Categorical course: Neoplasms of the central nervous system, pp 72-75. Presented by the American Society of Neuroradiology, Los Angeles, March 17-18, 1990.

Miller SJ, Daniels DL, Meyer GA: Gadolinium-enhanced magnetic resonance imaging in temporal bone lesions, *Laryngoscope* 99:257-260, 1989.

Sze G, Vichano LS III, Brant-Zawadzki M, et al: Chordomas: MR imaging, *Radiology* 166:187-191, 1988.

Vogl T, Bruning R, Schedel H, et al: Paragangliomas of the jugular bulb and carotid body, *AJNR* 10:823-827, 1989.

CHAPTER 54

Intracranial lesions (differential diagnosis by anatomic location): globe, optic nerve, and orbit

KEY CONCEPTS

1. Intraocular calcification in a child under 3 years of age should be considered retinoblastoma until proved otherwise.
2. In children over 3 years of age, intraocular calcification is seen with retinopathy of prematurity, larval granulomatosis, and optic nerve head drusen.
3. The most common causes of leukocoria in infants and young children are retinoblastoma and primitive hyperplastic vitreous. Retinopathy of prematurity, posterior cataract, coloboma, uveitis, larval granulomatosis, and Coats' disease are less common causes.
4. The most common intraocular neoplasm in an adult is probably metastasis, followed by uveal melanoma.
5. Differential diagnosis of enlarged optic nerve sheath complex:
   a. Common
      (1) Optic nerve glioma
      (2) Optic nerve sheath meningioma
      (3) Patulous subarachnoid space
   b. Less common
      (1) Optic neuritis
      (2) Metastases
      (3) Increased intracranial pressure
      (4) Perioptic hemangioma
      (5) Plexiform neurofibroma
6. The most common cause of an intraconal mass in adults is pseudotumor; the most common cause of proptosis in adults is thyroid ophthalmopathy. The most common orbital tumor is cavernous hemangioma.

An excellent detailed discussion of imaging the normal and pathologic orbit can be found in Chapter 14 of H. Ric Harnsberger's book *Head and Neck Imaging* in the Mosby–Year Book series "Handbooks in Radiology." The following is a summary of lesions affecting the eye and orbit with diseases subdivided into anatomic locations: globe, optic nerve sheath complex, and extraocular-intraconal. Extraconal lesions are primarily those of the lacrimal gland, extraconal fat, and bone and are not considered here.

I. Globe.
  A. Congenital.
    1. Anophthalmos.
      a. Rare.
      b. Usually associated with trisomy syndromes.
    2. Coats' disease.
      a. Pathology: retinal telangiectasia with retinal or subretinal exudates and retinal detachment.
      b. Radiology: variable depending on stage of disease.
        (1) Computed tomography (CT): normal-sized globe with dense vitreous, usually not calcified.
        (2) Magnetic resonance (MR): hyperintense vitreous with elevated, detached retina.
    3. Primitive hyperplastic vitreous.
      a. Pathology: persistence and hyperplasia of embryonic hyaloid vascular system.
      b. Radiology.
        (1) CT: retrolental noncalcific density, usually in small or normal-sized globe; sometimes persistent hyaloid canal courses from back of lens to posterior globe.
        (2) MR: posterior chamber usually hyperintense in all sequences, central hypointense band.
    4. Coloboma.
      a. Pathology: two types, iris and scleral. Latter is fusion defect of fetal choroidal fissure of optic stalk causing localized defect in sclera, uvea, and retina at junction of globe and optic nerve.
      b. Radiology: CT or MR shows normal or small globe with posterior scleral defect and outpouching of vitreous; can occur with or without a retroocular cyst.
    5. Retinopathy of prematurity (retrolental fibroplasia).
      a. Pathology: abnormal proliferation of retinal vascular buds, often associated with high oxygen concentration and prematurity.
      b. Radiology: bilateral, usually noncalcified vitreous densities, often in small globes.

    6. Microphthalmia.
      a. Pathology: small eye, unilateral or bilateral, occurring as isolated phenomenon or with other ocular-orbital abnormalities (see box, p. 345).
      b. Imaging: small shrunken globe that may be calcified (phthisis bulbi).
    7. Macrophthalmia (buphthalmos or "cow eye"): Most cases of true buphthalmos are congenital (see box, p. 345). Sometimes acquired staphyloma (elongated globe) can give appearance of large eye. Asymmetric positioning of patients within scanner can also make one globe look larger than the other on a given section.
B. Infectious and inflammatory.
    1. Larval granulomatosis.
      a. Pathology: infestation by nematode *Toxocara canis*.
      b. Radiology: small, dense, usually noncalcified globe without discrete mass.
    2. Visceral larva migrans.
    3. Congenital rubella (cause of microphthalmia).
    4. Scleritis.
C. Trauma.
    1. Repeated retinal detachments.
    2. Penetrating injury.
    3. Hemorrhage or choroidal effusion from blunt trauma.
    4. Dislocated lens.
    5. Metallic foreign bodies.
    6. Surgery.
D. Vascular.
    1. Choroidal hemangioma.
      a. Pathology: can occur as isolated phenomenon or in association with Sturge-Weber syndrome.
      b. Radiology.
        (1) CT: noncalcified vitreous mass with strong contrast enhancement.
        (2) MR: Hemangioma itself is hypodense on T1-weighted image (T1WI); chronic subretinal exudate may be hyperintense; hemangioma usually hyperintense on T2WI.
        (3) Differential diagnosis: uveal melanoma, metastasis.
    2. Coats' disease (see earlier discussion).
    3. Vitreous hemorrhage from diabetes or cardiovascular disease.
E. Neoplasms.
    1. Retinoblastoma.
      a. Incidence: most common primary intraocular malignant tumor of childhood; 10% familial.
      b. Age: 98% under 3 years of age.

    c. Pathology: calcified posterior chamber mass with characteristic Flexner-Wintersteiner rosettes. Between 25% and 40% are bilateral or multifocal within same eye. "Trilateral retinoblastoma" is bilateral retinoblastomas plus pineal tumor (usually pineoblastoma). Some pathologists consider all these to be primitive neuroectodermal tumors.

    d. Radiology.

      (1) CT: normal-sized globe with focal posterior chamber mass; more than 95% are calcified (either clumped or punctate). Meningeal dissemination can appear as diffuse meningeal enhancement, nodular masses, ependymal and subependymal enhancement, or ventricular dilatation.

      (2) MR: mass often hypointense on T2WI.

  2. Uveal melanoma.

    a. Incidence: most common primary intraocular neoplasm in adults.

    b. Age: 50 to 70 years.

    c. Pathology: 85% arise from choroid, 9% from ciliary body, 6% from iris.

    d. Radiology.

      (1) Ultrasonography: echodense posterior chamber mass.

      (2) CT: noncalcified posterior chamber mass most common.

      (3) MR: Pigmented tumors have short T1 (hyperintense on T1WI) because of paramagnetic effect of melanin; usually hypointense on T2WI.

      (4) Differential diagnosis: choroidal hemangioma, hemorrhage, effusion, retinal detachment, metastases. NOTE: Can be difficult to differentiate amelanotic melanoma from choroidal metastasis or hemangioma.

  3. Metastatic tumors.

    a. Pathology: lung and breast most common origins.

    b. Radiology.

      (1) CT: irregular hyperdense posterior chamber masses, usually along posterior wall of globe.

      (2) MR: signal varies.

      (3) Differential diagnosis: choroidal hemangioma, retinal detachment, uveal melanoma.

F. Miscellaneous lesions of globe.

  1. Cataract (imaging has limited role because these are easily diagnosed by ophthalmoscopy or slit-lamp examination).

  2. Drusen.

    a. Pathology: Cellular accretion of hyaline-like material on optic disc gives "pseudopapilledema" appearance.

   b. CT: focal calcification at optic nerve heads, 75% bilateral.
  3. Ocular hamartoma (retinal astrocytoma).
     a. Occurs with tuberous sclerosis and neurofibromatosis.
     b. Look for features of tuberous sclerosis in brain; CT appearance of retinal lesion can resemble retinoblastoma and other masses except is typically not calcified.
II. Optic nerve sheath complex.
  A. Congenital.
     1. Hypoplasia of optic nerve (septooptic dysplasia; see Chapter 28): small optic canal, absence or defects in septum pellucidum, prominent anterior recesses of third ventricle.
     2. Neurofibromatosis (see Chapter 29): Optic nerve gliomas and plexiform neurofibromas are associated with neurofibromatosis type 1.
     3. Widened subarachnoid space around optic nerve: occurs both as normal variant and occasionally with increased intracranial pressure.
  B. Inflammatory.
     1. Optic neuritis.
        a. Pathology: multiple sclerosis, pseudotumor, sarcoidosis, radiation therapy, viral neuritis; syphilis, toxoplasmosis, and tuberculosis occasionally affect optic nerve.
        b. Radiology.
           (1) CT: often normal.
           (2) MR: Optic nerve may be hyperintense on T2WI, enhanced after contrast material is administered.
  C. Traumatic and vascular.
     1. Hemorrhage and edema may cause focal or diffuse enlargement of optic nerve.
     2. Traumatic avulsion.
     3. Fracture (orbital floor, optic canal).
     4. Retinal vein occlusion.
     5. Orbital varix.
  D. Metabolic: Graves' disease occasionally causes optic nerve enlargement.
  E. Neoplasms of optic nerve and sheath.
     1. Optic nerve glioma.
        a. Incidence: most common primary neoplasm of optic nerve sheath complex (80%).
        b. Age: most common in children from 2 to 6 years. One third have neurofibromatosis type 1. Optic nerve gliomas can be seen
        c. Pathology: Childhood optic gliomas are usually low-grade malignancies, often pilocytic astrocytoma. Malignant optic glioma,

primarily seen in adults, is rare, often fatal disease that usually extends from intracranial glioma.
    d. Radiology.
        (1) CT: fusiform optic nerve enlargement typical, although occasionally tubular or eccentric configuration seen. Calcification rare. Some enhancement in 50%.
        (2) MR: isointense enlarged nerve on T1WI; typically hyperintense on T2WI. May extend intracranially and involve chiasm, both orbits, and retrochiasmatic optic pathways.
  2. Optic nerve sheath meningiomas.
    a. Incidence: second most common primary neoplasm of optic nerve sheath complex.
    b. Age: middle-aged women, children with neurofibromatosis.
    c. Pathology: arise either from arachnoid cells of nerve sheath or from orbital extension of intracranial meningioma.
    d. Radiology.
        (1) CT: tubular enlargement of optic nerve sheath. Calcification common. Enhancement usually strong and homogeneous around nonenhancing nerve ("tram track" appearance). Latter is not specific for meningioma (has also been reported with optic neuritis and pseudotumor).
        (2) MR: isointense tubular or rounded enlargement of intraconal optic nerve sheath; enhancement of thickened sheath (visible when T1WI with fat suppression is used); no retrochiasmatic extension.
  3. Other neoplasms of optic nerve sheath complex are rare.
    a. Posterior extension of retinoblastoma or uveal melanoma.
    b. Lymphoma and leukemia.
    c. Plexiform neurofibroma (orbital involvement from peripheral nerves).
    d. Schwannoma (usually from orbital branch of trigeminal nerve).
III. Retrobulbar space and muscle cone.
  A. Trauma.
    1. Hematoma.
    2. Foreign body.
  B. Vascular.
    1. Venous varix.
      a. Pathology: dilated vein(s) from intracranial or orbital arteriovenous malformation or arteriovenous fistula.
      b. Radiology.
        (1) CT: lobulated, intensely enhancing masses that often change size with Valsalva maneuver.
        (2) MR: flow voids or flow-related enhancement; thrombi with

blood degradation products may be present.
2. Superior ophthalmic vein (SOV) thrombosis.
   a. Pathology: usually occurs in conjunction with cavernous sinus thrombosis.
   b. Radiology.
      (1) CT: dense, enlarged SOV.
      (2) MR: thrombus in SOV.
3. Carotid-cavernous fistula (see Chapter 17).
C. Inflammatory.
  1. Pseudotumor (idiopathic orbital inflammation).
    a. Incidence: most common cause of intraorbital mass in adult.
    b. Pathology: variable histologic findings; often lymphocytic infiltrate.
    c. Location: Orbital pseudotumor may involve any of orbital contents alone or in combination (see following) and may mimic tumor or Graves' disease.
      (1) Retrobulbar (intraconal) fat (76%).
      (2) Extraocular muscle(s) (57%).
      (3) Optic nerve (38%).
      (4) Uvea and sclera (33%).
      (5) Lacrimal gland (5%).
      (6) Bilateral (10% to 15%).
    d. Radiology.
      (1) CT: "tumefactive" type seen as unilateral canal and intraconal enhancing mass; "myositic" type can involve muscles of cone, *including* tendinous insertions. Uveal-scleral and optic nerve involvement are sometimes seen. Diffuse orbital infiltration may occur.
      (2) MR: compared with fat, pseudotumor typically hypointense on T1WI, isointense on T2WI. May enhance strongly but heterogeneously. NOTE: Extraocular muscles themselves also normally enhance.
  2. Cellulitis.
    a. Incidence: uncommon complication of sinusitis, fracture, lid infection, foreign body.
    b. Pathology: *Staphylococcus aureus* and *Streptococcus* most common organisms.
    c. Location: extraconal and preseptal more common than intraconal.
    d. Radiology.
      (1) CT: can resemble pseudotumor. Look for evidence of ethmoid sinusitis and trauma. Strands of increased density in retrobulbar fat may be present.

      (2) MR: hypointense on T1WI, sometimes with SOV thrombosis.

  3. Abscess.

    a. Incidence: rare complication of sinusitis and orbital cellulitis.

    b. Location: subperiosteal most frequent followed by orbital fat.

    c. Radiology (CT): early in course may have nonspecific changes of orbital inflammation and cellulitis; later, focal low-attenuation collection with enhancing rim.

D. Metabolic and endocrine.

  1. Thyroid ophthalmopathy.

    a. Incidence: most common cause of exophthalmos in adults (most have hyperthyroidism); females/males 4:1.

    b. Pathology: lymphocytic and plasma cell infiltration of extraocular muscles with mucopolysaccharide deposition; spares tendinous insertions.

    c. Location.

      (1) In descending order of frequency: inferior, medial, and superior rectus muscles.

      (2) One isolated muscle belly involved in 10%.

      (3) Bilateral muscle involvement in 80%.

    d. Radiology.

      (1) CT: fusiform enlargement of one or more extraocular muscles that spares tendons. Contrast enhancement common. Increase in retrobulbar fat volume common.

      (2) MR: enlarged muscles; signal compared with that of fat is hypointense on T1WI, hyperintense on T2WI. Inhomogeneous enhancement following contrast administration.

E. Neoplasms.

  1. Cavernous hemangioma.

    a. Incidence: most common orbital tumor.

    b. Age: 20 to 40 years.

    c. Pathology: large vascular spaces, dense fibrous pseudocapsule.

    d. Location: intraconal most common but can have both intraconal and extraconal components or occasionally be entirely extraconal.

    e. Radiology.

      (1) CT: round, well-delineated, hyperdense intraconal mass that typically spares apex. Phleboliths may be present. Strong, uniform enhancement is rule.

      (2) MR: hypointense signal compared with that of fat on T1WI, hyperintense on T2WI.

  2. Capillary hemangioma.

    a. Age: neonates, infants less than 1 year.

    b. Pathology: proliferation of endothelial cells with multiple capillaries; tends to regress spontaneously.

    c. Location: extraconal (often eyelid) most common, but may be extensive and involve multiple compartments.

    d. Radiology.

        (1) CT: irregular, either well- or poorly marginated mass, enhancement with contrast.

        (2) MR: heterogeneous (hypointense signal compared with that of fat; flow voids) on T1WI.

3. Lymphoma.

    a. Incidence: third most common cause of proptosis after orbital inflammation (Graves' disease and pseudotumor) and hemangiomas. One percent of patients with systemic lymphoma have orbital involvement.

    b. Age: older adults (mean age 50 years).

    c. Pathology: non-Hodgkin (B cell) lymphoma in most cases.

    d. Location: can involve any part of orbit. In descending order of frequency:

        (1) Lacrimal gland.

        (2) Conal or intraconal space.

        (3) Optic nerve sheath complex.

    e. Radiology.

        (1) CT: spectrum from well-delineated high-density mass to diffuse infiltration of intraconal space, resembling pseudotumor. If bilateral, non-Hodgkin lymphoma is primary diagnosis; pseudotumor is bilateral in only 10% to 15%. Other considerations are sarcoid and myositis.

        (2) MR: variable; usually hypointense to fat on T1WI, but T2WI signal is variable. Can be hyperintense. Usually enhanced by contrast material; fat suppression techniques are helpful.

4. Lymphangioma.

    a. Incidence: relatively rare.

    b. Age: infant or young child.

    c. Pathology: dilated endothelial-lined vascular channels. Does not involute (unlike capillary hemangiomas). Propensity to hemorrhage.

    d. Radiology.

        (1) CT: lobulated, hypodense mass.

        (2) MR: multicystic, heterogeneous; often contains fluid-fluid levels with blood degradation products.

5. Rhabdomyosarcoma.

    a. Incidence: most common nonocular malignant tumor of orbit in

children (retinoblastoma is most common overall); third most common primary childhood malignancy of head and neck (after brain tumors and retinoblastoma).
b. Age: 8 to 10 years.
c. Pathology: by far most common primary extracranial tumor that invades cranial vault in children; orbit is most common site of head and neck rhabdomyosarcoma.
d. Radiology.
  (1) CT: isodense with brain on nonenhanced CT; usually enhances strongly and uniformly.
  (2) MR: variable. Contrast-enhanced scans useful for delineating intracranial extension.
6. Dermoid and epidermoid tumors.
  a. Incidence: most common benign orbital tumors of childhood.
  b. Location: usually between globe and orbital periosteum in extraconal space, but can be intraconal.
  c. Radiology: dermoid tumors usually have density and signal like fat and can erode bone, whereas epidermoid tumors, containing only squamous debris and cholesterol, have density of fluid on CT.
7. Metastases: Hematogeneous metastases and direct extension of sinonasal tumors each represent about 5% of orbital tumors.
8. Miscellaneous: Tolosa-Hunt syndrome.
  a. Clinical findings: painful ophthalmoplegia with variable intracavernous cranial nerve involvement; usually responds promptly to steroids.
  b. Pathology: nonspecific inflammatory process in cavernous sinus, often extending into orbital apex.
  c. MR: cavernous sinus–orbital apex mass isointense to brain on T1WI, often strongly enhanced by contrast media.
  d. Differential diagnosis: lymphoma, pseudotumor, meningioma, sarcoidosis.

SUGGESTED READINGS

Atlas SW: Magnetic resonance imaging of the orbit: current status, *Magnet Res Q* 1:39-96, 1989.
Bilanuik LT, Zimmerman RA, Newton TH: Magnetic resonance imaging: orbital pathology. In Newton TH, Bilanuik LT (eds): *Modern neuroradiology. Vol. 4. Radiology of the eye and orbit,* New York, 1990, Clavadell Press, pp 5.1-5.84.
Desai SP, Carter J, Jinkins JR: Contrast-enhanced MR imaging of Tolosa-Hunt syndrome: a case report, *AJNR* 12:182-183, 1991.
Graeb DA, Rootman J, Rohertson WD, et al: Orbital lymphangiomas: clinical, radiologic, and pathologic characteristics, *Radiology* 175:417-421, 1990.
Guy J, Mancuso A, Beck R, et al: Radiation-induced optic neuropathy: a magnetic resonance imaging study, *J Neurosurg* 74:426-432, 1991.

360 *Disease processes by anatomic location*

Guy J, Mancuso A, Beck R, et al: Radiation-induced optic neuropathy: a magnetic resonance imaging study, *J Neurosurg* 74:426-432, 1991.

Guy J, Mancuso A, Quistino RG, et al: Gadolinium-DTPA-enhanced magnetic resonance imaging in optic neuropathies, *Ophthalmology* 97:592-600, 1991.

Handler LC, Davey IC, Hill JC, Lauryssen C: The acute orbit: differentiation of orbital cellulitis from subperiosteal abscess by computerized tomography, *Neuroradiology* 33:15-18, 1991.

Hendrix LE, Kneeland JB, Haughton VM, et al: MR imaging of optic nerve lesions, *AJNR* 11:749-754, 1990.

Hosten N, Sander B, Cordes M, et al: Graves ophthalmopathy: MR imaging of the orbits, *Radiology* 172:759-762, 1989.

Just M, Kahaly G, Higer HP, et al: Graves ophthalmopathy: role of MR imaging in radiation therapy, *Radiology* 179:187-190, 1991.

Kaissar G, Kim JH, Bravo S, Sze G: Histologic basis for increased extraocular muscle enhancement in gadolinium-enhanced MR imaging, *Radiology* 179:541-542, 1991.

Langer BG, Charletta DA, Mafee MF, Spigos DG: MRI of the normal optic pathway. *Semin US, CT, MR* 9:401-412, 1988.

Lee DH, Simon JH, Szomowski J, et al: Optic neuritis and orbital lesions: lipid-suppressed chemical shift MR imaging, *Radiology* 179:543-549, 1991.

Mafee MF: Magnetic resonance imaging: ocular pathology. In Newton TH, Bilanuik LT (eds): *Modern neuroradiology. Vol. 4. Radiology of the eye and orbit,* New York, 1990, Clavadell Press, pp 3.1-3.45.

Meli FJ, Boccaleri CA, Manzitti J, Lylyk P: Meningeal dissemination of retinoblastoma, *AJNR* 11:983-986, 1990.

Peyster RG, Augsburger JJ, Shields JA, et al: Intraocular tumors: evaluation with MR imaging, *Radiology* 168:773-779, 1988.

Raymond WR, Char DH, Norman D, Protzko EE: Magnetic resonance imaging of uveal tumors, *Am J Opthalmol* 111: 633-641, 1991.

Ronami H, Tamamura H, Kimizu K, et al: Intraocular lesions in patients with systemic disease: findings in MR imaging, *AJR* 154:385-389, 1990.

Tien RD, Chu PK, Hesselink JR, Szumowski J: Intra- and paraorbital lesions: value of fat-suppression MR imaging with paramagnetic contrast enhancement, *AJNR* 12:245-253, 1991.

Yousem DM, Atlas SW, Grossman RI, et al: MR imaging of Tolosa-Hunt syndrome, *AJNR* 10:1181-1184, 1989.

SECTION VII

SPINE AND CORD

CHAPTER 55

Spine and cord: congenital malformations

KEY CONCEPTS

1. Diastematomyelia means "split cord," not duplicated cord.
2. Tethered cord may be occult and occasionally does not become symptomatic until adulthood.
3. Magnetic resonance (MR) is the procedure of choice in evaluating congenital malformations of the spine and cord.

I. Normal development of spine and cord.
 A. Neurulation.
   1. Embryonic ectodermal proliferation forms "primitive streak" along surface of embryo by day 15 of gestation.
   2. Primitive pit with nodule of proliferating cells (Hensen's node) at cephalic end.
   3. Migration of cells into pit forms notochord.
   4. Notochord induces formation of neural plate, a dorsal midline collection of neural ectodermal cells that is continuous laterally with cutaneous ectoderm.
   5. Cells at cutaneous neural ectodermal interface thicken and form neural crest.
   6. Cells along lateral neural plate thicken and form neural folds.
   7. Neural folds are bent toward each other.
   8. Closure of neural tube begins at cervical area.
   9. Overlying ectoderm separates from and closes over neural tube.
   10. Neural crest cells separate from neural tube and migrate laterally, eventually forming dorsal root ganglia (among other structures).
   11. Neural tube progressively elongates and, through process called retrogressive differentiation, forms conus and filum.

12. Mesenchyme forms into somites and sclerotomes; parts of these migrate to lie dorsally between neural tube and ectoderm, forming precursors of neural arches, meninges, and paraspinous muscles.
13. Parts of sclerotomes fuse to form vertebral bodies.
14. Notochordal remnants persist between developing vertebral bodies and become nuclei pulposi.

II. Congenital and developmental anomalies: Recent studies have shown that MR is procedure of choice in evaluating spinal dysraphism and other congenital anomalies. In only a few cases of great anatomic complexity is it necessary to perform myelography, computed tomography (CT), or myelo-CT.

A. Meningocele is extension of meninges outside bony spinal canal.
1. Embryology: probably results from localized failure of neural tube closure.
2. Pathology: protrusion of dura, arachnoid, and cerebrospinal fluid (CSF) *without containing intrinsic neural tissue.*
3. Bony abnormalities: range from absent spinous process to multi-level spina bifida.
4. Associated abnormalities: may include low-lying conus and filum insertion into mouth of meningocele.
5. Most common cause of simple meningocele is probably not congenital but postsurgical.

B. Myelomeningocele is meningocele containing cord or nerve roots or both.
1. Embryology: same as meningocele, except vertebral subarachnoid space expands and displaces neural placode posteriorly.
2. Pathology: dorsal midline protruding oval plaque (placode) of neural tissue plus meninges and CSF through widely dysraphic neural arch. Dura is deficient posteriorly; pia-arachnoid lines ventral (inner) surface of placode. Both dural and ventral roots arise ventrally from placode, which itself blends imperceptibly into surrounding skin margins.
3. Bony abnormalities: spina bifida aperta.
4. Associated abnormalities.
   a. Diastematomyelia in 30% to 45%.
   b. Hydromyelia in 30% to 75%.
   c. Developmental scoliosis.
   d. Most have Chiari malformation (90% Chiari II).

C. Diastematomyelia ("split cord"; diplomyelia is true double cord with each having a set of roots and vertebral column, extremely rare if it exists at all).
1. Embryology: possibly result of split notochord.
2. Pathology: two "hemicords," frequently asymmetric in size, each lined by its own pia; 90% reunite below cleft. Half of patients

have single arachnoid dural tube; half have local doubling of same. Location: between T9 and S1 in 85%. Purely thoracic in 20%, lumbar in 50%, both in 20%. Cervical extremely rare.

3. Bony abnormalities almost always present.
   a. Laminae abnormal in more than 90% (often intersegmental fusions).
   b. Spina bifida in 85% to 100%.
   c. Widened interpediculate distance.
   d. Abnormal vertebral bodies (hemivertebrae, block vertebrae) in 85%.
   e. Scoliosis or kyphosis in 50% to 60%.
   f. Bone spur: present in only 50% and not a necessary feature of diastematomyelia. May be partially cartilaginous. Levels:
      (1) L1-3 in 50%.
      (2) T7-12 in 25%.
      (3) L4-5 in 18%.
      (4) T1-6 in 5%.
      (5) Cervical rare.
4. Associated abnormalities.
   a. Low-lying conus in 75%.
   b. Tethered singly or doubly in 60%.
   c. Occurs in 30% to 45% of Chiari II malformations.
   d. Hydromyelia.

D. Hydrosyringomyelia: Classically, term "hydromelia" means dilatation of ependymal-lined central canal, whereas "syringomyelia" is used to designate spinal cord cavitations that are outside central canal, originating in and primarily involving cord parenchyma. Practically, it is difficult to distinguish these two entities, so they are often considered together as "hydrosyringomyelia."
   1. Embryology and etiology: many pathophysiologic theories. Can be congenital or acquired (e.g., posttraumatic).
   2. Pathology: See above.
   3. Bony anomalies: canal often widened and dysraphic.
   4. Associated anomalies: myelomeningocele in 50% to 80%; very common with Chiari II; can occur alone.

E. Intraspinal enteric cysts, dural enteric fistulas ("split notochord" syndrome): splitting or deviation of notochord with persistent communication between gut and skin, variable combination of fistulas, sinuses, diverticula, duplications, and cysts. Vertebral anomalies usually present.

F. Spinal lipomas: collection of mature fat plus connective tissue. Divided into three types.
   1. Intradural lipoma (4%).
      a. Location: cervical and thoracic most common (these usually lie

along dorsal or subpial surface of cord and may tether conus), but can occur anywhere in cord or cauda equina.

  b. Bony anomalies: focal spina bifida common, but canal can be normal or only focally expanded.

2. Lipomyelomeningocele (84%).

  a. Embryology: Like myelocele, lipoma lies dorsal (but is attached) to placode. Lipoma is in continuity with subcutaneous fat. Defect is covered by intact skin.

  b. Pathology: widely bifid canal with posterior herniation of neural placode to form dorsal subcutaneous mass composed of fat, fibrous tissue, neural tissue, and meningocele.

  c. Bony anomalies.

    (1) Spine becomes increasingly dysraphic from above downward.

    (2) Segmentation anomalies in approximately 40%.

    (3) Sacral anomalies in up to 50%.

  d. Associations: rare in Chiari II (but common in myelomeningocele).

3. Fibrolipomas of filum terminale (12%).

  a. Embryology: unknown.

  b. Pathology: can be in intradural or extradural portion of filum or in both. Can occur with or without tethered spinal cord.

  c. "Fatty" filum terminale: thin streak of fat in filum seen in approximately 1% of nonselected lumbosacral spine scans. Can be asymptomatic and incidental with normal conus. Can be associated with tether.

G. "Tight" filum terminale.

1. Pathology: short, thick filum terminale (more than 2 mm) with conus below L2-3 level (conus is at or above this level in 98% of people; L3 in 2%).

2. Bony anomalies.

  a. Kyphoscoliosis in 25%.

  b. Spina bifida occulta.

3. Associated anomalies: lipoma in 20% to 25%.

4. Radiology: 75% have low-lying conus with thickened filum or fibrolipoma or both, often with patulous dural sac. Cord stretched tightly across any kyphoscoliosis.

5. NOTE: Occasionally persons with occult tethered cord do not have symptoms until adulthood.

H. Neurofibromatosis: multiple manifestations (see Chapter 29).

1. Pathology: dyshistiogenesis of mesodermal and neuroectodermal tissue. Schwann cell is neoplastic element.

2. Bony anomalies.

  a. Scoliosis in 40% to 60%.

    b. Widened canal in 3%; ectatic patulous dura and posterior vertebral scalloping in 10%.
    c. Lateral thoracic and anterior sacral meningoceles.
    d. Cervical vertebral scalloping and enlarged foramina in 7%; alignment abnormalities in up to 25%.
  3. Spinal nerve sheath tumors.
    a. Pathology.
      (1) Neurofibromatosis type 1: neurofibromas.
      (2) Neurofibromatosis type 2: schwannomas.
      (3) Sarcomatous transformation of schwannoma very rare; 5% to 10% of neurofibromas become malignant.
    b. Location.
      (1) Extramedullary intradural in 70%.
      (2) Extradural in 15%.
      (3) Both ("dumbbell") in 15%.
I. Congenital neoplasms of the spine and cord (see Chapter 57).

SUGGESTED READINGS

Barkovich AJ: Congenital anomalies of the spine. In *Pediatric neuroimaging,* New York, 1990, Raven Press, pp 227-271.

Brophy JD, Sutlon LN, Zimmerman RA, et al: Magnetic resonance imaging of lipomyelomeningocele and tethered cord, *Neurosurgery* 25:336-340, 1989.

Davis PC, Hoffman JC Jr, Ball TI, et al: Spinal abnormalities in pediatric patients: MR imaging findings compared with clinical, myelographic, and surgical findings, *Radiology* 166:679-685, 1988.

Halliday AL, Sobel RA, Martuza RL: Benign spinal nerve sheath tumors: their occurrence sporadically and in neurofibromatosis types 1 and 2, *J Neurosurg* 74:248-253, 1991.

Isu T, Iwasaki Y, Akino M, Abe H: Hydrosyringomyelia associated with a Chiari I malformation in children and adolescents, *Neurosurgery* 26:591-597, 1990.

Merx JL, Bakker-Niegen SH, Thijssen HOM, Walder HAD: The tethered spinal cord syndrome: a correlation of radiological features and preoperative findings in 30 patients, *Neuroradiology* 31:63-70, 1989.

Naidich TP, McLone DG, Harwood-Nash DC: Spinal dysraphism. In Newton TH, Potts DG (eds): *Computed tomography of the spine and spinal cord,* New York, 1983, Clavadell Press, pp 249-253.

Oi S, Kudo H, Yamada H, et al: Hydromyelic hydrocephalus, *J Neurosurg* 74:371-379, 1991.

Okumura R, Minami S, Asato R, Konishi J: Fatty filum terminale assessment with MR imaging, *J Comput Assist Tomogr* 14:571-573, 1990.

Raghavan N, Barkovich AJ, Edwards M, Norman D: MR imaging in the tethered spinal cord syndrome, *AJNR* 10:27-36, 1989.

Samuelsson L, Bergstrom K, Thomas KA, et al: MR imaging of syringohydromyelia and Chiari malformations in myelomeningocele patients with scoliosis, *AJNR* 8:539-546, 1987.

Scatliff JH, Kendall BE, Kingsley DPE, et al: Closed spinal dysraphism, *AJNR* 10:269-277, 1989.

Sherman JL, Barkovich AJ, Citrin CM: The MR appearance of syringomyelia: new observations, *AJNR* 7:985-995, 1986.

Tartori-Donati P, Cama A, Rosa ML, et al: Occult spinal dysraphism: neuroradiological study, *Neuroradiology* 31:512-522, 1990.

CHAPTER 56

Spine and cord: trauma and degenerative disease

KEY CONCEPTS

1. Disc desiccation and degeneration are part of the normal aging process and begin around 20 years of age. Bulging discs and asymptomatic herniations are also common.
2. Overuse injuries occurring secondary to repetitive, unrepaired microtrauma are a common cause of low back pain in children and adolescents.
3. "Far lateral" or extraforaminal disc herniations can be overlooked if structures *outside* the canal are not carefully examined on spine computed tomography (CT) and magnetic resonance (MR).
4. Low thoracic and high lumbar disc herniations and occult conus lesions can have low back pain as the initial symptom and may be overlooked if MR scans do not routinely include the thoracolumbar junction.
5. Causes of "failed back" syndrome include persistent or recurrent herniated nucleus pulposus (HNP) at same level; HNP at nonoperated level; scarring and fibrosis; spinal, meningeal, or neural inflammation ("neuritis"); postoperative intraspinal hemorrhage; facet syndromes; remote phenomena unrelated to the spine (e.g., hip disease); and occult conus lesion.
6. As a general rule, scars are enhanced by contrast material and discs are not. Vascularized disc fragments are sometimes enhanced.

I. Trauma: Extensive discussion of spinal fractures and cord injury is beyond scope of this book. Following summarizes some important general considerations.

A. Spine: general mechanisms of injury and associated fracture types.

368

1. Flexion injury.
   a. Anterior wedging and comminuted body fracture.
   b. Posterior ligamentous disruption.
   c. Facet and body subluxation (anteroposterior).
2. Extension injury.
   a. Posterior element fracture.
   b. Anterior ligamentous disruption.
   c. Facet and body subluxation (anteroposterior).
3. Axial loading (compression) and vertical force injury.
   a. "Head down": diving.
   b. "Bottom up": jumping.
   c. Vertebral body compression and fracture.
   d. Lateral element fracture and compression.
4. Rotation injury (usually in combination with others).
   a. Lateral mass fracture.
   b. Unilateral or bilateral facet subluxation.

B. Spine: some specific fracture types.
   1. Jefferson fracture: "burst" fracture of C1 (axial loading). Cord damage rare.
   2. Hangman fracture: various types, but hyperextension or distraction injury leads to traumatic spondylolysis. Bilateral C2 pedicle fracture with separation of neural arch from C2 body with or without anterior subluxation. Cord damage rare.
   3. Odontoid fracture: odontoid bone alone or with lateral mass fracture. CAUTION: Odontoid fracture can be missed on axial CT without sagittal and coronal reformatting.
      a. Differential diagnosis: os odontoideum.
      b. Sequelae: subluxation and cord compression.
   4. Atlantooccipital dislocation: usually fatal.
   5. Atlantoaxial dislocation: usually accompanied by fractures and transverse ligament disruption. Nontraumatic causes of C1-2 subluxation include:
      a. Normally lax ligaments in child.
      b. Inflammation (tonsillitis, pharyngitis).
      c. Rheumatoid arthritis.
   6. "Clay-shoveler's fracture": spinous process fractures of lower cervical spine (sometimes accompanied by "teardrop" avulsion fracture of anterior vertebral body).
   7. Miscellaneous cervical fractures and dislocations.
   8. Thoracic "burst" fracture.
   9. Thoracolumbar junction fractures.
      a. Axial compression leads to vertebral body wedging.

> > > (1) "Burst" fracture with or without retropulsed fragment.
> > > (2) Traumatic disc herniation.
> > b. Facet distraction and subluxation.
> 10. Miscellaneous.
> > a. "Seat-belt" (Chance's) fracture: flexion injury with facet distraction and subluxation with or without vertebral body compression.
> > b. "Overuse injuries" occurring secondary to repetitive, unrepaired microtrauma cause low back pain in children and adolescents. Pars interarticularis and pedicle fractures are common. Routine CT or single photon emission computed tomography (SPECT) may be helpful in detecting occult lesions.

C. Cord and soft tissues.
> 1. Epidural hematoma (reported incidence with spine fracture varies from 0.5% to 7.5%, but condition is probably underdiagnosed).
> 2. Cord hemorrhage, contusion, edema, and compression.
> 3. Cord transection.
> 4. Root avulsion ("empty root sleeve" sign seen with myelography).
> 5. Sequelae.
> > a. Myelomalacia.
> > b. Syringomyelia.
> > c. Atrophy.
> > d. Meningocele.

II. Degenerative diseases.

A. Disc.
> 1. Changes with aging: dehydration, fissures, radial annular tears, asymptomatic herniations.
> > a. Between 20 and 40 years: 36% of people have degenerated discs on MR.
> > b. By age 50, 85% to 95% of adults have disc degeneration at autopsy.
> > c. Between 60 and 80 years: 98% have one or more degenerated discs on MR.
> > d. Up to 60 years of age: steady increase in disc degeneration occurs with age. About 20% of asymptomatic patients under age 60 have one or more frank HNPs.
> 2. Disc bulges and herniations.
> > a. Bulge: smooth, nonfocal, concentric expansion of disc outside margins of vertebral end-plate.
> > b. Herniation: focal protrusion of disc material.
> > c. "Free" fragments: fragments that migrate away from interspace and are discontinuous with parent disc. Fragments from donor disc move up and down in equal numbers. More than 90% are

off-midline in anterior epidural space (fragments rarely straddle the midline).

    d. May be enhanced by contrast material if chronic herniation with vascularized granulation tissue is present.

    e. Location of HNP: anterior, posterior, neural foraminal, "far lateral" (outside neural foramen). NOTE: Extraforaminal disc herniations can be easily overlooked if radiologist does not look *outside* canal on spine MR or CT.

    f. Level of HNP.

        (1) Lumbar: 85% to 90% at L4-5, L5-S1; 5% to 8% at L3-4; 2% at L2-3; 1% at L1-2, T12-L1.

        (2) Thoracic: with advent of MR, higher prevalence (one series found approximately 15% thoracic HNPs in series of cancer patients undergoing screening MR).

        (3) Cervical: most at C4-5, C5-6, C6-7.

B. Facet joints and degeneration.

    1. Articular cartilage loss normal after 20 years of age.

    2. Subchondral thickening and sclerosis.

    3. Bony overgrowth (osteophytes).

        a. Neural foraminal encroachment.

        b. Lateral recess narrowing.

        c. Spinal stenosis: Effect of congenitally small canal or "short pedicle" syndrome is to make small disc bulges and herniations more significant than they would be if canal were normal or capacious.

C. Ligamentum flavum "hypertrophy" (buckling is probably more accurate) can lead to:

    1. Spinal stenosis.

    2. Neural foraminal encroachment.

D. Vertebral body osteophytes can lead to:

    1. Spinal stenosis.

    2. Neural foraminal encroachment.

    3. Lateral recess syndrome.

E. Age-related marrow changes adjacent to vertebral end-plates common.

    1. Type I: decreased signal on T1WI, increased on T2WI. Can be enhanced. Caused by replacement of cellular marrow by fibrous marrow.

    2. Type II: increased signal on T1WI (fatty replacement of marrow), isointense to slightly hyperintense on T2WI. Caused by disruption and fissuring of end-plates with vascularized fibrous tissue; therefore can be enhanced somewhat.

    3. Type III: decreased signal on both T1WI and T2WI. Caused by extensive dense bony sclerosis.

F. Postoperative spine.
 1. Scar versus HNP on MR evaluation.
   a. Scar.
     (1) Obliterates epidural fat, conforms to epidural space.
     (2) Lacks mass effect, often not contiguous with disc.
     (3) On precontrast T1WI, isointense or slightly hypointense to thecal sac; hypointense to cerebrospinal fluid on T2WI. Signal lower than that of adjacent intraspinal or paraspinal fat.
     (4) After contrast administration: typically enhanced immediately; enhancement may or may not be uniform; maximum intensity usually within 5 minutes.
   b. HNP.
     (1) Mass effect.
     (2) Often contiguous with annulus.
     (3) Typically no enhancement immediately after contrast material is administered, although vascularized retained fragments may become enhanced with time. NOTE: Very occasionally, HNP enhancement occurs immediately.
     (4) May have retained fragment (low signal) surrounded by enhancing peridiscal scar.
   c. CAVEAT: In immediate postoperative spine (up to 12 weeks) may be difficult to distinguish postoperative changes from HNP.
 2. Normal postoperative disc.
   a. May lose height; signal consistent with dehydration.
   b. Following contrast administration, linear enhancement extending deep into disc is common.
 3. Arachnoiditis: variable findings.
   a. Clumped, thickened roots.
   b. "Empty" thecal sac (roots are laterally retracted and adhere to walls of thecal sac).
   c. Focal dural and meningeal thickening.
   d. Arachnoiditis usually does not show much enhancement following administration of contrast material.
 4. "Neuritis" (postoperative enhancement of individual inflamed nerve roots).
 5. Pseudomeningocele.
 6. Infection.
   a. Epidural abscess.
   b. Osteomyelitis.
 7. Causes of "failed back" syndrome.
   a. Persistent or recurrent HNP at same level.

      b. HNP at nonoperated level.

      c. Scar.

      d. Spinal, meningeal, or neural inflammation.

      e. Perioperative intraspinal hemorrhage.

      f. Facet syndrome.

      g. Remote phenomena unrelated to spine (e.g., hip).

      h. Occult conus lesion.

G. Avascular necrosis (AVN) of vertebral body.

    1. Plain films: centrally located, horizontally oriented radiolucent linear cleft within compressed vertebral body.

    2. MR: varies according to stage of AVN. Classic:

      a. Hypointense intravertebral cleft on T1WI that is strikingly hyperintense on T2WI.

      b. Peripheral hypointense zone on T2WI that surrounds hyperintense cleft ("double line sign") is due to peripheral sclerosis surrounding central granulation tissue.

    3. Differential diagnosis.

      a. Neoplasm: also hypointense on T1WI and hyperintense on T2WI, but hyperintensity usually more diffuse and less intense with tumor.

      b. Osteomyelitis: increased, more diffuse signal on T2WI in adjacent disc and end-plates.

      c. Multiple myeloma: intravertebral vacuum cleft reported in a few cases.

SUGGESTED READINGS

Afshani E, Kuhn JP: Common causes of low back pain in children, *Radiographics* 11:269-291, 1991.

Boden SD, Davis DO, Dina TS, et al: Abnormal magnetic-resonance scans of the lumbar spine in asymptomatic patients, *J Bone Joint Surg* 72A:403-408, 1990.

Brant-Zawadzki M, Post MJD: Trauma. In Newton TH, Potts DG (eds): *Modern neuroradiology. Vol I. Computed tomography of the spine and spinal cord,* New York, 1983, Clavadell Press, pp 149-186.

Grenier N, Kressel HY, Schiebler ML, et al: Normal and degenerative posterior spinal structures: MR imaging, *Radiology* 165:517-525, 1987.

Hueftle MG, Modic MT, Ross JS, et al: Lumbar spine: postoperative MR imaging with Gd-DTPA, *Radiology* 167:817-824, 1988.

Jinkins JR, Osborn AG, Garrett D, et al: Enhanced MR of spinal nerve radiculitis: relationship to the lumbosacral post-surgical syndrome, Paper presented at a meeting of the American Society of Radiology, Washington, DC, 1991.

Johnson CE, Sze G: Benign lumbar arachnoiditis, *AJNR* 11:763-770, 1990.

Kulkarni MV, Bondurant FJ, Rose SL, Narayana PA: 1.5 Tesla magnetic resonance imaging of acute spine trauma, *Radiographics* 8:1059-1082, 1988.

Naul LG, Peet GJ, Maupin WB: Avascular necrosis of the vertebral body: MR imaging, *Radiology* 172:219-222, 1989.

Ross JS, Masaryk TJ, Schrader M, et al: MR imaging of the postoperative lumbar spine, *AJNR* 11:771-776, 1990.

Ross JS, Modic MT, Masaryk TJ: Tears of the anulus fibrosus. *AJNR* 10:1251-1254, 1990.

Schellinger D, Manz HJ, Vidic B, et al: Disk fragment migration, *Radiology* 175:831-836, 1990.

Traughber PD, Havlina JM Jr: Bilateral pedicle stress fractures: SPECT and CT features, *J Comput Assist Tomogr* 15:338-340, 1991.

Williams MP, Cherryman GR, Husband JE: Significance of thoracic disc herniation demonstrated by MR imaging, *J Comput Assist Tomogr* 13:211-214, 1989.

Yamashita Y, Takahashi M, Matsuno Y, et al: Chronic injuries of the spinal cord: assessment with MR imaging, *Radiology* 175:849-854, 1990.

Yu S, Haughton VM, Ho PSP, et al: Progressive and regressive changes in the nucleus pulposus, parts I and II, *Radiology* 169:87-97, 1988.

CHAPTER 57

Spine and cord: neoplasms

With M. Judith Donovan Post

KEY CONCEPTS

1. Most cord neoplasms are gliomas; 95% are astrocytomas or ependymomas. Glioblastoma in cord is rare (contrast with brain gliomas).
2. In children 60% of cord tumors are astrocytomas, 30% ependymomas; in adults ependymoma is more common.
3. The most common malignant bony spine tumor is metastasis from primary neoplasm elsewhere.

I. Neoplasms of vertebral column: For more detailed discussion of skeletal neoplasms and tumorlike diseases of the spine, see Chapter 1 of B.J. Manaster's *Skeletal Radiology* in the Mosby–Year Book series "Handbooks in Radiology."
   A. Benign.
      1. Hemangioma.
         a. Incidence: 10% to 12% at autopsy.
         b. Age and sex: more common in females; occurs after puberty (in middle age).
         c. Location: anywhere, but most commonly lower thoracic: all or part of prevertebral body involved; occasionally almost completely extraosseous with extensive tissue mass within epidural space.
         d. Pathology: hamartoma, with thin-walled vessels, fibroadipose stroma, few but thick trabeculae.
         e. Computed tomography (CT): "polka-dot" vertebrae; soft tissue mass may or may not be present (best shown if intrathecal contrast material used).
         f. Magnetic resonance (MR): mottled and hyperintense on both T1-

and T2-weighted imaging (T1WI and T2WI); focal or diffuse involvement. Contrast-enhanced MR best delineates extent of epidural soft tissue mass and degree of cord compression.

2. Osteoid osteoma.
   a. Incidence: 6% of benign bone tumors.
   b. Age and sex: male/female 4:1; 5 to 20 years of age (rare after 30 years).
   c. Location: neural arch, transverse process.
   d. Pathology: variably mineralized central nidus, dense peripheral reactive sclerosis.
   e. CT: small radiolucent center, dense peripheral sclerosis; nidus may have dense calcification.
   f. MR: hypointense on T1WI and T2WI.

3. Benign osteoblastoma (giant osteoid osteoma).
   a. Incidence: less than 1% of bone tumors (nearly half of all osteoblastomas are found in axial skeleton).
   b. Age and sex: male/female 2:1; 70% in patients less than 20 years of age.
   c. Location: posterior elements (laminae, pedicles).
   d. Pathology: osteoclasts, foci of osteoid and mature bone.
   e. CT: well-defined solitary lytic expansile lesion; thin sclerotic rim; often contains mottled calcification.
   f. MR: mixed signal because of variably calcified fibrocartilaginous components.
   g. Differential diagnoses: aneurysmal bone cyst; giant cell tumor; eosinophilic granuloma; metastasis.

4. Osteochondroma.
   a. Incidence: 6% affect spine.
   b. Location: spinous processes or transverse processes; cervical or thoracic most common.
   c. Pathology: cartilaginous cap covering bony exostosis. Often multiple.
   d. CT: demonstrates entire lesion and shows its relationship to paraspinal and intraspinal tissues; intrathecal contrast enhancement shows extent of cord compression and thecal sac compromise.
   e. MR: mixed signal intensities because of variably calcified fibrocartilaginous portions of tumor.

5. Eosinophilic granuloma.
   a. Age: 5 to 10 years; extremely rare after 30 years.
   b. Location: vertebral body, usually cervical; often multiple.
   c. CT: lytic lesion with collapsed body; no sclerosis.
   d. MR: vertebral plana, cord compression.

6. Aneurysmal bone cyst.
   a. Incidence: less than 1% of primary bone tumors; 20% spinal.
   b. Age: 70% less than 20 years of age; 90% less than 30 years.
   c. Location.
      (1) Cervical or thoracic.
      (2) Posterior elements.
      (3) May extend into pedicles and body of vertebra.
      (4) May cross disc space into next vertebra.
   d. Pathology: thin-walled blood-filled cavities without endothelium or elastic layers.
   e. CT: expansile soft tissue mass; may involve several vertebrae; enhancement with contrast media.
   f. MR: well-defined, expansile, lobulated mass; low-signal rim on both T1WI and T2WI; contents septated and hyperintense on T2WI; fluid-fluid levels common.
7. Giant cell tumor.
   a. Incidence: 4% of primary bone tumors; 10% in spine. Malignant transformation in 10%.
   b. Age: second and third decades.
   c. Location: sacrum (rare elsewhere in spine); occasionally vertebral body.
   d. CT: lytic, destructive, expansile; no calcification.
   e. MR: hypointense on T1WI; mixed hypointense and isointense on T2WI; may be hyperintense foci of hemorrhage and cyst formation.
   f. Differential diagnoses: osteoblastoma, aneurysmal bone cyst.
B. Malignant: primary.
   1. Chordoma.
      a. Incidence: 1% to 4% of spinal tumors.
      b. Sex and age: male/female 2:1; any age.
      c. Location: Two thirds of CNS chordomas occur in spine, one third at base of skull; in spine, sacrococcygeal area affected most often.
      d. Pathology: originate from intraosseous notochordal remnants.
      e. CT.
         (1) Lytic, destructive.
         (2) One or more vertebral bodies and discs affected.
         (3) Soft tissue mass (may be almost entirely extraosseous).
         (4) Calcification 30% to 70%.
      f. MR: lobulated, septated mass with fibrous capsule. Contents:
         (1) Hypointense on T1WI.
         (2) Extremely hyperintense on proton density–weighted scan and T2WI.

2. Ewing's sarcoma.
   a. Incidence: rarely primary in spine; is usually metastatic from another site.
   b. Age: peak in second decade or first half of third decade.
   c. Pathology: arises from immature reticulum cells or primitive mesenchyme.
   d. Location: usually found in vertebral bodies but can spread to posterior elements (sacrum and lumbar region most common locations).
   e. CT: bone erosion, soft tissue mass.
   f. MR: low signal intensity on T1WI and very high signal intensity on T2WI.
3. Plasmacytoma and multiple myeloma (myelomatosis).
   a. Incidence: spine involvement with frequent pathologic compression fractures; vertebral collapse occurs in two thirds.
   b. Age and sex: fifth to seventh decades; male/female 3:1.
   c. Location: vertebral body usually involved first, then pedicle.
   d. Pathology: arises from hematogenous cells in bone marrow.
   e. CT: lytic expansile lesion, often with pathologic compression fractures; soft tissue mass with canal impingement best seen with intrathecal contrast material.
   f. MR: longer T1 and T2 relaxation values than normal marrow. High signal intensity on T1WI and T2WI secondary to hemorrhage may also be seen, as well as collapsed vertebrae and soft tissue mass.
4. Hodgkin disease.
   a. Age: 20 to 30 years of age; more common in men.
   b. Location: vertebral bodies, ribs, pelvis, and femurs.
   c. Plain films: "ivory vertebrae" often with vertebral body collapse; occasionally, scalloping anteriorly (from enlarged paraaortic nodes).
   d. CT: hyperdense vertebral bodies, paraspinal and epidural soft tissue masses; fusiform, lobulated paraspinal masses caused by enlarged lymph nodes.
   e. MR: variable signal but usually hypointense on T1WI. Look for preexisting marrow changes in irradiated spine (fatty marrow replacement).
5. Non-Hodgkin lymphoma.
   a. Age and sex: 40 to 60 years of age; more common in men.
   b. Location: vertebral bodies.
   c. CT: vertebral body hyperostosis and destruction, enlarged lymph nodes, epidural extension (best evaluated with intrathecal contrast enhancement).

    d. MR: hypointense on T1WI, hyperintense on T2WI; canal extension and lymphadenopathy may be demonstrated; inhomogeneous lesions may be seen.

6. Chondrosarcoma.
    a. Age and sex: mainly fourth to sixth decades; male/female 2:1.
    b. Location: posterior and anterior elements of spine may be involved, with local extension from one level to next.
    c. Pathology: malignant cartilage tumors arising from bone or preexisting exostosis.
    d. Radiology.
      (1) Lytic lesion.
      (2) Associated with soft tissue mass.
      (3) Often contains calcification.
      (4) CT demonstrates extent of vertebral destruction and calcification; soft tissue involvement and cord compression are delineated better with MR.

7. Osteogenic sarcoma.
    a. Age and sex: 10 to 25 years; slight male predominance.
    b. Location: spine rarely affected (25 recorded cases in literature).
    c. Pathology: mesenchymal origin with tumor osteophytic production; can develop after radiation (reported latent period ranges from 5 to 25 years).
    d. CT.
      (1) Osteogenic and osteolytic bone changes.
      (2) Radiation changes in adjacent vertebrae.
      (3) Defines soft tissue components and associated calcification.
    e. MR: Appearance varies according to subtype and presence of osteoid, bone, cartilage, calcification, and hemorrhage. Look for postirradiation marrow changes.

C. Malignant metastatic disease.
1. Spine.
    a. Incidence: most common malignant spine tumor.
    b. Age and sex: middle to late decades; equal prevalence in men and women.
    c. Location: spine most common osseous site; most frquently involves vertebral body but can affect any part of vertebra.
    d. Pathology: breast, prostate gland, lung, kidney, thyroid gland, and lymphoma most common primary sites.
    e. CT: multifocal lytic, destructive lesions, with or without sclerosis; paraspinal and epidural soft tissue masses common.
    f. MR: hypointense on T1WI, hyperintense on T2WI; soft tissue mass, pathologic fracture, and cord compression common. CAUTION: May become isointense with contrast material on T1WI.

MR imaging more sensitive than bone scintigraphy in detecting vertebral metastases.

II. Neoplasms of nerve roots, dura, and spinal cord.
  A. Benign spinal nerve sheath tumors.
    1. Two types.
       a. Neurofibromas.
       b. Schwannomas.
    2. Incidence and associations.
       a. Most common intraspinal tumors (15% to 30%).
       b. Can be sporadic (nearly all sporadically occurring nerve sheath tumors are schwannomas).
       c. Neurofibromatosis type 1 associated with neurofibromas.
       d. Neurofibromatosis type 2 associated with schwannomas.
    3. Location.
       a. Dorsal nerve roots.
       b. Extramedullary intradural in 70%.
       c. Extradural in 15%.
       d. Combined intradural and extradural ("dumbbell") in 15%.
       e. Intramedullary (in spinal cord) in less than 1%.
    4. Pathology.
       a. Schwannoma: Schwann cells.
       b. Neurofibroma: Schwann cells and fibroblasts.
    5. CT: extramedullary soft tissue mass, bony changes (expansion).
    6. MR: variable; isointense or hypointense on T1WI, often hyperintense on T2WI. May be inhomogeneous; schwannomas usually enhanced strongly.
  B. Meningioma.
    1. Incidence: 25% to 45% of intraspinal tumors (most common primary intraspinal tumor in some series); can be multiple (usually in von Recklinghausen's disease).
    2. Age and sex: fifth and sixth decades; 80% in women.
    3. Location: 65% to 80% thoracic, rest cervical (lumbar uncommon); 85% extramedullary intradural, 15% extradural ("dumbbell" rare).
    4. CT: isodense to hyperdense intradural mass; bone erosion; calcification rare (10%); cord displacement shown with intrathecal contrast enhancement.
    5. MR: variable but usually isointense; enhanced strongly: calcification seen as areas of signal absence.
  C. Spinal cord tumors.
    1. General.
       a. Gliomas constitute greater than 90% of cord tumors.
          (1) Children: astrocytoma in 60%, ependyoma in 30%.
          (2) Adults: ependyoma in 55% to 60%, astrocytoma in 30% to 40%.

b. Others (less than 10% of cord tumors).
   (1) Hemangioblastoma (1% to 3%).
   (2) Metastases (1% to 3%).
2. Ependymoma.
   a. Incidence: overall most common cord neoplasm (lower cord, conus, and filum most common locations).
   b. Age and sex: third to sixth decades; slight male preponderance.
   c. Pathology: often myxopapillary tumor of filum.
   d. CT: 15% to 35% have vertebral scalloping or canal expansion; expansile cord mass shown with intrathecal contrast enhancement.
   e. MR.
      (1) Enlarged cord or filum, often multilevel; expanded canal.
      (2) Irregular, poorly defined mass.
      (3) Hypointense on T1WI, typically hyperintense on T2WI; often inhomogeneous (blood degradation products and necrosis or cysts).
      (4) Strong, uniform enhancement.
3. Astrocytoma.
   a. Incidence: 20% to 30% of cord gliomas.
   b. Age: more common in children (60% of intramedullary tumors).
   c. Pathology: 75% low grade; glioblastoma and anaplastic astrocytoma rare (unlike in brain).
   d. Location: cervical or thoracic (rostral more common in children).
   e. CT and myelography: isodense to hypodense expansile cord lesion.
   f. MR: similar to ependymoma (cannot be distinguished on MR); associated cysts, hemorrhage, and contrast enhancement common.
4. Lipoma.
   a. Age and sex: first three decades; equal prevalence by sex.
   b. Location: 60% intradural (dorsal cord, filum), 40% extradural; thoracic more common than cervical.
   c. CT: homogeneously hypodense mass.
   d. MR: hyperintense on T1WI, hypointense on T2WI (like fat elsewhere).
5. Hemangioblastoma.
   a. Incidence: rare (1% to 3% of spinal tumors).
   b. Location: 60% intramedullary, 80% solitary; one third of patients have von Hippel–Lindau disease; thoracic 50%, cervical 40%.
   c. Radiology: solid 40%, cystic 60%.
      (1) CT: enlargement of interpediculate and anterior-posterior di-

ameters of spinal canals. Hypodense tumor enhances usually homogeneously; intrathecal contrast enhancement may reveal dilated veins.

(2) MR: vessels demonstrated as serpiginous areas of intermediate intensity signal on T2WI. Tumor sometimes associated with cyst or syrinx. Gadolinium enhances vascular portions of tumor but not associated cyst.

6. Acquired epidermoid tumor.
   a. Etiology: previous lumbar puncture (69% of nonstylet needles pick up epidermal tissue that could potentially be implanted into canal).
   b. CT and myelography: well-delineated extramedullary intradural lumbar mass.
   c. MR: variable but often isointense to cerebrospinal fluid.

7. Intramedullary metastases.
   a. Incidence: uncommon.
   b. Age: fifth to eighth decades.
   c. Pathology: breast, lung.
   d. Radiology: nonspecific intramedullary mass on MR; isointense on T1WI, often enhance strongly: cord edema may be seen on T2WI.

III. Congenital tumors of spine and cord: rare neoplasms, mostly teratomas, dermoid tumors, and epidermoid tumors.

A. Teratoma.
   1. Two types: sacrococcygeal and intraspinal.
      a. Sacrococcygeal teratoma.
         (1) Pathology: aberrant and persistent tissue from the three germinal layers; one third of sacrococcygeal tumors are immature or anaplastic.
         (2) Location: can be sacral alone (approximately 50%), sacral and pelvic, or entirely presacral.
         (3) Imaging: highly variable depending on composition. Usually both cystic and solid, often partially calcified. Most are lobulated, relatively well-delineated masses.
      b. Intraspinal teratoma.
         (1) Incidence: less than 1% of intraspinal tumors.
         (2) Pathology: See preceding.
         (3) Location: can be intramedullary or extramedullary.
         (4) Radiology: highly variable depending on composition; may have associated syrinx.

B. Dermoid and epidermoid tumors.
   1. Incidence: 1% to 2% of all intraspinal tumors but 10% of spine tumors in children.

2. Pathology: congenital lesions derived from dermal or epidermal rests, with (20%) or without (80%) associated dermal sinus. (CAUTION: Cutaneous aspect of sinus tract can be several segments away from intraspinal mass.) Vertebral anomalies common.
3. Location.
    a. Dermoid tumors mostly in lumbosacral area, rare above conus.
    b. Epidermoid tumors can be found at any level but are more common in lumbosacral area; 60% are extramedullary; 40% intramedullary.
4. Radiology: like dermoid and epidermoid tumors elsewhere; dermoid tumors behave more like fat. Epidermoid tumors usually isointense with CSF. Typically neither is enhanced.

SUGGESTED READINGS

Algra PR, Bloem JL, Tissing H, et al: Detection of vertebral metastases: comparison between MR imaging and bone scintigraphy, *Radiographics* 11:219-232, 1991.

Baker LL, Goodman SB, Perkash I, et al: Benign versus pathologic compression fractures of vertebral bodies: assessment with conventional spin-echo, chemical-shift, and STIR MR imaging, *Radiology* 174:495-502, 1990.

Barkovich AJ: Congenital tumors of the spine and neoplasms of the spine. In *Pediatric neuroimaging,* New York, 1990, Raven Press, pp 261-263, 273-291.

Briger RK, Williams AL, Daniels DL, et al: Contrast enhancement in spinal MR imaging, *AJNR* 10:633-637, 1989.

Carmody RF, Yang PJ, Sieley GW, et al: Spinal cord compression due to metastatic disease: diagnosis with MR imaging versus myelography, *Radiology* 173:225-229, 1989.

Ciapetta P, Salvati M, Capoccia G, et al: Spinal glioblastomas: report of seven cases and review of the literature, *Neurosurgery* 28:302-306, 1991.

Demachi H, Takashima T, Kadoya M, et al: MR imaging of spinal neurinomas with pathological correlation, *J Comput Assist Tomogr* 14:250-254, 1990.

Enzmann DR, DeLaPaz RL: Tumor. In *Magnetic resonance of the spine,* St Louis, 1990, Mosby–Year Book, pp 301-422.

Feider HK, Yuille DL: On epidural cavernous hemangioma of the spine. *AJNR* 12:243-244, 1991.

Fruehwald FXJ, Tscholakoff D, Schwaighofer B, et al: Magnetic resonance imaging of the lower vertebral column in patients with multiple myeloma, *Invest Radiol* 23:193-199, 1988.

Halliday AL, Sobel RA, Martuza RL: Benign spine nerve sheath tumors: their occurrence sporadically and in neurofibromatosis types 1 and 2. *J Neurosurg* 74:248-253, 1991.

Hilseth A, Mork SJ: Primary intraspinal neoplasms in Norway, 1955-1986, *J Neurosurg* 71:842-845, 1989.

McCormick PC, Torres R, Post KD, Stein BM: Intramedullary ependymoma of the spinal cord, *J Neurosurg* 72:523-532, 1990.

Munk PL, Helms CA, Holt RG, et al: MR imaging of aneurysmal bone cysts, *AJNR* 153:99-101, 1989.

Nemoto O, Moser RP Jr, Van Dam BE, et al: Osteoblastoma of the spine. *Spine* 15:1272-1280, 1990.

Parizel PM, Balerizux D, Rodesch G, et al: Gd-DTPA-enhanced MR imaging of spinal tumors, *AJNR* 10:249-258, 1989.

Post MJD: Tumors of the spine and spinal cord, First Annual Categorical Course in Neuroimaging, Chicago, 1988, American Society of Neuroradiology.

Ross JS, Masaryk TJ, Modic MT, et al: Vertebral hemangiomas: MR imaging, *Radiology* 165:165-169, 1987.

Sze G, Krol G, Zimmerman RD, Deck MDF: Malignant extradural spinal tumors: MR imaging with Gd-DTPA, *Radiology* 167:217-223, 1988.

Williams AL, Haughton VM, Pojunas KW, et al: Differentiation of intramedullary neoplasms and cysts by MR, *AJR* 149:159-164, 1987.

Yuh WTC, Flickinger FW, Barloon TJ, Montgomery WJ: MR imaging of unusual chordoma, *J Comput Assist Tomogr* 12:30-35, 1988.

Yuh WTC, Zachar CK, Barloon TJ, et al: Vertebral compression fractures: distinction between benign and malignant causes with MR imaging, *Radiology* 172:215-218, 1989.

CHAPTER 58

Spine and cord: vascular disease, infection, and miscellaneous

KEY CONCEPTS

1. Isolated spinal cord aneurysms are rare but occur in up to 50% of arteriovenous malformations (AVMs).
2. Most spine and cord vascular malformations are AVMs.
3. Infectious spondylitis typically involves disc space and entire bodies of two or more contiguous vertebrae but spares posterior elements. (Neoplasm usually is more focal, spares the disc, and often involves pedicles and neural arch.)
4. Cord multiple sclerosis (MS) can mimic neoplasm (both can expand cord, enhance, and be hyperintense on T2-weighted image [T2WI]); brain magnetic resonance (MR) is helpful if changes suggestive of MS are identified.
5. Fifteen percent of patients with chronic cord compression have intramedullary signal abnormalities (hyperintense on T2WI) adjacent to compressive lesions.

I. Vascular disease.
  A. Saccular aneurysm (rare except with AVM, in which these are relatively common and are flow related).
  B. Vascular malformations.
    1. Capillary telangiectasias (20% of spinal vascular malformations): See Chapter 14.
    2. Cavernous angiomas (5% to 15% of spinal vascular malformations).
    3. Venous angiomas: uncommon; can occur in cord or vertebral body.
    4. AVMs.
      a. Most common spinal vascular malformation.
      b. Can be dural or intradural; 40% of intradural vascular malforma-

tions are intramedullary, 60% extramedullary (dorsal cord most common).

    c. Intradural AVMs can be manifest as with subarachnoid hemorrhage (10% to 30%) or progressive myelopathy; children with dural AVMs may have cardiomegaly with high output failure.

  5. Radiology.

    a. MR.

      (1) Serpentine areas of high-velocity signal loss.

      (2) Acute or subacute thrombi, hemorrhage.

      (3) Cord edema (enlarged, hyperintense cord on T2WI).

      (4) Sequelae: myelomalacia (small gliotic cord often with hyperintense foci on T2WI and evidence of old hemorrhage) and cord atrophy.

    b. Myelography: serpiginous filling defects; typically over dorsal surface of cord (characteristic "hairpin" configuration of anterior spinal artery may be seen).

    c. Angiography.

      (1) Enlarged spinal, medullary, and radicular arteries and prominent draining veins.

      (2) Flow-related aneurysm present in up to 50%.

C. Infarction.

  1. Cord infarcts are difficult to diagnose and verify.

  2. Acute infarcts are typically isointense on T1WI, hyperintense on T2WI, with variable extent of involvement. Late changes are atrophy and myelomalacia.

  3. Can occur with surgery, infection, or trauma or spontaneously.

II. Infection and inflammation: Infections of spine and cord can involve vertebral body, paravertebral musculature, intervertebral discs, epidural space, leptomeninges, and rarely cord itself.

A. Spine and disc.

  1. Routes of spread: direct (e.g., surgery) and hematogenous. Latter can be either arterial or venous (via Batson's plexus).

  2. Initial infectious nidus is probably subchondral vertebral body from which spread to discs, adjacent vertebrae, soft tissue, and epidural space can occur.

  3. Radiology.

    a. CT (progressive infection).

      (1) Often two adjacent vertebral bodies plus disc involved.

      (2) Diffuse osteolytic involvement of entire vertebral body.

      (3) Sparing of posterior elements is typical.

      (4) Extensive prevertebral soft tissue involvement (in contrast to more focal with neoplasm).

      (5) Gas may be present within both bone and soft tissue (al-

though intrabody gas is *far* more common with avascular necrosis than infection).

    (6) Occasionally extremely aggressive, mimicking tumor.

  b. MR (pyogenic infection).

    (1) Normal marrow signal replaced (typically appears abnormally hypointense on T1WI), hyperintense on T2WI.

    (2) Disc narrowed and hyperintense on T2WI.

    (3) May show enhancement (CAUTIONS: Can be enhanced to isointensity with marrow on T1WI; marrow in children under 10 years of age is normally enhanced; enhancement can persist long after clinical resolution of infection).

    (4) Adjacent soft tissue planes obscured (lack of sharp fat-muscle interface).

    (5) Anterior vertebral body destruction (loss of normal low-signal cortical margin).

    (6) Focal lytic bone involvement, often with marginal sclerosis, is common.

    (7) Pott's disease (tuberculosis of spine): thoracic location; slow progression, typically with relative preservation of disc; calcification and psoas abscess may be present; later, angular kyphosis may develop. MR findings may be more suggestive of neoplasm than infection.

    (8) Brucellosis: lumbar location most common; bone destruction limited to end-plates; disc collapsed.

B. Epidural space.

  a. Incidence: uncommon; usually secondary to infection elsewhere, spondylitis, or paravertebral abscess.

  b. Imaging findings vary from clearly identifiable, focal or extensive, enhancing extradural mass with high signal on T2WI (abscess pattern) to extensive homogeneous collections difficult to distinguish from adjacent meningitis (cellulitis pattern).

  c. Can extend over several spinal segments.

  d. Osteomyelitis and epidural abscess more common in patients with substance abuse.

C. Meningitis: imaging findings usually nonspecific; may consist of thickened meninges and nerve roots (smooth or, less commonly, nodular pattern); enhancement on T1WI. If secondary cord edema or infarction is present, hyperintense areas may be present in cord on T2WI.

D. Cord abscess: Very rare.

E. Transverse myelitis and AIDS myelopathy: nonspecific findings of diffuse increase in cord signal intensity on T2WI, typically over many segments. Differential diagnosis: infiltrating neoplasm, sarcoidosis, less commonly MS. (MS tends to be more focal.)

III. Miscellaneous.
  A. MS: similar to MS in brain (see Chapter 39). Cord lesions can be focal, rounded areas of increased signal on T1WI or more extensive, somewhat "feathered" or poorly marginated lesions that can mimic neoplasm (cord expansion can be present in acute stage as can enhancement by contrast material). Brain MR may be helpful if characteristic lesions of MS are identified. Cord atrophy can be seen with long-standing MS.
  B. Sarcoidosis.
    1. Central nervous system involvement in 5% of patients, primarily of leptomeninges and hypothalamus and infundibular area of brain.
    2. Spine or cord sarcoid is rare; can involve leptomeninges, cord, or both.
    3. MR.
      a. Cord expansion with patchy, multifocal, peripheral enhanced areas that appear broad based toward surface of cord; T2WI shows nonspecific increased signal of cord.
      b. Leptomeningeal thickening and enhancement.
  C. Cord compression: 15% of patients with chronic compressive lesions of cervical cord have abnormal high signal intensity of cord adjacent to extradural lesion. Probably reflects focal demyelination secondary to chronic pressure; more extensive areas of gliosis, necrosis, and diffuse demyelination can occur with marked compression and long-standing disease.

SUGGESTED READINGS

Angtuaco EJC, McConnell JR, Chaddock WM, Flanigan S: MR imaging of spinal epidural sepsis, *AJNR* 8:879-883, 1987.

Barakos JA, Mack AS, Dillon WP, Norman D: MR imaging of acute transverse myelitis and AIDS myelopathy, *J Comput Assist Tomogr* 14:45-50, 1990.

Barnwell SL, Dowd CF, Davis RL, et al: Cryptic vascular malformation of the spinal cord: diagnosis by magnetic resonance imaging and outcome of surgery, *J Neurosurg* 72:403-407, 1990.

Dickman CA, Harrington TR, Sonntag VKH, et al: Magnetic resonance imaging in the diagnosis of disk space infection, *BNI Q* 5:14-18, 1989.

Elksnis SM, Hogg JP, Cunningham ME: MR imaging of spontaneous spinal cord infarction, *J Comput Assist Tomogr* 15:228-232, 1991.

Endress C, Buyot DR, Fata J, Salciccioli G: Cervical osteomyelitis due to IV heroin use, *AJR* 155:333-335, 1990.

Enzmann DR: Infection and inflammation. In Enzmann DR, DeLaPaz RL, Rubin JB (eds): *Magnetic resonance imaging of the spine,* St Louis, 1990, Mosby–Year Book, pp 260-300.

Larsson E-M, Holtas S, Nilsson O: Gd-DTPA-enhanced MR of suspected spinal multiple sclerosis, *AJNR* 10:1071-1076, 1989.

McCormick PC, Michelson WJ, Post KD, et al: Cavernous malformations of the spinal cord, *Neurosurgery* 23:459-463, 1988.

Minami S, Sagoh T, Nishimura K, et al: Spinal arteriovenous malformation: MR imaging, *Radiology* 169:109-115, 1988.

Nesbit GM, Miller GM, Baker HL Jr, et al: Spinal cord sarcoidosis: a new finding at MR imaging with Gd-DTPA enhancement, *Radiology* 173:839-843, 1989.

Post MJD, Quencer RM, Montalvo BM, et al: Spinal infection: evaluation with MR imaging and intraoperative US, *Radiology* 169:765-771, 1988.

Sharif AS, Aideyan OA, Clark DC, et al: Brucellar and tuberculous spondylitis: comparative imaging features, *Radiology* 171:419-425, 1989.

Smith AS, Weinstein MA, Migushima A, et al: MR imaging characteristics of tuberculous spondylitis vs. vertebral osteomyelitis, *AJNR* 10:619-625, 1989.

Takahashi M, Yamashita Y, Sakamoto Y, Kojima R: Chronic cervical cord compression: clinical significance of increased signal intensity on MR images, *Radiology* 173:219-224, 1989.

Van Lom KJ, Kellerhouse LE, Pathria MN, et al: Infection versus tumor in the spine: criteria for distinction with CT, *Radiology* 166:851-855, 1988.

Index

Page numbers followed by *t* indicate tables.

Neoplasm(s)—cont'd
of ventricular ependyma,
contrast-enhanced studies of,
224-225
of vertebral column, 375-380
Neoplastic arteriopathy, 114
Neoplastic disease, calvarial thickening
from, 153
Nerve(s)
abducens (VI), anatomy and function of,
134
cranial
lower, 135-138
skull base and, 133-138
tumors of, in von Recklinghausen's
disease, 190
upper, 133-135
facial (VII), anatomy and function of,
135-136
glossopharyngeal (IX), anatomy and
function of, 136
hypoglossal (XII), anatomy and function
of, 137-138
oculomotor (III), anatomy and function of,
133-134
olfactory, anatomy and function of, 133
optic (II), anatomy and function of, 133
spinal accessory (XI), anatomy and
function of, 137
trigeminal (V), anatomy and function of,
134-135
trochlear (IV), anatomy and function of,
134
tumors of, involving external carotid
artery, 13
vagus (X), anatomy and function of,
136-137
vestibulocochlear (VIII), anatomy and
function of, 136
Nerve cell tumors, 295-296
Nerve sheath tumors, 298-300
involving external carotid artery, 13
Neural organization and alignment in brain
embryology, 171
Neural sheath tumors of skull base, 141
Neural tube closure, disorders of, 178-182
cephaloceles as, 180-181
Chiari malformations as, 178-180
corpus callosum anomalies as, 181
Dandy-Walker complex as, 181-182
Neurinomas, acoustic, bilateral,
neurofibromatosis with, 191-192
Neuritis, 349
optic, 354
Neuroblastoma, cerebral, primary, 295
Neurocutaneous syndromes, 187-192,
196-197
neurofibromatosis as, 188-192

Neurocutaneous syndromes—cont'd
ocular findings in, 189
vascular narrowing/occlusion from, 74-75
von Recklinghausen's disease as, 188-191
Neurodegenerative diseases, 263-269; *see
also* Degenerative brain disorders
Neuroectodermal tumor, primitive,
intraventricular masses from, 220
Neuroepithelial cysts, intraventricular,
216-217,
Neuroepithelial tumors, 316-317
Neurofibromas, 299-300
plexiform, in von Recklinghausen's
disease, 190
Neurofibromatosis, 188-192, 366-367
with bilateral acoustic neurinomas,
191-192
intracranial calcifications in, 159
vascular narrowing/occlusion from, 74
Neurohypophysis
choristoma of, 342
granular cell tumor of, 342
Neuronal heterotopias, 184
Neurosarcoidosis, contrast-enhanced
meningeal studies in, 229-230
Neurulation, 363-364
Nonglial tumors, 292-318
leukemia as, 309
of lymphoreticular system, 308-309, 310
of maldevelopmental origin, 311-318
of mesenchymal tissue, 302-306
of nerve cells, 295-296
of nerve sheath, 298-300
of primitive bipotential precursors,
292-295

O

Occipital artery, areas of supply of, 9
Occipital sinus, 57
Occlusions of middle cerebral artery, 46
Occlusive cerebrovascular disease, collateral
blood flow in, 102-104
Ocular hamartoma, 354
Oculomotor (III) nerve, anatomy and
function of, 133-134
Odontoid fracture of spine, 369
Olfactory nerve, anatomy and function of,
133
Oligodendroglioma, 289-290
intracranial calcifications from, 161
Ophthalmic artery, 22, 23
Ophthalmopathy, thyroid, 357
Optic canal, 130
Optic (II) nerve
anatomy and function of, 133
glioma of, 354-355
in von Recklinghausen's disease,
189-190